PDA Connections
Mobile Technology for Health Care Professionals

Frances H. Cornelius, PhD, MSN, RN, CNE
Assistant Professor
Drexel University
College of Nursing and Health Professions
Philadelphia, Pennsylvania

Mary Gallagher Gordon, MSN, RN, CNE
Clinical Assistant Professor
Drexel University
College of Nursing and Health Professions
Philadelphia, Pennsylvania

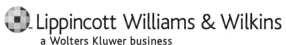
Lippincott Williams & Wilkins
a Wolters Kluwer business
Philadelphia • Baltimore • New York • London
Buenos Aires • Hong Kong • Sydney • Tokyo

Senior Acquisitions Editor: Jean Rodenberger
Managing Editor: Betsy Gentzler
Editorial Assistant: Marivette Torres
Production Project Manager: Cynthia Rudy
Director of Nursing Production: Helen Ewan
Senior Managing Editor / Production: Erika Kors
Art Director: Joan Wendt
Manufacturing Coordinator: Karin Duffield
Production Services / Compositor: Black Dot Group
Printer: R.R. Donnelley–Crawfordsville

Copyright © 2007 by Lippincott Williams & Wilkins.

All rights reserved. This book is protected by copyright. No part of it may be reproduced, stored in a retrieval system, or transmitted, in any form or by any means—electronic, mechanical, photocopy, recording, or otherwise—without prior written permission of the publisher, except for brief quotations embodied in critical articles and reviews and testing and evaluation materials provided by publisher to instructors whose schools have adopted its accompanying textbook. Printed in the United States of America. For information write Lippincott Williams & Wilkins, 530 Walnut Street, Philadelphia, PA 19106.

Materials appearing in this book prepared by individuals as part of their official duties as U.S. Government employees are not covered by the above-mentioned copyright.

Microsoft product screen shots are reprinted with permission from Microsoft Corporation.

9 8 7 6 5 4 3 2 1

Library of Congress Cataloging-in-Publication Data
PDA connections : mobile technology for health care professionals / [edited by] Frances
H. Cornelius, Mary Gallagher Gordon.
    p. ; cm.
  Includes bibliographical references and index.
  ISBN 0-7817-5999-4 (alk. paper)
  1. Medicine—Data processing. 2. Medical informatics. 3. Pocket computers. I. Cornelius, Frances
H. II. Gallagher Gordon, Mary. [DNLM: 1. Computers, Handheld. 2. Medical Informatics.
W 26.5 P348 2007]
R858.P43 2007
610.285—dc22

                    2006007929

Care has been taken to confirm the accuracy of the information presented and to describe generally accepted practices. However, the authors, editors, and publisher are not responsible for errors or omissions or for any consequences from application of the information in this book and make no warranty, express or implied, with respect to the content of the publication.

The authors, editors, and publisher have exerted every effort to ensure that drug selection and dosage set forth in this text are in accordance with the current recommendations and practice at the time of publication. However, in view of ongoing research, changes in government regulations, and the constant flow of information relating to drug therapy and drug reactions, the reader is urged to check the package insert for each drug for any change in indications and dosage and for added warnings and precautions. This is particularly important when the recommended agent is a new or infrequently employed drug.

Some drugs and medical devices presented in this publication have Food and Drug Administration (FDA) clearance for limited use in restricted research settings. It is the responsibility of the health care provider to ascertain the FDA status of each drug or device planned for use in his or her clinical practice.

LWW.com

Dedication

To my husband, John, who was my anchor and sounding board throughout this endeavor. To my children, Ryan and Janis, who provided inspiration and a strong desire to be a good role model. To my mother, who was always there, quietly in the background doing whatever it took to instill some semblance of order in our chaotic lives. To my sister, Gabe, who provided much-needed mini mental health breaks by sending me humorous e-mails as well as inspirational messages. Finally, to my dad, who taught me early on that I should always aim high and that there is nothing one cannot achieve through hard work and perseverance. Thank you all. Without you, this book would not have been possible.

Frances H. Cornelius

To Freddy, who is always there, filled with love and patience. To my children, who never complained about unmade lunches, the lack of homemade cookies, or sporadic dinners, and always provided a constant source of support, encouragement, and belief. A special thanks to my parents, who have given me the guidance, support, and love to get here. Thank you all—I love you.

Mary Gallagher Gordon

Contributors

Jennifer Angat
Student, Graphic Design
Old Dominion University
Norfolk, Virginia

Judith L. Draper, MSN, APRN, BC
Assistant Professor
Drexel University
College of Nursing and Health Professions
Philadelphia, Pennsylvania

Francine Gelo, RN, BSN
Director of Outreach and Health Education
11th Street Family Health Services of
    Drexel University
Philadelphia, Pennsylvania

MaryCate Gordon
Student, Technical Writing and
    Political Science
Old Dominion University
Norfolk, Virginia

H. Lynn Kane, RN, MSN, MBA, CCRN
Cardiac Clinical Nurse Specialist
Thomas Jefferson University
 Hospital–Methodist Division
Philadelphia, Pennsylvania

Faye A. Pearlman, RN, MSN, MBA
Clinical Assistant Professor
Drexel University
College of Nursing and Health Professions
Philadelphia, Pennsylvania

Patricia Dunphy Suplee, PhD, CS, RNC
Assistant Dean of Special Projects
Drexel University
Philadelphia, Pennsylvania

Magdeleine Vasso, MSN, RN, CS
Clinical Assistant Professor
Drexel University
College of Nursing and Health Professions
Philadelphia, Pennsylvania

Roberta Waite, EdD, RN, MSN, CS
Assistant Professor
Drexel University
College of Nursing and Health Professions
Philadelphia, Pennsylvania

Linda Wilson, RN, PhD, CPAN, CAPA, BC
Assistant Professor
Drexel University
College of Nursing and Health Professions
Philadelphia, Pennsylvania

Reviewers

Samira Ali, RN, MSN(NI), BSN
Lecturer
King Saud University for Health Sciences
Riyadh, Saudi Arabia

B. Amy Clouse
Educational Program Manager
Maryland General Hospital
Baltimore, Maryland

Brandie Dawson, RN, BSN
Independent Legal Nurse Consultant
Towson State University
Towson, Maryland

Martha S. Gallagher, PhD, MSN, RN, CNS
Associate Professor
Lourdes College
Sylvania, Ohio

Sylvia Suszka Hildebrandt, BS, MN, ARNP, CCNI
Owner/Editor, PDAcortex.com
Consulting Nurse, Group Health Cooperative
Seattle, Washington

Eleanor Hunt, MSN, RN, BC
Clinical Informatics Analyst
Misys Healthcare Systems
Raleigh, North Carolina

Rhonda Hutton, MSN, RN
Practical Nursing Program Coordinator
State Fair Community College
Sedalia, Missouri

Tracey Ann Jensen, RN, MSN, MBA, MMIS
Nursing Instructor
Merced College
Merced, California

Eileen Kaslatas, MSN, RN
Professor, Nursing Faculty
Macomb Community College
Clinton Township, Michigan

Pamela Young Mahon, PhD, RN
Associate Professor of Nursing
Kingsborough Community College
    of the City University of New York
Brooklyn, New York

Lauren E. O'Hare, EdD, RN
Chair, Department of Nursing
Wagner College
Staten Island, New York

Catherine Richmond, RN, MSN
Professor of Nursing, Lead Teacher Nursing III
Alfred State College
Alfred, New York

Mary Ann Smeltzer, BSN, MSN, RN
Director of Clinical Operations
NetHealth Systems, Inc.
Pittsburgh, Pennsylvania

Janet Spinks, BSN, MSML, CPHQ, CAAMA, CQM
Health Care Consultant
Spinks & Associates LLC
Frederick, Maryland

Sara Breckenridge Sproat, MSN, RN, BC
Lieutenant Colonel, United States Army
  Nurse Corps and Deputy Director,
  Division of Regulated Activities
Walter Reed Army Institute of Research
Silver Spring, Maryland

James Templin, BSN, RN
Education Coordinator
Mountain States Health Alliance
  HomeCare Services
Johnson City, Tennessee

Jason M. Thorton, RN, BSN
Staff II, CICU, ICU, IS Clinical Lead
Children's Hospital
Boston, Massachusetts

Patricia Whelan, PN, RN, BbCN
Instructor of Nursing
Grant MacEwan College, University of Alberta
Edmonton, Alberta

Bruce Wilson, RN, MSN, PhD
Professor, Department of Nursing
University of Texas–Pan American
Edinburg, Texas

Michelle Woodbeck, RN, BSN, MS
Associate Professor of Nursing
Hudson Valley Community College
Troy, New York

Preface

Health care professionals practice in a dynamic environment in which technology and innovation are the norm. Information is essential to guide clinical practitioners in all health care disciplines, and it is increasing exponentially. Health care is increasingly driven by information; consequently, the delivery of patient care demands effective management of information. The ability to manage information effectively and efficiently at the point-of-care is a core skill that health care professionals must master.

PDA Connections: Mobile Technology for Health Care Professionals provides a structured introduction to the PDA and its use in clinical practice. Readers will have opportunities to learn new strategies to incorporate the PDA into their clinical practices as they develop professional competencies. The goal of the text is to promote PDA skills, which will enable the user to access and retrieve information effectively and efficiently, as the need arises or changes, for the purpose of guiding interventions in various clinical practice settings. If such proficiencies can be developed, they have the potential to revolutionize health care practice and, consequently, outcomes.

Organization of the Text

PDA Connections is divided into three units. The first unit, Learning to Use Your PDA, introduces the novice to the PDA and the standard functionalities of these powerful devices. The second unit, Case Scenarios and Learning Activities, provides opportunities to practice point-of-care information access, using real-life case studies to engage the student. This unit contains General Case Studies, with questions that can be answered using the free trial versions of Lippincott Williams & Wilkins' electronic references for the PDA. The Advanced Case Studies require the complete version of these references, to be purchased by the student. More information about the case studies is given in the introduction to Unit 2. The third unit, Advanced Functionalities—Letting the Technology Do the Heavy Lifting, provides an overview of tools, software, and accessories that further expand the use of the PDA for the health care professional.

Special Features

The chapters in Units 1 and 3 contain several features to enhance learning. **Key terms** are defined at the beginning of each chapter and are in bold type at their first appearance in the chapter. For easy reference, these key terms are also listed in the glossary at the end of the book. Many of the chapters include **Test Drive** exercises, strategically placed to support mastery of the content. Each chapter includes **Tips From the Experts** that will help readers avoid common pitfalls in using a PDA. **Learning Activities** at the end of each chapter provide readers with the opportunity to demonstrate competence. Also, each chapter contains **WebLinks** for additional resources and learning activities.

thePoint

Lippincott Williams & Wilkins offers an online course and content manager called thePoint at **http://thePoint.LWW.com/cornelius**, where readers can download free trial versions of the PDA references used in the General Case Studies and purchase any full-version PDA references needed to complete the exercises in the Advanced Case Studies.

Frances H. Cornelius

Mary Gallagher Gordon

Acknowledgments

Writing a book is an intensive experience and cannot be accomplished without the support of others. We would like to acknowledge the support that we received from our colleagues. In addition, we would like to thank Lippincott Williams & Wilkins for the opportunity to write this book and for the support provided throughout this project.

F.H.C.

M.G.G.

Contents

Unit 3   Advanced Functionalities—Letting the Technology Do the Heavy Lifting   313

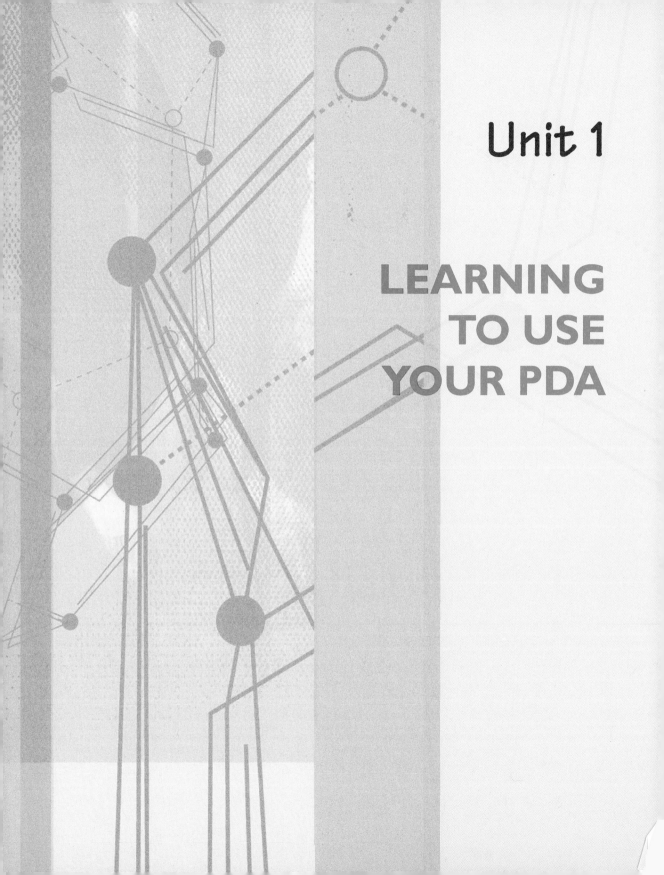

Unit 1

LEARNING TO USE YOUR PDA

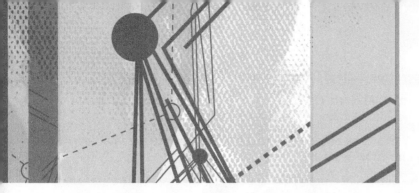

Introduction
to the PDA

Frances H. Cornelius

Key Terms

Beam (Beaming) • To send information via the infrared port between two PDAs or to a printer or other infrared-enabled device

Bluetooth • A short-range (about 33 feet or 10 meters) wireless connection protocol for cellular phones, mobile PCs, and other portable devices; it can also be used to send information between two PDAs or to send information to a printer

Compact Flash (CF) • Memory chips enclosed in a small plastic case that retain data after they are removed from the system; commonly used in handheld computers, cell phones, digital cameras, and audio players to expand memory and functionality

Infrared (IR) port • A sensor that allows exchange of data between PDAs, a PDA and a printer, or a PDA and another IR-enabled device; the range capability is about 3 feet

Linux • A very stable, open source version of UNIX operating system, available at no charge

Operating System (OS) • Software that is the foundation enabling programs to run on a PDA, for example, Palm OS and Pocket PC OS

Palm • An operating system for PDAs created by Palm, Inc.

Personal Digital Assistant (PDA) • A small handheld computer that organizes information; also known as handheld, palmtop

Pocket PC • A Windows-based operating system for PDAs created by Microsoft; also known as WinCE

RAM (Random-Access Memory) • Temporary storage of PDA files that enables PDA applications to run

ROM (Read-Only Memory) • Used for static memory on a PDA; typically the space where the operating system is stored or where fixed Personal Information Data applications are shipped with the standard PDA OS

Secure Digital (SD) card • Memory chips enclosed in a small plastic case that retain data after they are removed from the system; for memory data storage only

Secure Digital Input/Output (SDIO) card • An interface, similar to CF cards, that extends the functionality of devices with SD card slots by allowing data to be transmitted both into and out from a device

Stylus (Stylus pen) • The input device for a PDA—the user touches the screen with a stylus to execute commands

Universal Serial Bus (USB) • An interface between a computer and add-on devices, serving as a way to connect peripheral devices to computers; allows you to connect multiple devices concurrently and replaces the functionality of serial and parallel ports, including keyboard and mouse ports

Wi-Fi • An abbreviation for "wireless fidelity;" a high-frequency wireless local area network (WLAN) that uses radio signals to transmit and receive data over an area of about 200 feet; allows handhelds, desktops, and other wireless devices to exchange information at up to 11 mbs (megabytes/sec) at several hundred feet; also known as 802.11a, 802.11b, 802.11g

Personal Digital Assistants (PDAs) have much to offer. These handy devices store, organize, process, and permit instant retrieval of important clinical and business information. PDAs have emerged as useful, and often indispensable, tools to guide professional practice. These small computers have the capacity to store several clinical reference books, which literally places the resources in the palm of your hand, easily accessible, while delivering care in various settings, including the bedside. In addition, other features, such as database input and management and wireless technology, offer the health care provider additional resources while saving time and may provide a means to deliver "just enough information, just in time." Increasingly, health professionals are using PDAs to improve accuracy, save time, and streamline their paperwork. PDAs are fast becoming as essential as one's stethoscope.

PDAs replace bulky reference note cards and outdated manuals. PDAs move policies, references, and standards of care from the shelf into the hands of the health professional at the bedside, in the office, and in the home (Hunt, Kearns, & Bailey, 2002). According to VanDenKerkhof, Goldstein, Lane, Rimmer & Van Dijk (2003), patient assessments performed while using a PDA were more likely to contain documentation regarding pain and side effects (e.g., nausea, pruritus, and hypotension) than the paper assessments. The PDA may even enhance the efficiency of the patient assessment process through the provision of more comprehensive digital data for research, clinical, and administrative needs (VanDenKerkhof et al., 2003).

A Growing Trend for Health Professionals

PDA use in health care is on the rise. There is limited information about the use of PDAs in health care, but in 2000, a survey of PDA use found that 20% of physicians and 1% of nurses used the devices. A more recent survey, released in September 2003, indicates that these numbers have increased to 47% of physicians and 18% of nurses currently using PDAs in health care settings (Stolworthy, 2003).

Handheld computers are being used increasingly to "extend the human mind's capacity to recall and process large numbers of relevant variables and to support information management, general administration and clinical practice" (Stolworthy & Suszka-Hildebrandt, 2002). PDAs are currently used in the clinical setting primarily for decision support and error reduction, checking drugs, dosages, and compatibilities (McGowen, 2003; Stolworthy & Suszka-Hildebrandt, 2002).

The use of this technology has brought with it some criticism and the concern that it will result in "de-skilling" of the health care profession. Critics wonder whether having so much information on such a small device will result in decreased analytical, problem-solving, and clinical skills among health care providers (De Ville, 2001; Martinsons & Chong, 1999). In fact, when first introduced to the capabilities of PDAs, students have asked, "If I have so much information in my PDA, why should I bother to study or prepare for clinical?" This is a reasonable question. Indeed, there is concern that embracing this technology will result in a health care professional who is dependent upon the small handheld device, unable to make even the most mundane clinical decision without first consulting it. This concern has been raised before. In fact, Socrates voiced a similar concern more than two thousand years ago about the advent of written documents. He thought that having written documents to refer to would lead to forgetfulness in the learner. De Ville (2001) maintains that this technology merely provides "information that is already available in a more convenient form . . . if clinicians give electronic versions of standard research tools no more or less respect than they have given their previously available hard copy versions, there is little reason for concern" (p. 454).

Undoubtedly, information is valuable—often essential—in helping health care professionals do their jobs; however, too much information can be a detriment to practice. "An overabundance of information can actually keep an individual from finding the information needed. While drowning in information, the individual may starve for knowledge" (Young, 2000, p. 15). Information is only useful when it meets the following criteria: it must be the right information, given to the right person, at the right time, in the right place, and in the right amount. It is only when these five criteria are met that adequate decision support is available (Thede, 2003; Young, 2000).

Information is critical in order to make sound decisions, and decision support information is essential when working with patients. An effective, efficient information retrieval system that supports accessing information that is both relevant and timely is essential. The key is to use technology to make the right information available when the person needs it, with minimal effort, in an amount that answers the question without being overwhelming—"just enough, just in time." Today's health care professional must develop skills to access and retrieve information in the currently cluttered information age. A PDA is one tool to help achieve this goal. By adopting handheld technology, the health care professional can empower his or her practice by providing high-quality care based on current information and resources. When one has up-to-the-minute, patient-specific information, care is more likely to be appropriate, timely, effective, efficient, and safe (Hunt et al., 2002).

History of the PDA

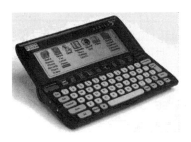

Figure 1.1 Series 3a by Psion. (Courtesy of http://www.bioeddie. co.uk.)

Handheld technology is a fairly recent development. The world's first handheld computer, Psion I, was introduced in 1984. Only slightly bigger than a pack of cigarettes, this device performed basic organizer functions. It had 8-bit technology, 10 K character storage, and a 16 character LCD display screen—quite innovative for the time. Soon, the Psion II was released containing 64 K ROM and 32 K RAM, and then a rapid succession of newer versions with greater capacity. The Series 3a by Psion, shown in Figure 1.1, was the first handheld device that users could link to their desktop PC for data transfers. This was a major innovation. In addition, this device had more memory (16-bit) and an LCD screen with twice the display capacity of its predecessor, as well as a 58-key keyboard. The Series 5 offered users even more capacity (32-bit), increased LCD screen size (640 x 240 pixels), and a larger keyboard.

The success of Psion drew considerable attention. In 1983, Apple, hoping to have similar success, launched the Newton MessagePad, depicted in Figure 1.2. The Newton was the first to use touch-sensitive screens and handwriting recognition software. The Newton was not well received by consumers because it was too large (in both size and weight), its handwriting software did not function properly, and the device was loaded with features that consumers didn't really use at that time.

In 1996, US Robotics introduced the Palm Pilot (Pilot 1000 and Palm 5000), a new handheld device that used a data entry system by means of a stylus and the Graffiti handwriting software program, which uses a simplified alphabet

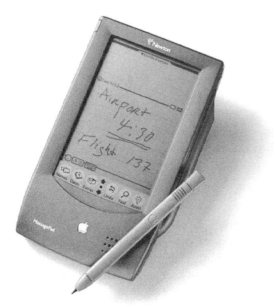
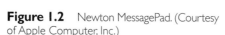

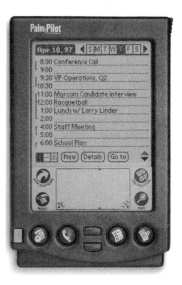

Figure 1.2 Newton MessagePad. (Courtesy of Apple Computer, Inc.)

Figure 1.3 Palm Pilot 3 Com. (Photo by http://www.ixbt.com)

for handwriting recognition. In 1997, US Robotics was bought by 3Com and a new generation of handhelds that were smaller and lighter was introduced. These new Palm devices featured a graphical user interface and desktop docking cradle for PC transfers (see Figure 1.3). Palm Pilot sold over 1 million units during its first year, besting Sony's Walkman, which took one and a half years to reach 1 million worldwide sales. By 1999, Palm was leading the industry with the Palm V and its Graffiti software.

Several factors contribute to Palm's success. First, **Palm** has an open hardware and software architecture that encourages independent development of third-party add-ons and software for the Palm devices—the more accessories and applications, the greater the versatility and hence greater demand for the devices. Leong (2001) explained this growth as follows:

> "In 1997 there were 2,000 developers working on innumerable third-party add-ons and software. In January 2001, the numbers of developers increased to 140,000. All these features endeared them to gadget freaks and have so far ensured their domination of the market. Perhaps, the clearest indication of their success can be seen by the fact that the product name given to a revolutionary product, Palm, has become recognized as the generic term for describing Palmtops—much like how the Sony product name Walkman has become synonymous with cassette tape players" (Leong, March 9, 2001, p. 2).

Since the late 1990s, Microsoft's Windows-based **Pocket PC** devices have been gaining in popularity. In 2000, Pocket PCs comprised only 11% of the market share. In April 2004, Palm and Pocket PC were virtually neck-and-neck with 40.7 and 40.2% of the market sales, respectively.

Standard Components: Getting to Know Your PDA

Basic A&P of the PDA

No matter which PDA you select, the following are universal characteristics shared by all PDAs:

- LCD screen
- Stylus
- Battery
- Memory
- Infrared (IR) port

LCD Screen

The LCD (liquid crystal display) screen on a PDA is similar to that of a laptop or PC screen but is different in that it has input capabilities (a touch screen). This allows the user to not only view data on the PDA screen, but also enter data by tapping on the screen using a stylus.

Stylus

The stylus is a plastic, pen-like device that permits the user to tap on the LCD screen without marring the surface. The tap of the stylus alters the small electrical current in the screen and transmits the command.

Battery

The battery is important. You will lose all data stored in the RAM of your PDA, including references, if the battery runs down. Some PDAs use alkaline (AAA) batteries. Most PDAs now have rechargeable alkaline batteries (lithium, nickel-cadmium, or nickel-metal hydride), which are good for six or more hours. Batteries are greatly improved these days; many cannot be overcharged, so it is safe to plug your device into a charger on a daily basis. Several factors will decrease your battery life:

1. Operating system (OS)—Pocket PC OS will use more power due to its increased memory requirements
2. More memory—the more memory you have, the more power is needed to support it
3. Color LCD display
4. Use of audio features, including voice recording and MP3 player
5. Use of wireless features such as Wi-Fi or Bluetooth.

Memory

PDAs have two kinds of memory: read-only memory (ROM) and random-access memory (RAM). Because a PDA doesn't have a hard drive, it stores basic programs such as your address book, calendar, and operating system in the ROM chip. This will keep all data intact, even if your PDA loses power. Anything you add—data or other software—is stored in the RAM. If your device loses power, all applications installed and data stored in the RAM will be lost. Having programs stored on the system's RAM is advantageous, because when you turn on your PDA, your applications/data are instantly available and you don't have to wait for applications to load. Another benefit is that when you enter data (make changes to a file), the information is stored automatically, so there is no need to use a *Save* command. Even when the device is turned off, the data remains intact because your PDA continues to draw a small amount of power from the batteries.

Infrared (IR) Port

Most PDAs have an infrared (IR) port that uses infrared light to beam (transmit) information to a PC, printer, or another PDA. For example, you can easily transmit a contact name and phone number to a colleague by using the infrared communications port. The infrared transmission range is limited, effective for beaming data across a distance of about 3 feet. This topic will be discussed in more detail in Chapter 6.

Operating Systems (OS)

An important consideration is the operating system (OS) or platform. There are currently four operating systems on the market: Palm OS, Pocket PC, Linux, and Symbian. As stated in the previous section, the handheld market is currently dominated by Palm and Pocket PC. While there are many different brands of PDAs, most run on either Palm OS or Pocket PC OS. Simply stated, the difference between operating systems is similar to the difference between Windows and Macintosh computers: programs are not compatible or interchangeable.

In general, your major consideration in selecting an operating system is which OS your colleagues and your health care system use because using the same one will allow you to exchange information more easily. Some prefer the Palm OS because of its functionality, ease of use and simplicity. Others prefer the Pocket PC/Windows OS because of the familiar interface resembling the PC and the ability to work in programs such as Word or PowerPoint. However, it is important to note that similar programs are available in Palm.

Two other operating systems, Linux and Symbian, are not as common but are building a contingent of strong advocates. Linux is a version of UNIX operating system. It has become popular because it is a very stable operating platform, and it is an open source software system that is available at no charge. The Symbian OS is an alternate OS for phones and PDAs. It is less well known than its counterparts, but it is also acquiring a strong following due to its stable phone/PDA interface. Currently, only a few PDAs can operate using the Linux or Symbian OS, but you can expect that to change in the future.

Standard (Integrated) Applications and Features

All PDAs come with some kind of personal information management (PIM) software. PIM software usually has the capability to perform the following time-saving tasks:

- Store contact information (names, addresses, phone numbers, e-mail addresses)
- Make task or to-do lists
- Take notes
- Write memos
- Keep track of appointments (date book, calendar)
- Remind you of appointments (clock, alarm functions)
- Plan projects
- Do calculations
- Keep track of expenses (Freudenrich, 2003)

It is important to note that not all of these functions are included in every PDA, so it is useful to first review your needs and then make sure the device has the necessary applications. Also, it is important to make sure that your PC has similar software so that you can easily exchange information between your PDA and PC. Sometimes, the associated PIM software for your PC is included with the PDA software. Many of the standard PIM applications will be discussed in greater detail in Chapter 4.

Optional Components, Features, and Accessories

It is important to purchase a PDA that has enough memory for the references and applications you wish to use and the capability to add more memory. A good rule of thumb is to get twice as much memory as you think you will need. In addition, it is important to make sure your PDA has the capability for expansion. As you become more experienced in using your device, you will want to add and use more features. Just like a computer, your PDA needs to have free memory to allow the programs to operate more efficiently; otherwise, the programs will be slow and may freeze. The key is to get a PDA that has enough memory for the references/programs you wish to use.

Memory Cards

Many PDAs come with external expansion slots to accommodate additional storage in the form of Compact Flash (CF) cards, Secure Digital (SD) cards, or Memory Sticks (MS), as depicted in Figure 1.4. You can keep most references and applications on these external storage cards, which frees up your PDA's RAM, allowing the programs to run more quickly and smoothly. In addition, the expansion slots provide you with the capability to extend your PDA by adding wireless networking capability, Bluetooth, serial, Universal Serial Bus (USB), infrared, modems, cameras, and much more.

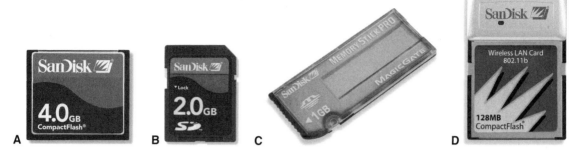

Figure 1.4   **A** Compact Flash card. **B** Secure Digital card. **C** Memory Stick. **D** Dual card. (Courtesy of SanDisk, Inc.)

CF is the most commonly used because it has been around the longest and has the most options available for expansion. They can expand the memory on your PDA as well as increase its functionality by allowing you to add accessories like a camera or barcode scanner. It is important to note that CF comes in two different sizes: Type I and Type II. Because Type I is thinner than Type II, devices that support only Type I CF cannot use Type II CF because it will not fit in the slot. Type II devices, however, can use Type I cards.

SD is often referred to as a *Multimedia* card. There are two types of SD cards: basic and Secure Digital Input/Output (SDIO). The basic SD card can be used as memory only. The SDIO card is a secure digital card with input and output capability. An SDIO card can function similarly to a CF card, allowing expansions like cameras, network adaptors, and so on. In this case, it is important to note that your PDA must have an SDIO slot to use any of the available SDIO expansion accessories. All CF slots can use memory or expansion cards; however, SD slots can use memory only, whereas SDIO slots can use both memory and expansions.

Usually, only Sony products use an MS card. Unlike the SD card, the MS slot can support an expansion device for either memory or accessories.

Dual Cards (Memory/Wireless)

Some manufacturers offer dual cards, which provide both additional memory and wireless capability. An example is depicted in Figure 1.4D. Dual cards are available in both CF and SD and further expand the functionality of the PDA, especially if there is only one expansion slot available, which is often the case in many PDAs. Thus, the user is not forced to decide between additional memory and connectivity. For more about this topic, see Chapter 6.

On an ongoing basis, new extensions, accessories, and software become available to further enhance and extend the functionality of your PDA. These new items include advanced organizational tools, programs, and applications, as well as accessories that allow you to do more with your device. Most of the newer devices come with one or more expansion slots, which permit you to add additional memory and accessories, such as a camera, GPS mapping antenna, MP3 player, phone, scanner, or modem (see Figure 1.5). These advanced features and specialty software—maps, video games, and photo editing software—will be discussed in more detail in Chapters 16 and 17.

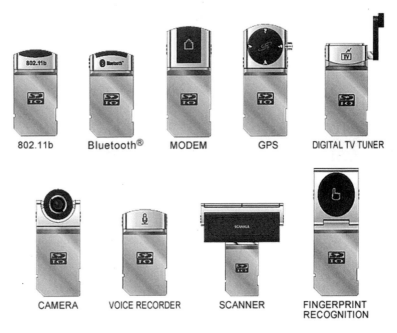

| 802.11b | Bluetooth® | MODEM | GPS | DIGITAL TV TUNER |

| CAMERA | VOICE RECORDER | SCANNER | FINGERPRINT RECOGNITION |

Figure 1.5   SDIO expansion cards. (Courtesy of SD Card Association.)

Wireless/Bluetooth

Many PDAs have built-in features that allow you to access and transmit data wirelessly. The two major wireless capabilities are Bluetooth and Wi-Fi (802.11b, 802.11a, and 802.11g). Bluetooth and Wi-Fi expansion cards are shown in Figure 1.6.

Bluetooth operates only at about 33 feet from another device and is the wireless equivalent of USB. Bluetooth is commonly used to connect directly to a computer (for syncing) or between multiple Bluetooth devices (as to a mobile phone). Bluetooth allows for a connection to the Internet only through another device, which means that you must be connecting to a device that has Internet capabilities to access the Internet through the PDA. Bluetooth capability can be a built-in feature, or you can add it using an external expansion slot.

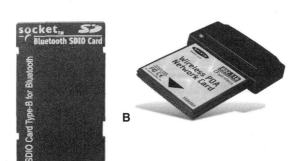

Figure 1.6 A External Bluetooth. (Courtesy of Socket Communications, Inc.) **B** Wireless expansion. (Courtesy of Belkin Corporation.)

Wi-Fi is the wireless equivalent of Ethernet or a local area network (LAN). Like Ethernet, Wi-Fi networks can be set up in a similar fashion, or established networks can be accessed. Access points can be deployed onto a wired network directly (via a wireless router) or simply connected to a specific machine. Wi-Fi allows for connection to the Internet through an established connection. If the network (or computer) that the Wi-Fi card is connected to has an Internet connection, the device can also use the Internet. Some devices may include Wi-Fi (most often 802.11b) integrated into them. If your PDA does not have built-in Wi-Fi capability, CF or SD Wi-Fi expansions are the only way of connecting a PDA to a Wi-Fi network.

In addition to Bluetooth and Wi-Fi, there is a long-range wireless solution for PDAs. Two of the major long range wireless providers are Global System for Mobile/General Packet Radio Service (GSM/GPRS) and Code Division Multiple Access (CDMA). Long-range wireless solutions for PDAs are based upon the same technology used by cell phones, allowing the user to access e-mail and the Internet anywhere and at anytime. Consequently, enhancing the mobility and connectivity of the PDA greatly increases its functionality. As stated earlier, these features will be discussed in more detail in Chapter 6.

Summary

You have had a broad introduction to the PDA and its significance for the health care professional. In the brief overview of the history of these powerful tools, you have learned that this is relatively new technology that has much to offer the health care professional. You have learned about the basic features of PDAs as well as some additional options that can greatly expand your PDA's functionality and use.

Tips From the Experts

Which PDA is best for you?

- First, consider how you will be using the device. If you plan to use it as a clinical reference and for patient record keeping (and not just for keeping your phone numbers and calendar), you should choose one with sufficient memory. It is important to get a PDA that has enough memory for the references and applications you wish to use and the capability to add more memory. So, expansion slots (SDIO and CF) are a must!
- It is important to get the *features* and *memory* that you will need for what you want to do. Go to Best Buy or a similar store and check out the PDAs. Take a look at the screen and features. Are they a good fit for you? That is the key.
- If wireless access is important to you, invest in a device that has an internal wireless card. This will free up your expansion slot for other accessories or more memory.

(Continued)

• Freeware is offered for both Pocket PC and Palm PDAs. Freeware is nice but should not be the major deciding factor for purchasing a device. Free programs for both operating systems are being offered by eager techies, but this may change in the future because they may start charging for these programs after they get you "hooked." To clarify this point, I use the example of the telephone feature *69, which was offered free of charge for years to telephone customers. However, after the public became accustomed to this convenient feature, the phone companies began to charge for the service.

LEARNING ACTIVITIES

1. Describe the differences between the four operating systems discussed in this chapter.
2. What is the difference between ROM and RAM?
3. What programs or applications might one expect to see stored on the ROM of a PDA? What programs or applications might one expect to see stored on the RAM of a PDA?
4. Describe the functionality and limitations of the four wireless features available to PDAs. (*Hint:* infrared, Bluetooth, Wi-Fi, and long-range wireless)

Visit http://thePoint.LWW.com/cornelius for supplemental information and activities.

References

De Ville, K. A. (2001). The ethical and legal implications of handheld medical computers. *The Journal of Legal Medicine, 22*, 447–466.

Freudenrich, C. (2003). How PDAs work. Retrieved on August 10, 2003 from http://electronics.howstuffworks.com/pda.htm/printable.

Hunt, E. C., Kearns, L. E., & Bailey, D. (2002). PDA use in nursing. Reference Hearing Proposal submitted by: Council on Nursing Informatics Action Proposal #1. Accepted at 2002 NCNA Annual Convention, Raleigh, NC. Retrieved May 20, 2003, from http://www.unc.edu/~dbailey1/CONI/CoNIRefHearProposal2002.doc.

Leong, D. (March 9, 2001). History of PDA—The beginning, PDAWear.com. Retrieved on August 10, 2003 from http://www.pdawear.com/news/article_pda_beginning.htm.

Martinsons, M. G., & Chong, P. K. C. (1999). The influence of human factors and specialist involvement on information systems success. *Human Relations, 52*(1), 123–152.

McGowen, K. (November 1, 2003). Trends in mobile computing in healthcare, PDA cortex. Retrieved November 4, 2003, from http://www.pdacortex.com/Trends_Mobile_Computing_Healthcare.htm.

Stolworthy, Y. (2003). RNs are mobilizing, PDA cortex. Retrieved January 6, 2004, from http://www.pdacortex.com/RNs_are_Mobilizing.htm.

Stolworthy, Y., & Suszka-Hildebrandt, S. (2002). Mobile information technology at the point-of-care, PDA cortex. Retrieved June 2, 2003, from http://www.pdacortex.com/mitatpoc.htm.

Thede, L. Q. (2003). *Informatics and nursing: Opportunities and challenges.* Philadelphia: Lippincott Williams & Wilkins.

VanDenKerkhof E., Goldstein D., Lane J., Rimmer M., & Van Dijk J. (2003). Using a personal digital assistant enhances gathering of patient data on an acute pain management service: A pilot study. *Canadian Journal of Anaesthesia (Journal canadien d'anesthesie), 50*(4), 6811.

Young, K. M. (2000). *Informatics for healthcare professionals.* Philadelphia: F. A. Davis.

2

Getting Started

Linda Wilson

Key Terms

ActiveSync • Computer program by Microsoft used to synchronize a Windows-based handheld device with a computer

Cradle • The base that the handheld device can be set in for the process of synchronization or charging

Palm Desktop • Palm computer program for use with Windows operating system

Serial port • A port on the computer where an external modem, a serial printer, or other device that uses a 9-pin serial connector can be attached

Syncing • Establishing a connection/partnership between the PDA and the computer in which files and programs are shared

USB port • A port on the computer where devices that require a Universal Serial Bus connection, such as a mouse, a scanner, a printer, or a PDA, can be attached

This chapter introduces the setup and basic functions of your handheld device and covers the differences for both a Windows CE-based handheld device and a Palm device. The chapter begins by reviewing the setup of your handheld device, including charging the device, with or without the use of a cradle. The step-by-step process for setting up your computer for synchronization is reviewed, including the installation of necessary computer programs and the process of how to make changes to your synchronization settings. The final topic of this chapter is a review of the purpose and selection of a Personal Information Management (PIM) system for your handheld device and the method of configuring the settings of the PIM for your personal preferences.

Setup: Before You Use Your PDA

Charging Your Device

Several methods can be used to charge your handheld device. Selection of a method will vary based on personal preference or whether you are at home or traveling. For example, while traveling, you may find it very cumbersome to carry the cradle with you due to its size and shape, and, instead, you might find it easier to just bring along the power cord and USB adapter.

It is important to maintain the charge on your handheld device so that you do not lose any data or installed programs. Today's batteries are very advanced; not only do they hold a charge longer, but also you no longer have to worry about overcharging the handheld device (see Chapter 1). Your handheld device will need to be charged at least 30 to 60 minutes per day based on use. Before you can do anything with your new PDA, you must charge it. Step-by-step instructions for various methods of charging your Windows CE/Pocket PC and Palm devices are presented in Box 2.1.

Box 2.1	**CHARGING YOUR PDA**

Windows CE/Pocket PC—Charging With a Cradle

1. Connect the power cord to the cradle.
2. Plug the power cord into the outlet.
3. Place your handheld device into the cradle.
4. While the device is charging, the charge light will be flashing.
5. When the device is fully charged, the light will be on but not flashing.

Windows CE/Pocket PC—Charging Without a Cradle

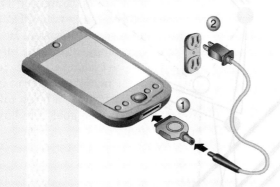

1. Connect the power cord to the USB port adapter.
2. Plug the power cord into the outlet.
3. While the device is charging, the charge light will be flashing.
4. When the device is fully charged, the light will be on but not flashing.

* *Do not* connect your PDA to your computer at this point.

Palm—Charging With a Cradle

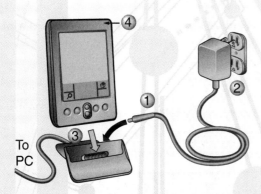

1. Connect the power cord to the cradle.
2. Plug the power cord into the outlet.
3. Place your handheld device into the cradle
4. While the device is charging, the charge light will be flashing.

5. When the device is fully charged, the light will be on but not flashing.

* Please note that in some models of the Palm handheld devices, the light does not flash while charging.

* *Do not* connect your PDA to your computer at this point.

Palm—Charging Without a Cradle

To charge your Palm without the cradle, you will need an adapter that will allow you to plug the power directly into your device. This adapter is usually an optional accessory so you may have to purchase this separately.

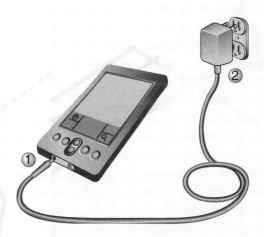

1. Connect the power cord to the PDA port adapter
2. Plug the power cord into the outlet
3. While the device is charging, the charge light will be flashing
4. When the device is fully charged, the light will be on but not flashing

* In some models of the Palm handheld devices, the light does not flash while charging. Images redrawn and modified with permission from Dell, Inc., and Palm, Inc.

Cables, Cradles, and Ports

Cables, cradles, and ports all accomplish the same task—allowing your PDA to synchronize (transfer information) with your desktop or laptop computer. The difference between the cable and cradle is that the cradle will allow the PDA to be displayed at an angle comfortable for viewing from a seated position. Both the cradle and cable allow for charging your PDA when plugged into the electronic cord. PDAs come with sync cable with a **USB port** alone or a **serial port** to connect to your desktop. The USB port allows for faster transfer of information than the serial port; however, unless you are installing a large software program, you may not notice the difference in speed. The goal is to have the PDA connect to the desktop, as shown in Figure 2.1.

Initial Setup/Configuration Before Connecting to a PC

It is always a good idea to read the installation instructions that come with your PDA. These instructions will take you through a step-by-step process for connecting your hardware (PDA, cables, cradles, and more) and provide detailed instructions for installing your software. After charging your PDA, you will be asked to initially set up your PDA. The setup process consists of working through a few screens that guide you through aligning your screen, setting the time and date, as well as entering owner information. You can follow these steps:

1. Turn on your handheld device.
2. Follow steps to align the screen.
3. Set up the date and time.
4. Enter your owner/contact information.

Please refer to Figure 2.2 for Pocket PC devices and Figure 2.3 for Palm devices for clarification.

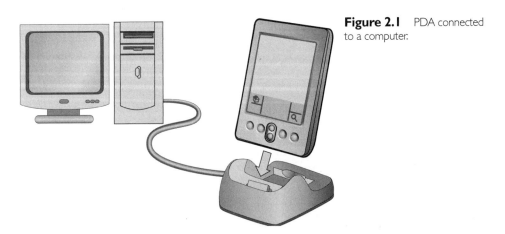

Figure 2.1   PDA connected to a computer.

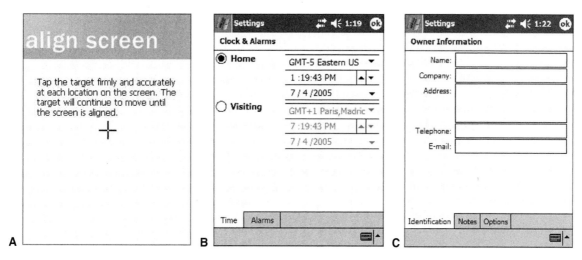

Figure 2.2 Pocket PC setup: **A** Align the screen. **B** Date and time screen. **C** Owner information screen.

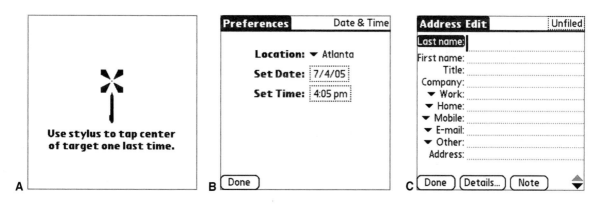

Figure 2.3 Palm setup: **A** Align the screen. **B** Date and time screen. **C** Owner information screen.

Syncing—Connecting Your PDA to Your Desktop

This section will review the programs needed for synchronization, or syncing, of your handheld device with your computer. You must install this software to your computer *before* connecting your PDA to the computer. Synchronization provides many benefits for your handheld device, such as providing a means to (1) install software, (2) back up all data to your PC, and (3) obtain automatic updates if available (and desired). Both the Windows CE/Pocket PC and Palm devices require specific software to accomplish these functions.

Syncing Windows CE/Pocket PC: Microsoft ActiveSync

Microsoft (MS) ActiveSync, the connecting software for PCs, allows your Pocket-based PDA to synchronize with your desktop computer and the MS program Microsoft Outlook.

If you have Microsoft Outlook on your computer, you will be able to synchronize your calendar, contacts, e-mail, tasks, and notes between your computer and PDA. Synchronizing means that both your computer and PDA will have the same up-to-date information, saving you the inconvenience of entering information separately into each device. Pocket PC software *does not* sync with Outlook Express, so before you go any further, you must determine which type of Outlook you have on your computer. To do this, follow these instructions:

1. Open your Outlook program.
2. Click on Help located on the toolbar at the top of your screen.
3. Click on About Microsoft Outlook (see Figure 2.4).

If you do not have Microsoft Outlook on your computer, you will need to install it to share calendar and other functions with your PDA. Many times with the purchase of a new PDA, the CD included contains both ActiveSync and MS Outlook software. The current version of MS ActiveSync can also be downloaded from the Internet. To download from the Internet, go to http://www.microsoft.com and click on Downloads; in the Keywords block, type in "activesync." At this site, you will be able to download and install the latest version of MS ActiveSync.

Before installing ActiveSync, be sure your PDA is not connected to the computer. It is okay to have your cradle connected, but *do not* place your PDA in the cradle before you have installed ActiveSync. When installing ActiveSync, whether you are installing from the CD or downloading from the Internet, you

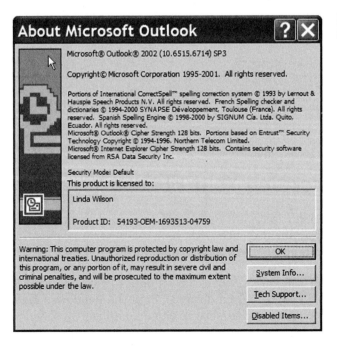

Figure 2.4   About Microsoft Outlook.

will receive a prompt asking whether you wish to open or save the file; choose Open. Although you may choose to save onto your computer, it is not necessary to do so. The application will function properly if you select Open.

As you proceed with the installation, you will be prompted to answer a few questions as to where to install the software on your C drive. You will be asked to develop a partnership between your computer and PDA. You will have a choice to set up a "standard partnership" or a "guest partnership." The standard partnership should be set up with the computer that you will be using on a regular basis. You can set up a standard partnership with up to two computers. A guest partnership would be set up when you are using a computer in a location in which you are working temporarily, such as in a library or public facility.

To simplify the process, all you really need to do is choose the default suggestions. Read carefully; at one point, you will be asked to connect your PDA cradle to your computer and place the PDA in the cradle. The sequence of steps is as follows:

1. Locate the USB port on your computer.
2. Plug the USB connector into a USB port on your computer.
3. Place the program CD into the CD-ROM drive of your computer or locate the appropriate version of software on the Internet.
4. The program will launch automatically if using a CD. If using the Internet to download the software, you will need to select Download and Run to install the software.
5. Follow the onscreen instructions.
6. Place your handheld in the cradle.
7. During the initial sync process, you will need to select the items you want to synchronize.
8. When the sync is completed you will see a message on your desktop computer that reads "device synchronized."

Modify Sync Settings on Your PDA

You can modify your sync settings by pressing on tools *on your PDA* in the Active Sync setting as shown in Figure 2.5. Try this yourself in the following exercise.

Test Drive . . . .

1. From the Today screen tap on Start.
2. Select Programs from the drop-down menu.
3. Select ActiveSync.
4. Select Tools in the bottom left of the screen (Figure 2.5A).
5. Select Options (Figure 2.5B). At this point, you are defaulted to the PC synchronization options screen.
6. Select the PC name for which you want to change the sync settings.

(Continued)

7. Select Server at the bottom of the page, which will take you to the server synchronization screen.
8. Select the items you would like synchronized (e.g., calendar, contacts, inbox), as shown in Figure 2.5C.
9. Select Mobile Schedules at the bottom of the screen, which will take you to the mobile schedule options screen.
10. Select your choices for syncing wirelessly for both peak and off-peak times (Figure 2.5D).

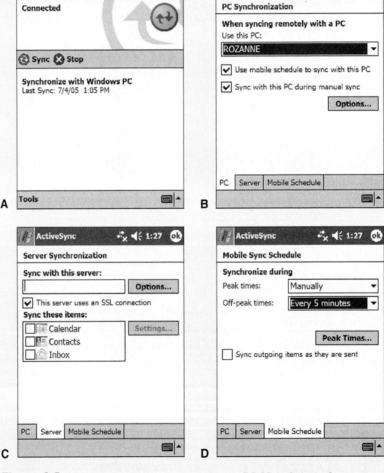

Figure 2.5   Modify sync options on your Pocket PC PDA: **A** ActiveSync screen. **B** Select options on your PDA. **C** Sync items select screen on your PDA. **D** Sync times option screen on your PDA.

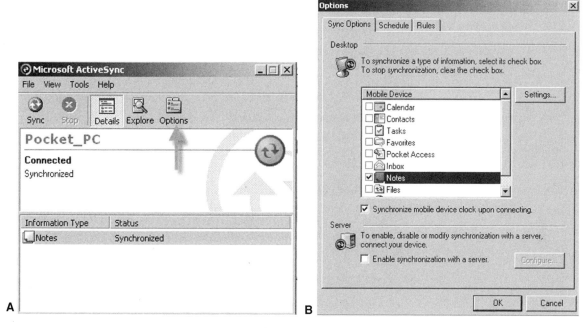

Figure 2.6 **A–B** Modify sync options on your PC.

Modify Sync Settings on Your PC

You can also modify sync options on your PC, using the ActiveSync box on your desktop. To begin, select Options located on the upper toolbar (see Figure 2.6A). In the next screen, you will see the list of PDA applications available for synchronization. Placing a check in the box next to a particular application will mark that application for synchronization with your PC (see Figure 2.6B).

You can also modify the settings for each item you are syncing with your PC. For example, if you wish to change the settings for your calendar, first you must highlight Calendar and then select Settings (Figure 2.7A). The next screen will provide options that will allow you to further personalize your sync settings (Figure 2.7B).

Tapping on the Options icon and selecting the tab Schedule, as depicted in Figures 2.8A and 2.8B, will allow you to further modify your sync settings. In this window, you can determine when you want synchronization to occur and adjust the sync schedule accordingly.

The Rules option, as shown in Figures 2.9A and 2.9B, allows you to decide what action will be taken when there is a conflict between the information housed on each device (PC and PDA). If there is a conflict between the desktop and the PDA, you can set up a rule that determines which machine wins.

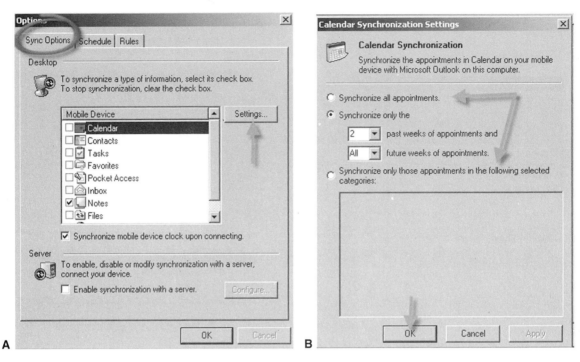

Figure 2.7   A–B Sync options screen on your PC: Settings.

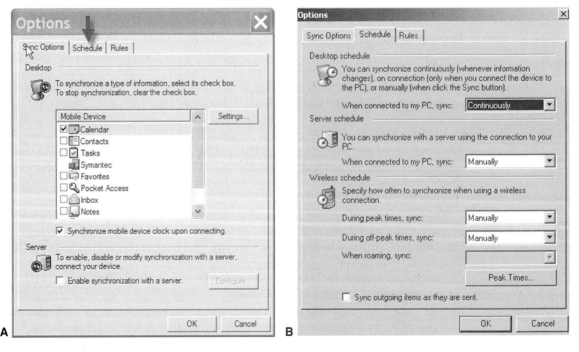

Figure 2.8   A–B Sync options screen on your PC: Schedule.

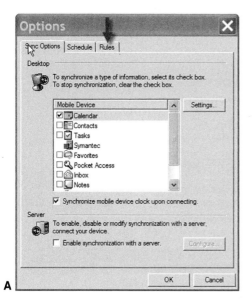
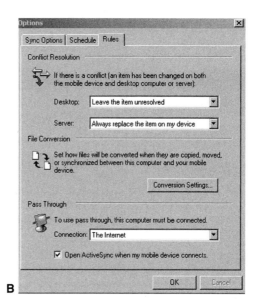

Figure 2.9 **A–B** Sync options screen on your PC: Rules.

Syncing Palm: Installing Palm Desktop/HotSync

The Palm uses a different software called Palm Desktop, which includes a feature called HotSync. This program allows you to install applications and to synchronize data between your Palm and desktop software, as well as a calendar/ PIM program, such as Microsoft Outlook or Palm Desktop. To complete the synchronization, you must connect your PDA and computer either directly or indirectly. Direct methods would include placing your handheld in the cradle with the cable attached to your computer or using infrared or Bluetooth technology. Indirect methods for connecting could include using a modem accessory or network HotSync technology.

To sync your Palm PDA, follow these steps:

1. Locate the USB port on your computer.
2. Plug the USB connector into a USB port on your computer.
3. Connect the power adapter cable to the back of the cradle to maintain charge.
4. Plug the adapter into an electrical outlet.
5. Place the program CD into the CD-ROM drive of your computer or locate the appropriate version of software on the Internet.
6. The program will launch automatically if using a CD. If using the Internet, you will need to select Download and Run to install the software.
7. Follow the onscreen instructions.
8. Place your handheld in the cradle when instructed to do so.
9. The first time you synchronize your data you will need to enter user information on the Palm desktop software. For future syncs the HotSync

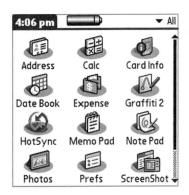

Figure 2.10 Select HotSync from main menu screen.

manager will recognize your handheld and will not ask for this information again.

10. When the sync is completed you will see a message on your desktop computer that states device is synchronized.

11. For future sync events you can select the HotSync option from the main menu on your handheld device (see Figure 2.10).

Modifying Your Connection Settings

You can modify your HotSync settings by clicking on the HotSync icon in the Windows system tray on your PC. Try modifying your settings in this exercise:

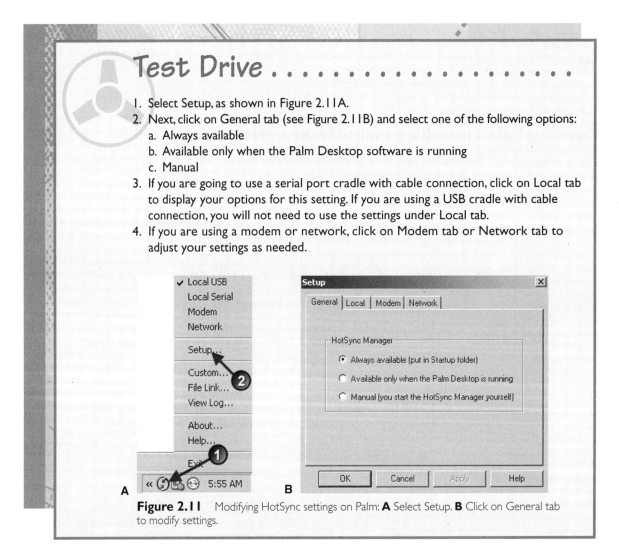

Test Drive . . . .

1. Select Setup, as shown in Figure 2.11A.
2. Next, click on General tab (see Figure 2.11B) and select one of the following options:
   a. Always available
   b. Available only when the Palm Desktop software is running
   c. Manual
3. If you are going to use a serial port cradle with cable connection, click on Local tab to display your options for this setting. If you are using a USB cradle with cable connection, you will not need to use the settings under Local tab.
4. If you are using a modem or network, click on Modem tab or Network tab to adjust your settings as needed.

Figure 2.11 Modifying HotSync settings on Palm: **A** Select Setup. **B** Click on General tab to modify settings.

All Palm models come with a calendar, address book, memo pad, to-do list, and some other basic programs installed and ready to use. Additional Palm software can be installed in various ways, including a download from the Internet or a software disk with an installer that will walk you through the process when synchronized with your computer. Downloading software is discussed in more detail in Chapter 5.

For each of the programs that you are using for your Palm handheld, you can customize your program settings to determine how files are handled during synchronization. For most Palm handhelds, these settings are called a *conduit*. The default setting allows all files to be synchronized between the Palm handheld and the desktop software. Some of the most common programs for the Palm handheld that have individual conduits are the Date Book, Address Book, Note Pad, To Do List, Memo Pad, and Palm Photos; Palm Desktop software also includes a specific system conduit and a specific install conduit.

To personalize the HotSync program settings, begin by clicking on the HotSync icon ⊘ in the Windows system tray in the lower right corner of your PC screen. You can also click on the HotSync command button on the Palm Desktop software menu bar. From the HotSync manager menu, select Custom. Next, you would select the appropriate user name from the list, as shown in Figure 2.12A (in this example, the user is FC), and then select a specific program from the list of conduits. In the example shown in Figure 2.12B, Datebook was the specific program selected. Then select Change to view modification settings available. Click on the changes you want to make and then click on OK to finish. Next, to save your settings, click on Done, as shown in Figure 2.12C.

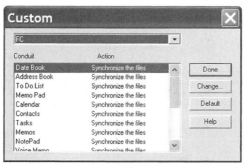

A

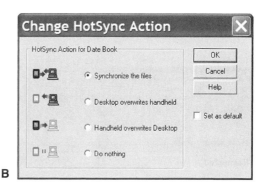

B

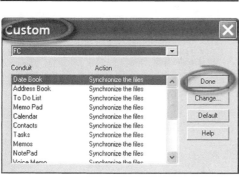

C

Figure 2.12 **A** Custom screen tool system manager. **B** HotSync action change screen. **C** Click on Done to complete.

Personal Information Management System

An important feature of handheld devices is the PIM System that they provide. Both Palm and Pocket PC offer PIM. Because Pocket PC devices function in a Windows-based environment, only Microsoft Outlook is available. Palm users have the option of using Palm Desktop or Microsoft Outlook. The process will be described in the next section.

PIM on Windows CE/Pocket PC

The Windows-based handheld device uses Microsoft Outlook as the PIM System. This program can help you manage all of your appointments, contacts, memos, and to-do lists. You must first install the Microsoft Outlook program to your computer from the CD that came with your handheld device. After the program is installed and you synchronize your handheld with your computer, you can configure the specific Microsoft Outlook settings for synchronization. To configure the settings, follow these steps:

1. Synchronize your handheld device with your computer.
2. On the synchronization dialog box, select Options, as shown in Figure 2.13A.
3. Select (highlight) Calendar, as shown in Figure 2.13B.
4. Select Settings.

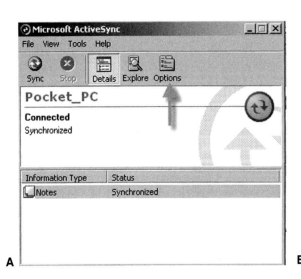
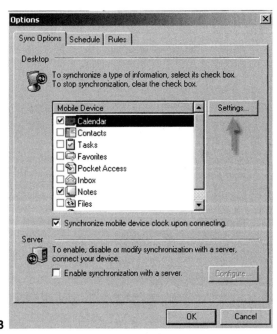

Figure 2.13 Configuring PIM settings for Pocket PC: **A** Sync dialog box. **B** Select Calendar.

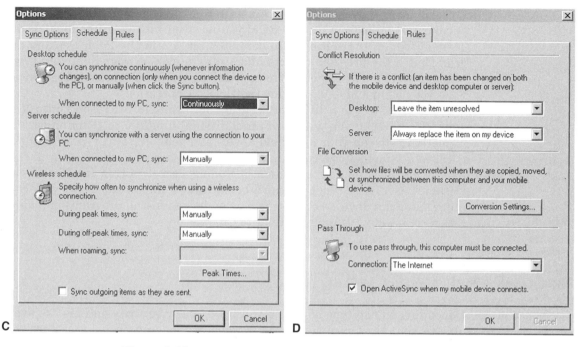

Figure 2.13 (Continued) **C** Schedule screen. **D** Select Rules screen.

5. Set the synchronization settings as desired for your appointments.
6. Select OK to save settings.
7. Select Schedule tab located at the top of the ActiveSync window.
8. Select how often you want the device to synchronize your calendar while connected to your PC (see Figure 2.13C).
9. Select OK to save settings.
10. Select the Rules tab located at the top of the ActiveSync window, as shown in Figure 2.13D.
11. Select the process for resolving conflicts in your calendar.
12. Select OK to finish.

PIM on Palm

The Palm device comes with the Palm Desktop program. The Palm Desktop is a very intuitive program that lets you quickly add or update your contacts, appointments, to-dos, and memos at your desktop computer, and then with a quick touch on the HotSync button synchronize the information with your PDA. If you are using this program as your PIM System, your handheld device will communicate automatically with the Palm Desktop program every time you HotSync your device.

The Palm Desktop program provides you with all of the essential personal management tools that you need, such as a calendar, contacts, and to-do list.

To begin using this software, you must first install the Palm Desktop software on your computer from the CD-ROM you received with your handheld device. The majority of the settings are defaulted for you in the Palm Desktop program, but if the program detects Microsoft Outlook on your computer, it will prompt you to make a selection as to which personal information program you want your handheld to use during the HotSync operation.

If you want to use a different program, for example, Microsoft Outlook, as your PIM System, you will need an additional program to communicate information between your handheld device and your PC. This type of program is called a sync tool or a conduit, and there are several to choose from for use with a Windows operating system, including Pocket mirror, Intellisync, and DesktopToGo. These programs must be purchased and installed onto your computer and Palm device. For instructions on how to install programs and applications onto your PDA, please refer to Chapter 5.

Security for Your PDA

Depending on the type of device you have, many security options are available to you. Most commonly, the options are logging on using a password (see Figure 2.14), a four-digit personal identification number (PIN), a fingerprint, or any combination of these security options. Additional protection can also be provided by setting a maximum number of attempts to log on to the device.

Since 2003, HIPAA regulations require that all electronic applications comply with current standards. These standards require that files containing patient health information on a handheld device be secure and/or encrypted. In addition, if information is going to be transmitted or stored, there must be measures in place to ensure privacy and confidentiality.

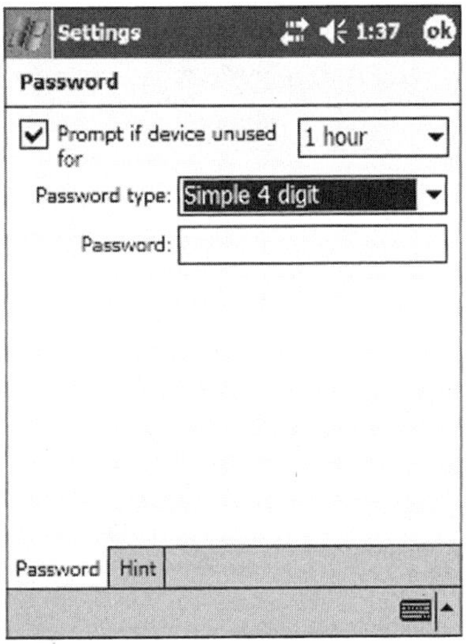

Figure 2.14   Selecting password settings.

Security for Windows CE/Pocket PC

To select security options for your Windows CE/Pocket PC PDA, follow the steps outlined here and illustrated in Figure 2.15.

1. Turn on your handheld device.
2. Tap on Start.
3. Select Settings.
4. Select Password from the menu (see Figure 2.15A).
5. Select the type of security you want, as shown in Figure 2.15B–C (No password; simple four-digit PIN; PIN and fingerprint [if available]; strong alphanumeric password; pin or fingerprint [if available]; password and fingerprint [if available]; password or fingerprint [if available]; fingerprint only [if available]).

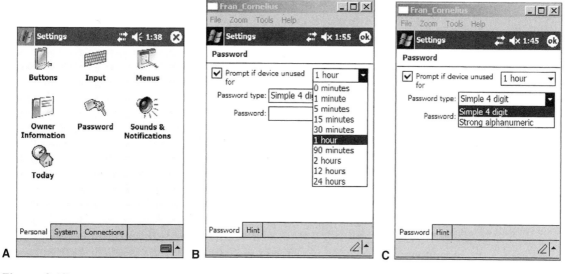

Figure 2.15 Security options for Windows CE/Pocket PC: **A** Setting password screen. **B** Select time after which PDA will prompt for password if device is unused. **C** Select type of password.

6. If selecting a password or PIN, you will be prompted to enter it at that time.
7. Select OK to save settings.

Security for Palm

To select security options for your Palm PDA, follow the steps outlined here and illustrated in Figure 2.16.

1. Turn on your handheld device.
2. Select Menu.
3. Select Preferences.
4. Select Security from the menu shown in Figure 2.16A.

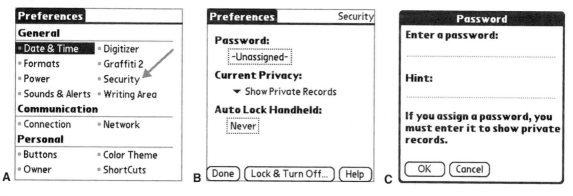

Figure 2.16 Security options for Palm: **A** Select security screen. **B** Select password screen. **C** Enter password and hint screen.

5. Select Password (see Figure 2.16B).
6. Enter a password (see Figure 2.16C).
7. Enter a hint for the password, in case you forget it.
8. Select OK to finish.
9. Some handhelds also have the option to auto lock the handheld device.

Summary

We have reviewed the steps involved in getting you "up and running" with your PDA. You have learned how to charge your PDA via your cradle or directly through a power outlet. You have also learned how to set up a partnership between your PDA and PC to synchronize information between the two devices, using a PIM system, such as Microsoft ActiveSync or Palm Desktop. In addition, you have learned how to modify the synchronization settings to accommodate your individual needs as well as steps to take to protect your information. Now you are ready to move on to Chapter 3, where you can learn how to enter information quickly and proficiently.

Tips From the Experts

Windows CE

When synchronizing and establishing a partnership with more than one computer, only one computer should synchronize with the Inbox (your e-mail). Your PDA cannot manage e-mail from more than one computer. In addition, your pocket PC has a default setting that limits the number of partnerships you can establish—that is, you can only establish a partnership with two computers. After you have had the PDA on a third computer, when you return to one of the original two computers, you will get a cue to delete a partnership and develop a new partnership with that computer.

Windows CE and Palm

When your PDA is not in use for extended periods of time or when it is at home or in the office, you should keep it in the cradle. Keeping it plugged in will ensure that when you are "off and running," you can grab your PDA with the confidence that it is fully charged and ready for use.

LEARNING ACTIVITIES

1. Modify your sync options as follows:
   A. Palm: HotSync your handheld device with the computer. From the custom dialog box on your PC, change the items that you want the handheld device to HotSync with that computer.

   B. Windows CE/Pocket PC: Sync your handheld device with the computer. From the synchronization box on your PC, change the items that you want the handheld to sync with that computer.

2. Set up the security system in your handheld, using a strong alphanumeric password. (Make sure it is a password that you can remember!)

 Visit http://thePoint.LWW.com/cornelius for supplemental information and activities.

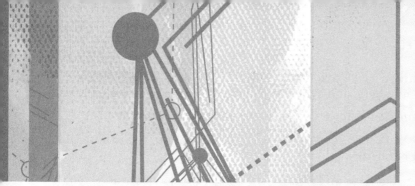

3

Getting Down to Basics: Data Entry Options

Mary Gallagher Gordon

Key Terms

Block Recognizer • A Pocket PC/Windows CE tool that mimics Palm Graffiti as a means for entering text or data, using the same unique shorthand alphabet developed by Palm

Configure • Setting options of built-in tools/features to user preferences

Foldable external keyboard • A device that attaches to your PDA either directly or via infrared (IR) and allows you to type as you would on your desktop

Graffiti • Palm's original Graffiti writing software that provides a quick way to enter text or data, using a unique shorthand alphabet

Keyboard • Built-in data entry tool for both Palm and Pocket PC/Windows CE devices that resembles a miniature keyboard. Using a stylus, you can tap on the letters to form the word

Letter Recognizer • A Pocket PC/Windows CE tool using conventional printed letters, numbers, and symbols to enter information into the PDA

Mode • The function or form used to enter information into the PDA

Transcriber • A Pocket PC/Windows CE tool that allows you to enter data, using your own handwriting

Writing area • The area on Palm devices, below the screen, where you enter data (text, numbers, or symbols)

K eeping notes of daily tasks is part of everyone's day. Yet remembering where the notepaper is placed, its note contents, and which tasks remain all add up to a waste of time and talents! Having all of the information in one place, in the palm of your hand, would be the ideal situation. This chapter addresses the technique of writing with the PDA.

All PDAs offer the user a choice regarding which mode or method to use to input information into the device. The Palm device offers users two choices: Graffiti and a built-in miniature keyboard. Graffiti is Palm's signature writing software, which provides a quick way to enter information into a handheld device. In addition to input modes similar to Palm's, Pocket PC/Windows CE devices offer two other options: letter recognizer and transcriber. Palm does offer a limited transcriber feature used for jotting down quick notes on Palm Note Pad.

Data Entry for Pocket PC/Windows CE

As stated earlier, Pocket PC/Windows CE devices offer four options for inputting information. These input methods are block recognizer (like Graffiti), keyboard, letter recognizer, and transcriber, as shown in Figure 3.1.

To configure your preferred data entry method, tap the Start button on the top left corner of the screen. In the drop-down panel, tap Settings and then select Input. At the bottom of the screen three options are listed. The Input Method option allows you to configure each input method. By tapping on the ▼ on the drop-down menu in the upper right side of the screen, you have the option of selecting one of the four input methods to configure (see Figure 3.2). To change input method, tap on the arrow and choose from the options offered. Tap on the input selected and the menu will diminish. Each of the modes offered has unique features while still maintaining some basic similarities. It would be a good idea to become familiar with each mode and to find the one that works best for you. The question mark within each mode brings up the Help file for assistance.

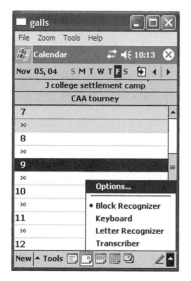

Figure 3.1 Pocket PC data entry options.

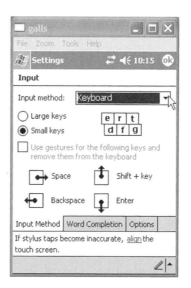

Figure 3.2 Configuring Pocket PC input methods: keyboard options.

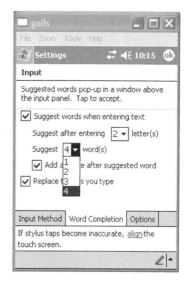

Figure 3.3 Options for Word Completion on Pocket PC.

Word Completion

Another feature offered with the PDA is the word completion feature. Remaining in the input settings, look on the bottom of the screen. Tap on Word Completion. The Word Completion option helps speed up data entry by suggesting words when you have entered only a few letters. The suggestions pop up as you enter text, and, if you tap on the suggested word, it will automatically be entered into the text you are creating. If the suggested word is not the one you want, you can ignore the suggestion and continue to enter the desired text. Additional options available include setting how many letters must be entered before a suggested word pops up, as well as choosing whether to have the device suggest more than one word at a time, as shown in Figure 3.3. This feature gives the option of the PDA to suggest anywhere from one to four words when letters are entered. This is a great time-saver!

Remaining in the Input menu, note the third section on the bottom right. This is the Options section, which allows you to change the default zoom level for both typing and writing. There is also the option that enables the PDA to capitalize the first letter of the sentence and to scroll upon reaching the last line.

Note the following sentence at the bottom of the screen: "If the stylus taps become inaccurate, align the touch screen." On occasion, you may notice that stylus taps onto your PDA screen are not accurate, that is, the device does not respond in the exact location of the tip of your stylus. In this event, you should realign your screen, which is easily done by going into your system settings. First, close all windows on your PDA screen so that you are back to your start page (Today screen). Then try the following exercise:

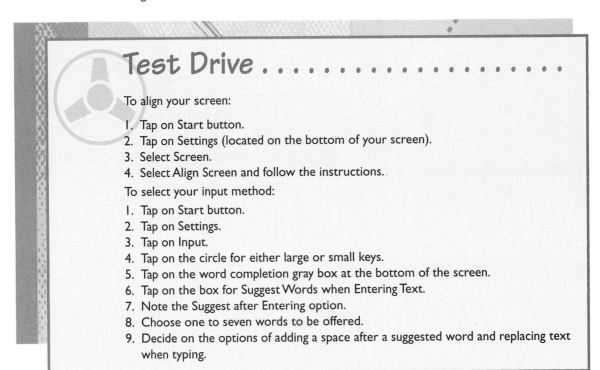

Test Drive...........................

To align your screen:

1. Tap on Start button.
2. Tap on Settings (located on the bottom of your screen).
3. Select Screen.
4. Select Align Screen and follow the instructions.

To select your input method:

1. Tap on Start button.
2. Tap on Settings.
3. Tap on Input.
4. Tap on the circle for either large or small keys.
5. Tap on the word completion gray box at the bottom of the screen.
6. Tap on the box for Suggest Words when Entering Text.
7. Note the Suggest after Entering option.
8. Choose one to seven words to be offered.
9. Decide on the options of adding a space after a suggested word and replacing text when typing.

Keyboard Option

The keyboard selection offers the ability to use the stylus to tap on each letter or symbol to complete a word. As discussed earlier, you have the option to change the default input method according to your preference (keyboard, block recognizer, letter recognizer, or transcriber) by going to the system settings. To get there on your PDA, go to Start → Settings → Input. The Input method drop-down menu lists all of the options available. When you select Keyboard, you have the option to change the size of the keys to either large or small (see Figure 3.2). To work with the keyboard, open Pocket Word by pressing Start → Programs → Pocket Word. In the bottom right corner of the screen, a small keyboard icon is shown.

The keyboard defaults to the lowercase letter mode, with the numbers at the top. To switch to capital letters, tap on the CAP tab, as shown in Figure 3.4. To see the numeric mode, tap on 123 in the top left corner or tap the shift key. To visualize special characters, tap on the *áü* button near the bottom left of the keyboard. Practicing switching to these different keyboard options makes for increased speed.

Pocket Word has many of the features that Microsoft Word offers. Tips to assist with inputting text into a document can be easily accessed. Pocket Word has four options located in the gray bar at the bottom of the screen: New, Edit, View, and Tools.

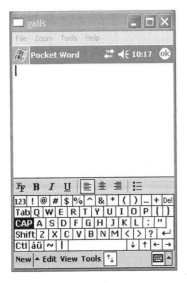

Figure 3.4 Switching to upper-case letters by pressing the CAP tab. Note that the CAP tab also changes the numbers to symbols.

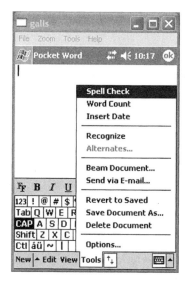

Figure 3.5   Pocket Word tool options such as Spell Check.

Tapping on New will begin a new word document. The arrow-up option beside New opens the drop-down menu for writing meeting notes, a new memo, phone memo, to-do list, or note.

Tapping on Edit offers users four options that are similar to those available to users of Microsoft Word. The Select All option allows you to select all of the text in the document and perform any number of word processing activities on your PDA. For example, you can copy and paste the text to another document or select Format to change the font and pen weight or to use bold, underline, italic highlight, or strikethrough. Other options available include paragraph alignment, text indent or bullet, and find and replace.

The View option allows you to choose the toolbar, wrap text to the window, or use the scroll button. You can make use of utilities such as drawing, writing, typing, or recording. If you need to zoom in, use the view selection. The view is presented in a word format. The Wrap to Window choice gives the writer the ability to toggle the document back and forth or to have the document fit to the screen. In the Writing option, the format shows lines on which to write the document; the Drawing option shows blocks in which to draw the work; the Typing option brings up a blank document; and Recording gives the option to voice the work to be saved.

In the Tools section of Pocket Word, there are more similarities to Microsoft Word on a desktop computer. As shown in Figure 3.5, options include Spell Check, Word Count, and Insert Date. Under Tools, a document may be saved, sent as an e-mail, or beamed. Under Options, the default template is a blank document; however, you may wish to set the default to another template to speed things up when you are entering data. You may choose to use one of the standard templates or create your own. The possibilities here are endless.

A final option is saving your important documents to a specific area and choosing how to display the document in the list of saved documents. You can save your document to a preestablished file folder, which can be on the PDA's Main Memory, iPAQ File Store, or an external memory card (SD or CF).

The blue up-and-down arrows on the bottom right, beside the Tools option in Figure 3.6, are a quick way to bring up or remove a tool bar. Which tool bar is available depends upon which view option has been selected from the View menu. For example, if Writing is bulleted, the blue arrows bring up the pencil with a choice of thickness from fine to thick; the left arrow will return the work from which it came; and F will format the work.

If Drawing is the view option bulleted, the pencil and thickness stay the same. The pencil with a colored line under it brings up the colors to use to draw; the paint will give background color options; the arrow back option is next; and the triangle brings up the format.

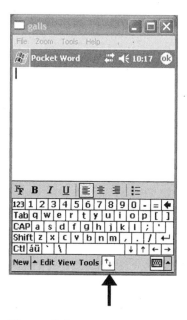

Figure 3.6   The blue arrow options in Pocket Word to change font, alignment, and bullets.

In the Typing view, the blue arrows ⬆ show the typical Windows Word toolbar that includes format, bold, italic, underlining, and aligning or bulleting. Again, these tools will speed up some of the word processing activities that you wish to perform on these handy little devices.

In the Recording view, the toolbar shows recording, stop, and the toggle of the document. You can reverse, forward, or adjust the volume. To minimize these toolbars, just tap on the blue arrows ⬆ again. This will enable you to record notes or instructions that will be linked to that particular document. Recording is a very handy feature for later jogging your memory when you have the time and opportunity to complete your documentation (data entry) onto that particular document.

Test Drive . . . .

1. Tap on Start, Programs, and Pocket Word.
2. In the bottom left corner, press New.
3. In the bottom right corner, press the arrow-up key and select Keyboard.
4. Type out the following: "Penny spent $1.00 (she used it all for candy!)."
5. Document the word count.
6. Insert the date.
7. Save the document as "Penny" to the main memory.

Block Recognizer

On the bottom right corner, tap on the arrow-up ▲ and choose the block recognizer. The block recognizer defaults to lowercase letters. To write a letter or symbol in the block recognizer, write between the two small dashes on the panel; the letters go to the left and the numbers to the right of the dashed line. To enter an uppercase letter, use the shift mode. Activating the shift mode requires drawing a straight line from the bottom of the screen halfway up the input box on the left side of the screen. If there is a change in the *abc* to *Abc* or *ABC,* the shift mode has been activated. *Abc* will capitalize the first letter of the word you are entering. You must engage the shift mode to display *Abc* for each word. The *ABC* mode will lock in capital letters so that all text you enter is uppercase.

The bold, black arrow on the right side of the screen will move the cursor back and erase the work in progress; the left or right arrow will move the cursor to the specified direction; the arrow that appears to go down to the next level will move the cursor down a row; *Spc* is the space tool; the question mark (?) key is the help mode; and the @$ key will bring up punctuation and symbol options.

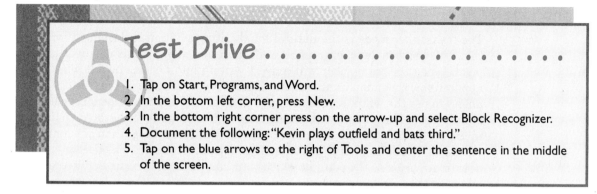

Test Drive . . . .

1. Tap on Start, Programs, and Word.
2. In the bottom left corner, press New.
3. In the bottom right corner press on the arrow-up and select Block Recognizer.
4. Document the following: "Kevin plays outfield and bats third."
5. Tap on the blue arrows to the right of Tools and center the sentence in the middle of the screen.

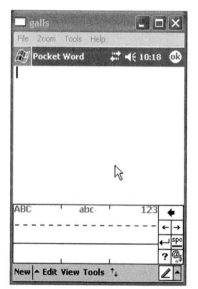

Figure 3.7 The Pocket PC Letter Recognizer input screen is divided into three sections.

Letter Recognizer

Letter Recognizer, also located at the bottom of your screen, has the same options as Block Recognizer. As shown in Figure 3.7, the input section is divided into three sections: the far left for capital letters, the middle for lowercase, and the far right for numbers. The dashed line in the middle is used to help you accurately place letters so that they can be correctly translated by the PDA. It is reminiscent of the paper used when you first learned penmanship in elementary school. All letters are entered in lowercase; the location in which you enter the letter determines whether it will be lowercase or uppercase.

The toolbar at the bottom of the screen is a consistent view in all of the inputting methods. You see New, Edit, View, and Tools. If you press the blue arrows ⬆ key in the bottom tool bar, you will see similar icons as you do with Word for Windows.

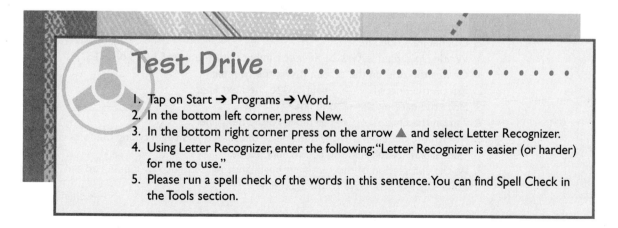

Test Drive . . . .

1. Tap on Start → Programs → Word.
2. In the bottom left corner, press New.
3. In the bottom right corner press on the arrow ▲ and select Letter Recognizer.
4. Using Letter Recognizer, enter the following: "Letter Recognizer is easier (or harder) for me to use."
5. Please run a spell check of the words in this sentence. You can find Spell Check in the Tools section.

Transcriber

The transcriber mode is the natural handwriting solution to document information. This mode is available on Pocket PC only and allows a mix of cursive and/or print. Using the transcriber will convert writing into text in the following notes applications: Calendar, Contacts, and Tasks. One advantage of Transcriber is the ability to use the whole screen as opposed to only the input section on the bottom of the screen. The writing will be converted to text from the integrated dictionary in the Pocket PC. A letter recognizer tutorial facilitates recognition of your handwriting style. Although it is not difficult to master, it requires a moderate amount of patience to get to the point at which your handwriting is accurately recognized by the PDA.

When looking at the screen, you will see that the first row of the toolbar is the same as in any of the other modes. The second row has tools specifically for the Transcriber application. Although the order of these icons and the symbols used may vary from PDA to PDA, all possess the same functionalities. Usually, the first icon on the left side of the screen (it may be a dark arrow or another symbol) controls the writing direction—that is, the angle at which you will be writing on the screen. This feature offers a bit more flexibility for individual writing styles as well as accommodating left-handed writers. Writing should be perpendicular to the direction selected.

Moving to the right, the next icon is the Letter Shapes programming tool, which allows you to "train" the tool to recognize your individual handwriting. The third icon is the Microsoft Transcriber keyboard. When tapped, it will display a selection of punctuation and other symbols to facilitate text entry. The fourth icon is the recognition mode. The option of uppercase, lowercase, or number mode is chosen here.

Now you can work on which documenting option you will want to use.

Test Drive . . . .

In this Test Drive, you will begin with the keyboard option.

1. Open Word.
2. Open a new document.
3. Writing in capital letters, begin a document with the title: CLASS NOTES.
4. Center the title on the screen (using the tool bar).
5. Tap on the Enter key (◁) to move to the next line.
6. Place the date on the second line.
7. Tap on the Enter key (◁) to move to the next line.
8. Realign the document to the left side of the screen and begin typing the following: "James plays baseball in the community league."
9. At the completion of the sentence, begin another sentence by tapping on the Enter key (◁) to move to the next line.

(Continued)

10. Change to the Block Recognizer and enter the following: "The rain is heavy and we may get 2 inches."
    (Did you remember to use the left side for the letters and the right side for the numbers?)
11. Again, begin another sentence by tapping on the Enter key (◁) to move to the next line.
12. Use the Letter Recognizer and enter the following: "MC is the goalie and there were 27 shots on goal!"

As stated earlier, the Transcriber allows you to type text in your own handwriting anywhere on the screen.

Test Drive . . . .

Using Transcriber, do the following:

1. Open the document, CLASS NOTES.
2. Select Transcriber as the input mode, tapping on the ▲ located in the lower right corner of the screen.
3. View the brief tutorial before tapping on OK. (A Help button on the lower left corner of the screen is used for more information. For the time being, do not place a check mark in the box beside "Don't show this.")
4. Type the following: "MaryCate's field hockey team won their last 5 games."

Transcriber takes a bit of time to become proficient, but, with a little practice, you may find that this option for entering text is right for you.

Using Transcriber Features to Create a Quick Note

You can easily create a quick note with a diagram or map, using Notes in your Windows-based device. Locate Notes by tapping on Start → Programs → Notes (you may need to scroll down to locate the Notes icon). To create a new note in Notes, tap on New on the lower left side of the screen. The default name for your new note will be Note. All subsequent notes will have a number added to the title: Note1, Note2, Note3, and so on. Clearly, it will be more useful to give the note a title that is more meaningful. To give your note a name, tap on the ▲ in the lower right corner of your new note and select a method to enter the title (Block Recognizer, Keyboard, or Letter Recognizer). Then after tapping on the pencil icon located on the bottom center of the screen, you can draw your diagram or map or jot a quick note. Your entry will be recorded and will resemble a hastily scrawled note on a memo pad.

Test Drive . . . .

1. Access Notes by tapping on New at the bottom of your Today screen.
2. Select Note.
3. Draw the following map, using your stylus on the PDA screen:

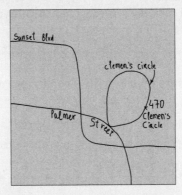

4. Tap on OK on the upper right corner of the screen.
5. Press and hold your stylus on Note1. You will see a pop-up menu that offers the Rename/Move option.
6. Highlight Rename/Move and, using Block Recognizer, Keyboard, or Letter Recognizer, type the following title: "Directions to Sue's house"
7. You have the option to save this document to a specific folder or to your storage card or the iPAQ File Store.
8. Tap on OK to finish.

Data Entry for Palm

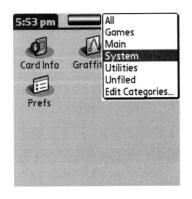

Figure 3.8 Palm showing All categories.

In Palm devices the **writing area** is located at the bottom of the PDA and is usually visible. In some of the newer Palm devices, a sliding cover conceals the writing area until the user needs it. As stated earlier, the Palm offers users two methods of data entry: Graffiti and Keyboard.

Graffiti

To access the writing tool in Palm, locate and tap on the "house" or home, 🏠, and then in the top right corner, tap on All, as shown in Figure 3.8. On the drop-down bar menu, tap on System and then select Graffiti 2. Using the tutorial provided, you can learn the Graffiti method for documentation. In the tutorial you will learn how to access the keyboard. The keyboard tutorial will show how the input section is divided into two areas;

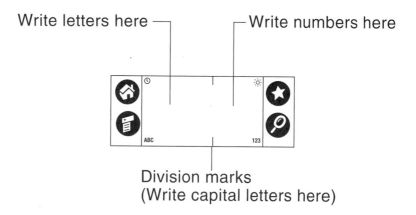

Figure 3.9 Palm input section tutorial.

the left side of the input panel is for letters and the right side is for numbers and symbols (see Figure 3.9). Tapping on "Try It!" will take you through a brief interactive tutorial, orienting you to Graffiti techniques of entering data, as shown in Figure 3.10.

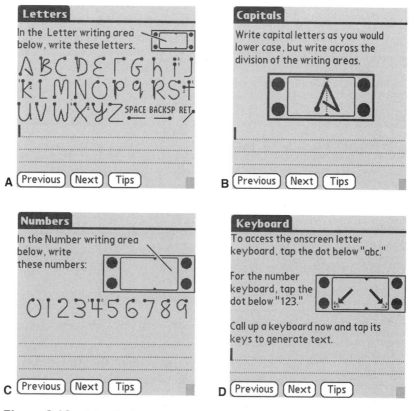

Figure 3.10 Palm Graffiti tutorial: **A** Writing all letters with tips. **B** Writing uppercase letters. **C** Writing numbers. **D** Accessing the on-screen keyboards.

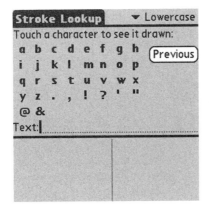

Figure 3.11 Palm Stroke Lookup for lowercase letters.

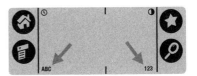

Figure 3.12 ABC and 123 links to Keyboard and Stroke Lookup.

Another useful feature within Graffiti is Stroke Lookup. While in the Stroke Lookup section of the tutorial, you can select a letter and view a demonstration of several techniques to enter that particular letter (see Figure 3.11). The quickest way to get to Stroke Lookup is to tap on either ABC or 123 located at the bottom left and right corners of the writing area of your PDA (see Figure 3.12). Now, try it yourself.

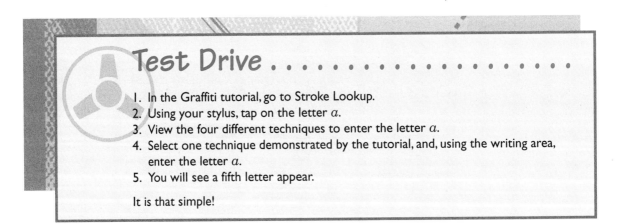

Test Drive . . . .

1. In the Graffiti tutorial, go to Stroke Lookup.
2. Using your stylus, tap on the letter a.
3. View the four different techniques to enter the letter a.
4. Select one technique demonstrated by the tutorial, and, using the writing area, enter the letter a.
5. You will see a fifth letter appear.

It is that simple!

In the Stroke Lookup screen, note the drop-down menu in the top left corner. Tap on ▼ the to see all of the options available for looking up a particular stroke: uppercase and lowercase letters, numbers, gestures, symbols, accents, and shortcuts (see Figure 3.13). You can review the different options offered for

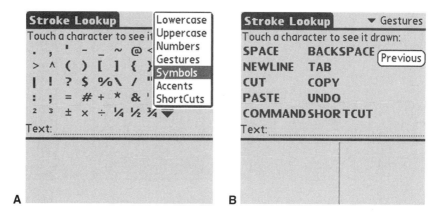

Figure 3.13 **A** Options under Stroke Lookup (symbols shown in background). **B** Gestures.

each letter, number, or symbol in this area. These are all important characters to learn and will speed up your data entry.

Keyboard

The writing area is divided into four sections, as you can see in Figure 3.14. Tapping on ABC on the bottom left corner of the panel (see Figure 3.12) will bring up the keyboard screen. Remember that to use the ABC or 123 links, you must be in an application that allows you to enter data, for example, Memo or Address.

When in Keyboard mode, in the bottom center of the screen, note the *abc, 123,* and *int'l* buttons, highlighted in Figure 3.15A. This keyboard is similar to the keyboard you use with your personal computer. Tapping on the *shift* key will capitalize just one letter (see Figure 3.15B). Tapping on the *cap* key, as shown in Figure 3.15C, will lock the capitalization function so that all letters selected will be capitalized. The key above the *cap* key will tab over on the page (see Figure 3.15D). The bold arrow on the right top row will delete text to the left of the cursor (i.e., backspace or delete), as shown in Figure 3.15E. The bold return arrow on the third row on the right will take you down a row (see Figure 3.15F).

Figure 3.14 The Palm writing area has four input areas.

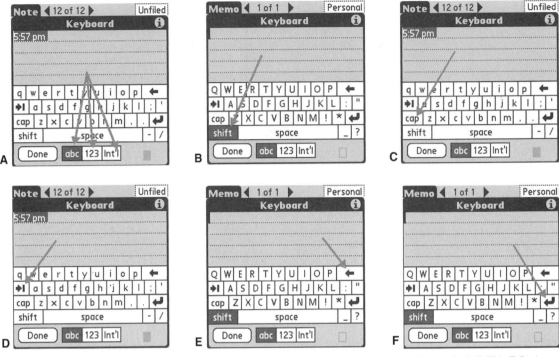

Figure 3.15 The Palm keyboard: **A** Letter, number, and international buttons. **B** Shift. **C** Caps lock. **D** Tab. **E** Backspace or delete. **F** Enter.

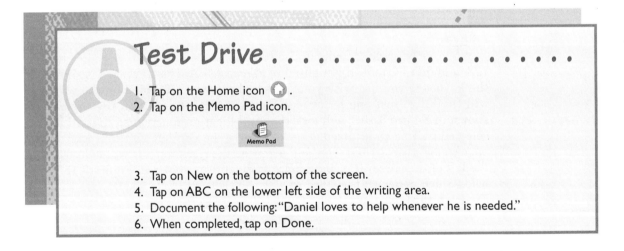

Test Drive . . . .

1. Tap on the Home icon 🏠.
2. Tap on the Memo Pad icon.

Memo Pad

3. Tap on New on the bottom of the screen.
4. Tap on ABC on the lower left side of the writing area.
5. Document the following: "Daniel loves to help whenever he is needed."
6. When completed, tap on Done.

Return to the note section by tapping on the Home 🏠, and scroll to locate the Memo Pad icon. Tapping on the *123* button located in the right lower corner of the writing area will bring up the screen for the numbers and symbols. The *int'l* button takes you to the international symbol section (see Figure 3.15A). Pressing on the information button 🛈 at the top of the note screen takes you to the tip section, which is beneficial to read.

Transcriber for Note Pad

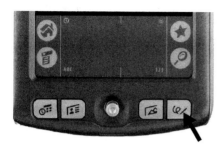

Figure 3.16 Quick link to Notes on Palm. (Image courtesy of Palm, Inc.)

When beginning a note, you can go directly to the Note section by pressing on the button located on the lower right face of the PDA that shows what looks like a pen writing (see Figure 3.16). This button opens the Notes page, where all notes previously saved are listed first. To write a new note, tap on New located at the bottom left of the screen. After pressing New, your entry is automatically tagged with the time and date. You can opt to delete the time and enter a more meaningful title for the document, using either the Graffiti or Keyboard input methods.

If using the Graffiti method to document, begin writing on the input panel at the bottom of the Palm. If you want to use the keyboard, use the stylus and tap on ABC at the bottom left of the writing area. The ability to use either capital or lowercase lettering for your note is an option. When the title of the note is completed, you can quickly jot your note or draw a picture/diagram on the screen, using the stylus. Your movements on the screen will be captured and imbedded in the note. When finished, tap on Done to save the note.

Test Drive . . . .

1. Press on the button located on the lower right face of the PDA (see Figure 3.16).
2. Using Graffiti on the writing area, type the following title: "Directions to Sue's house."
3. Draw the following map, using your stylus on the PDA screen:

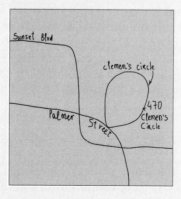

4. Tap on Done to save.
5. Tap on the title "Directions to Sue's house . . ." to view your document again.

You can organize your notes into categories (files) that will enable you to more quickly access your information. To place a note into a particular category, tap on the ▼ located at the top right corner of the screen. In this window, you can select a preset category (Business or Personal) or create a new category. To create a new category (or file folder), select Edit Categories from the drop-down menu. Select New, add the new category, and select OK to finish. Now you try it.

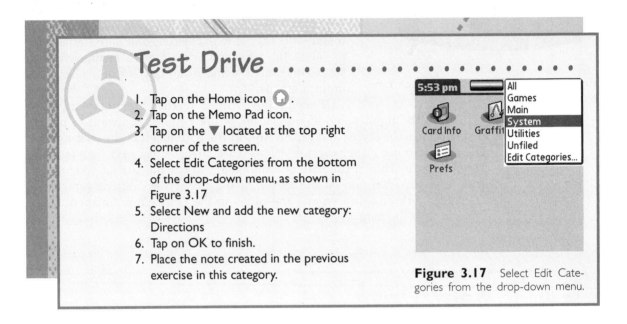

Test Drive . . . .

1. Tap on the Home icon ⌂.
2. Tap on the Memo Pad icon.
3. Tap on the ▼ located at the top right corner of the screen.
4. Select Edit Categories from the bottom of the drop-down menu, as shown in Figure 3.17
5. Select New and add the new category: Directions
6. Tap on OK to finish.
7. Place the note created in the previous exercise in this category.

Figure 3.17 Select Edit Categories from the drop-down menu.

External Keyboards—Another Way to Enter Data

Both Palm and Windows CE/Pocket PC devices can be used with a **foldable external keyboard** that helps you enter a large amount of information more easily than the built-in keyboard or Graffiti method. These portable external keyboards can attach easily to the base of the PDA or can connect wirelessly via IR. The advantage is that the input speed with the portable keyboard is very similar to the keyboard on a desktop. These devices will be discussed in more detail in Chapter 18.

Summary

PDAs offer users several choices in data entry methods. The Palm devices offer users a choice of either Graffiti or Keyboard methods for data entry, and the Windows CE/Pocket PC devices offer similar options as well as Letter Recognizer and Transcriber. The underlying principle with each option is that these methods provide users a quick and efficient way to input the information and are easy to learn and reliable. Nevertheless, as with all new things, there is a learning curve. Only by practicing and embracing this technology will one become comfortable and develop a level of mastery.

Tips From the Experts

Keeping the Screen Like New

- "I use a small amount of car wax on my Palm screen every few weeks and it does a great job at keeping the screen clean, scratch free, and feeling like new. When the pen seems to start to drag, I just wax the Palm and it is as good as new." (Art Graham@accraply.com, March 5, 1998, http://www. thepalmtree.com/tips.htm)
- "Clear Post-it flags make a great Graffiti overlay to protect from scratches." (William Hungerford. Retrieved September 4, 2005, from http://palmtops. about.com/od/pdatipsandtricks/l/bltips.htm)
- "Instead of expensive screen protectors, buy clear vinyl tablecloth from a fabric store, usually under $2.00 a yard. Cut to fit your screen, then add a few drops of water on your screen and attach and smooth out bubbles. Costs about a nickel per cover." (William Hungerford. Retrieved September 4, 2005, from http://palmtops.about.com/od/pdatipsandtricks/l/bltips.htm.)

LEARNING ACTIVITIES

1. Using Graffiti (Palm) or Block Recognizer (Pocket PC), enter the entire alphabet into a document (using Palm Note Pad or Pocket PC Word).
2. Open Notes in a Windows-based device or Note Pad in a Palm-based device. Give the note the title: "Map to the Johnson's House." Using the Transcriber function, enter the following information:

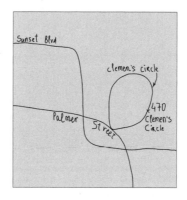

Visit http://thePoint.LWW.com/cornelius for supplemental information and activities.

4

Getting Comfortable With Organizational Features

Faye A. Pearlman • Frances H. Cornelius

Key Terms

Calendar button • A button located on the lower right side of the handheld device that, when pressed, provides quick access to the calendar

Categories • Organizing tools that enable the user to sort information into separate folders to help locate information (appointments or contacts) quickly

Contacts button • A button located on the lower right side of the handheld device that, when pressed, provides quick access to the contacts

Drop-down text menu • A list of preset text options available to speed up text entry on the PDA

Highlight • A technique of using the stylus to select specific text to be quickly deleted and permitting cutting and pasting text from one area to another

Search tool • Imbedded program that enables users to quickly locate information on the device; both the calendar and contact manager offer this feature

T
he earliest PDAs were not very sophisticated and had limited applications. They were initially marketed as devices that would assist in the organization and management of personal data, such as appointments, contacts, notes, and tasks. Advances in technology have greatly expanded the capabilities of handheld computers, yet the organizational features remain among the most universally used applications today.

Time management and organizational skills are critical elements of success in today's fast-paced world. Most people find that they access these programs frequently throughout the day and quickly become dependent upon the organizational features that PDAs provide. Pocket calendars, handwritten address books, notepads, collected business cards, and scattered snippets of paper are being replaced with a single device that stores information efficiently and can be updated with ease. This important information can be shared with your desktop PC, and both calendars will be kept up to date by using a simple automated software application such as Microsoft ActiveSync or Palm Desktop. Calendar and contact information can be integrated with e-mail and beaming functions to share information and communicate with others more effectively. This chapter introduces you to the built-in features of your PDA that help you get organized.

Contacts: The "New and Improved" Address Book

How many times have you had to copy information from one address book to another? How often have you crossed out information and tried to insert new information in a very limited space? Do you have a special family member or friend who has changed addresses, jobs, phone numbers, or contact information so many times that you have lost count? Do you have trouble sorting personal, professional, and business contacts? Have you ever uttered the words, "I know I wrote that address somewhere," "Where did I put that guest list?" or "I really meant to call you, but I lost the number"?

In our fast-paced, information-driven world, organized, readily accessible contact information is not a luxury; it is a necessity. PDAs have proven to be an excellent tool for keeping individuals "in touch" and "up to date" with important contact information in an efficient and organized manner. Throw away the tattered, old-fashioned, handwritten address books and worn-out excuses. Input the data into the address book of your PDA and experience the "latest and greatest version" of your personal "little black book."

Entering Contact Information

Like its handwritten predecessors, contact information can be manually entered into your PDA address book, using various input options available. As discussed in Chapter 3, PDAs, whether Palm or Windows-based, typically have various input mechanisms. Input mechanisms for Windows-based applications include a built-in keyboard, block recognizer, letter recognizer, and transcriber, as shown in Figure 4.1. Palm OS PDAs typically have two methods of input: a built-in keyboard and graffiti, as shown in Figure 4.2A and B.

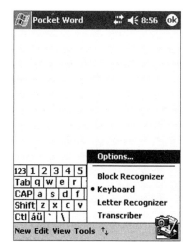

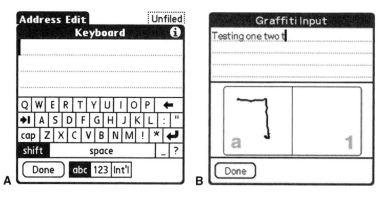

Figure 4.2 Palm input methods: **A** Built-in keyboard. **B** Graffiti.

Figure 4.1 Pocket PC input methods.

Pocket PC/Windows CE

In Windows-based applications, you can access your contact information several ways; the quickest way is to press the contacts button on the front of your PDA. This shortcut will take you directly to the opening screen of your contact information, as shown in Figure 4.3. You can also access this application by tapping on the Start button and selecting Contacts on the Start menu.

To input information, tap on New on the bottom left of the screen. You will be taken to a data entry screen that is similar to the one pictured in Figure 4.4. If you scroll down using the toolbar on the right side of the screen, you will be able to visualize all of the different fields available for data entry. Enter your data and select OK. When the information is displayed, only the fields that you have entered will appear.

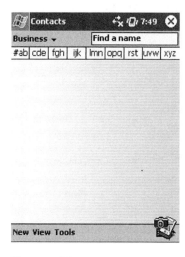

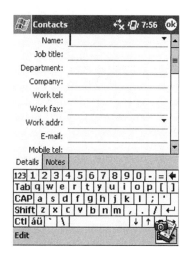

Figure 4.3 Pocket PC opening screen for contacts.

Figure 4.4 Pocket PC new contact entry.

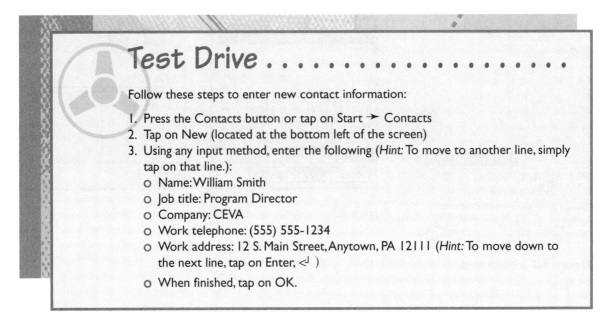

Test Drive . . . .

Follow these steps to enter new contact information:

1. Press the Contacts button or tap on Start ➤ Contacts
2. Tap on New (located at the bottom left of the screen)
3. Using any input method, enter the following (*Hint:* To move to another line, simply tap on that line.):
   o Name: William Smith
   o Job title: Program Director
   o Company: CEVA
   o Work telephone: (555) 555-1234
   o Work address: 12 S. Main Street, Anytown, PA 12111 (*Hint:* To move down to the next line, tap on Enter, ↵)
   o When finished, tap on OK.

When you finish, your new contact information will appear, as shown in Figure 4.5. If you make a mistake while entering the information, simply **highlight** that area and reenter the correct information. If, at a later date, you find that you have made a mistake or want to modify this contact-specific information, you can use the edit function to correct the mistake.

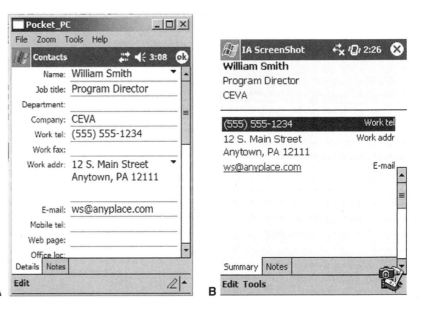

Figure 4.5   Test Drive: **A** Entering William Smith. **B** Completed new entry.

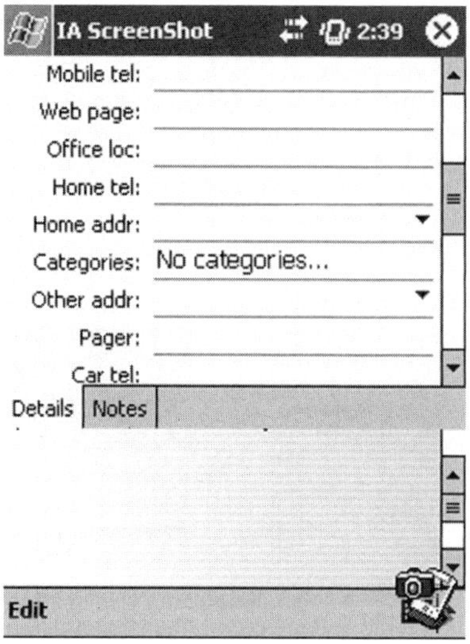

Figure 4.6 Pocket PC contact categories entry point.

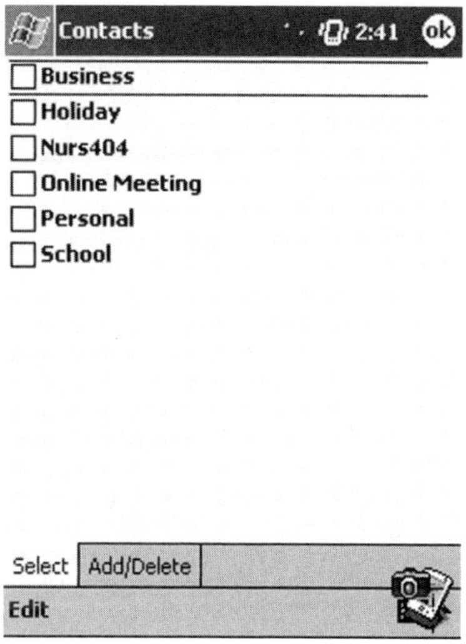

Figure 4.7 Pocket PC contact categories list.

While you are in the area that allows you to enter or edit a contact, you will notice a useful item called **Categories**, as you scroll down (see Figure 4.6). Tap on Categories, and you will be given the opportunity to add this contact to one or more of the default subject headings listed: business, personal, or holidays. To add an additional category, choose the Add/Delete tab at the bottom of the screen, name the new subject heading, and select Add to create a new category of contacts. Examples of standard and new categories are shown in Figure 4.7.

Test Drive . . . .

To organize your contact according to categories, follow the steps outlined here and illustrated in Figure 4.8:

1. Press the Contacts button or tap on Start ➤ Contacts.
2. Tap on Smith, William (the contact you entered in the earlier activity).
3. Tap on Edit located on the bottom of the screen.
4. Using the scroll bar located on the right side of the screen, scroll down and tap on Categories to display category options, as shown in Figure 4.8A.
5. Select Business.

(Continued)

6. Tap on OK to place William Smith in your business contacts (see Figure 4.8B).

To add a new category:

1. Repeat steps 1–3.
2. Tap on Add/Delete, located on the bottom of the screen, as shown in Figure 4.8C.

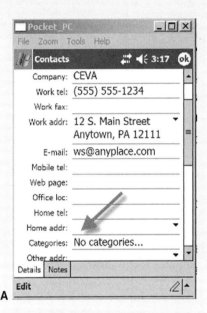

A

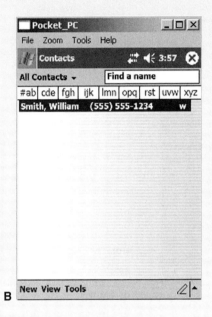

B

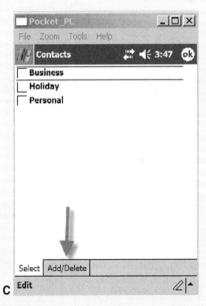

C

Figure 4.8 Pocket PC: **A–B** Placing a contact into a category. **C–F** Adding a new category.

(Continued)

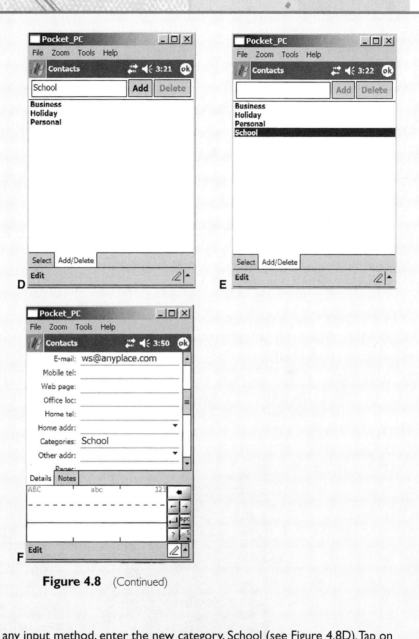

Figure 4.8 (Continued)

3. Using any input method, enter the new category, School (see Figure 4.8D). Tap on Add and you will see that this new category has been added to the options listed (see Figure 4.8E).
4. Tap on OK, located at the upper right corner of the screen.
5. You will notice that your contact has been automatically placed in the newly created category (see Figure 4.8F).

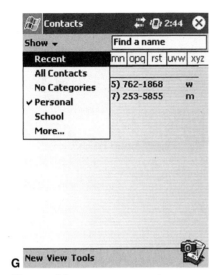

Figure 4.8   (Continued) **G** Available category options for sorting contacts.

Whenever you open the Contacts application, a contact list category will appear at the top left of your screen with a drop-down arrow next to it. Tapping on this arrow will reveal a drop-down menu, as shown in Figure 4.8G, which lists all of the available category options for sorting your contacts database. You can choose to view a complete list of all contacts or select from a more defined preselected group of contacts.

You can also enter information into your contact list or share your contacts with other PDA users by using the infrared beam function. See the Infrared section in Chapter 6 for more information on this topic. Contact information can also be shared between your desktop and the PDA using the synchronization function. More information on synchronization is provided in Chapter 2.

Palm

In Palm devices all of your contacts are in a section called Address or Contacts, depending on which Palm OS you have on your device. To facilitate further discussion throughout this chapter, we will be using the term Address. To access your contacts in a Palm-based PDA, you can push the Address button located on the front of your PDA, as shown in Figure 4.9A. You can also access your contacts by tapping on 🏠 and then tapping on the Address icon, as shown in Figure 4.9B.

To add a new contact, tap on New on the lower right-hand side of the screen. The next screen will be a data entry screen that is similar to the one pictured

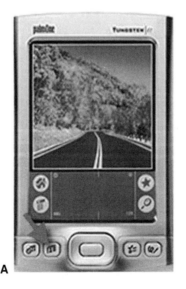

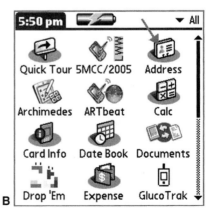

Figure 4.9   Accessing Palm contacts.

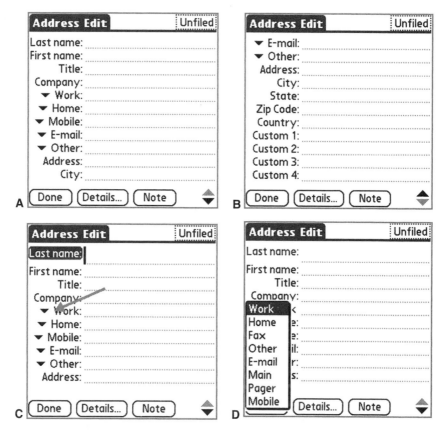

Figure 4.10   A–B Palm contact information fields. **C–D** Modifying field name options.

in Figure 4.10A. If you tap on the arrow ▼ located in the lower right-hand corner of the screen, you will be able to scroll down and see all of the different fields available for data entry, as shown in Figure 4.10B. Additional arrows located on the left side of the screen allow you to change the field name (work, home, fax, e-mail, main, pager, mobile, or other), as depicted in Figure 4.10C and D.

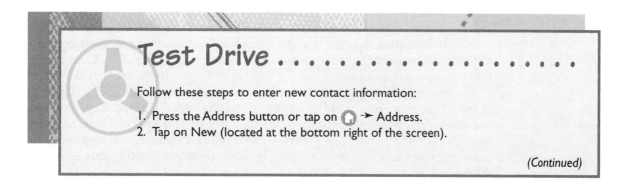

Test Drive . . . .

Follow these steps to enter new contact information:

1. Press the Address button or tap on 🏠 ➤ Address.
2. Tap on New (located at the bottom right of the screen).

(Continued)

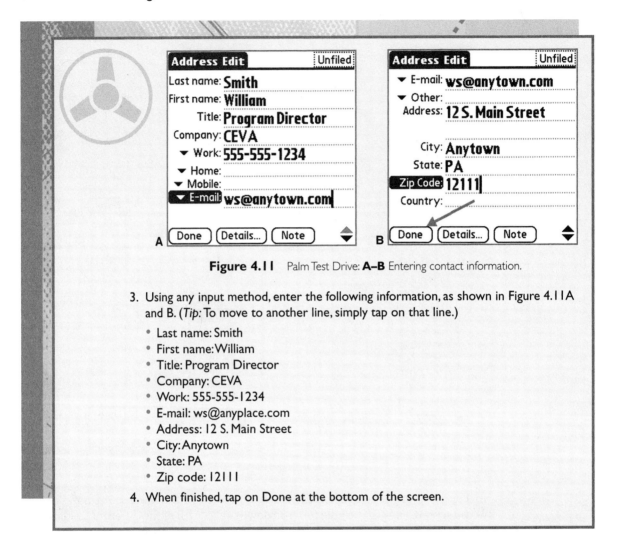

Figure 4.11 Palm Test Drive: **A–B** Entering contact information.

3. Using any input method, enter the following information, as shown in Figure 4.11A and B. (*Tip:* To move to another line, simply tap on that line.)

* Last name: Smith
* First name: William
* Title: Program Director
* Company: CEVA
* Work: 555-555-1234
* E-mail: ws@anyplace.com
* Address: 12 S. Main Street
* City: Anytown
* State: PA
* Zip code: 12111

4. When finished, tap on Done at the bottom of the screen.

If you make a mistake while entering the information, you can highlight that area and reenter the correct information, as shown in Figure 4.12A. If, at a later date, you find you have made a mistake or want to modify this contact-specific information, you can use the edit function to correct the mistake. Simply open the contact information you wish to edit by tapping on it. Then tap on Edit and make the changes from the screen, as shown in Figure 4.12B.

You also have the option to organize your contacts into categories. Located in the upper right corner of the screen is an item called Unfiled. Tap on it and you will be given the opportunity to file this contact in a category such as Business, Family, or Friends (see Figure 4.13A). You can also select the option Edit Categories and create a new category, rename, or delete existing categories, as shown in Figure 4.13B.

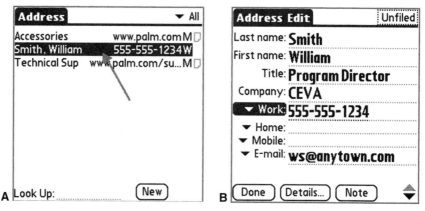

Figure 4.12 Palm: **A–B** Editing contact information.

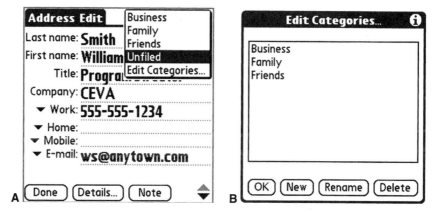

Figure 4.13 Palm: **A** Organizing contacts into categories. **B** Editing categories screen.

Test Drive . . . .

To organize your contacts according to categories, follow the steps outlined here and illustrated in Figure 4.14:

1. Press the Address (or Contacts) button, or tap on 🏠 ➜ Address.
2. Tap on Smith, William (the contact you entered in an earlier activity) to open the contact.
3. Tap on Edit, located on the bottom of the screen (see Figure 4.14A).
4. Tap on Details, also located on the bottom of the screen (see Figure 4.14B).
5. Tap on the ▼ next to Category (see Figure 4.14C).

(Continued)

6. Select Business to place William Smith in your business contacts.
7. Tap on OK.
8. Tap on Done, located on the bottom left of the screen, to save your changes. You will notice that William Smith is now in the Business category, as depicted in Figure 4.14D.

To add a new category:

1. Press the Address button or tap ⬒ ➙ Address.
2. Tap All, located at the upper right corner of the screen (see Figure 4.14E).
3. Tap on Edit Categories (see Figure 4.14F).
4. Tap on New, located on the bottom of the screen (see Figure 4.14G).
5. Using any input method, enter the new category School, as shown in Figure 4.14H.
6. Tap on OK and you will see that this new category has been added to the options listed.
7. Tap on OK again to finish.

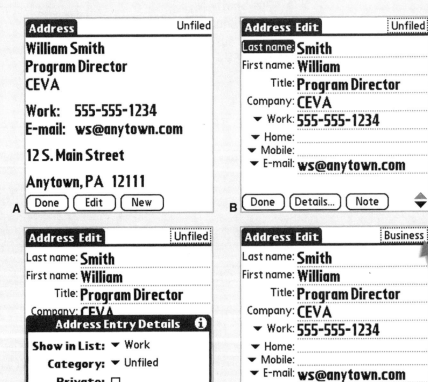

Figure 4.14 Palm Test Drive: **A–D** Placing a contact into a category.

(Continued)

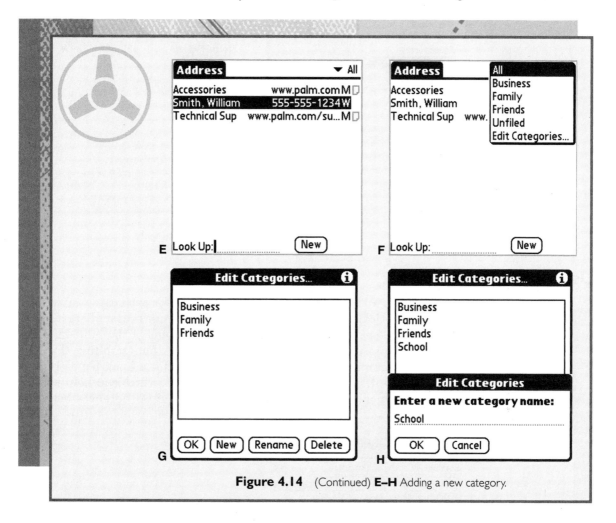

Figure 4.14 (Continued) **E–H** Adding a new category.

Whenever you open your address application, you will see your entire contact list. If you tap on the ▼ next to the word All you will see a **drop-down text menu** of all available categories for sorting your contacts database. As depicted in Figure 4.15A, you can choose to view a complete list of all contacts or select from a more defined preselected group of contacts. For example, if you select Business, you will see William Smith only, the contact you filed in that category in an earlier activity (see Figure 4.15B).

You can also enter information into your contact list or share your contacts with other PDA users by using the infrared beam function. See the Infrared section in Chapter 6 for more information.

Contact information can also be shared between your desktop and the PDA using the synchronization function. For more information, see the Synchronization section in Chapter 2.

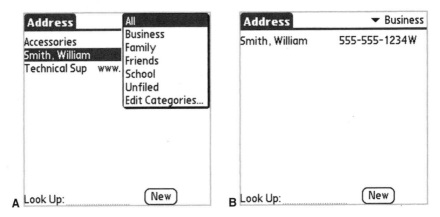

Figure 4.15 **A–B** Contacts category filter.

Using Contacts

In both Windows and Palm-based devices, contacts for each category will be listed in alphabetical order, based on last name. As your contact lists become longer, it may be easier and more efficient to use some of the built-in time-saving components that these devices offer rather than scrolling through the entire list. Both devices (Palm and Windows) offer a Look Up or Find a Name **search tool**, as shown in Figure 4.16A and B, which can help you locate a contact quickly. As you can see, there are slight differences between

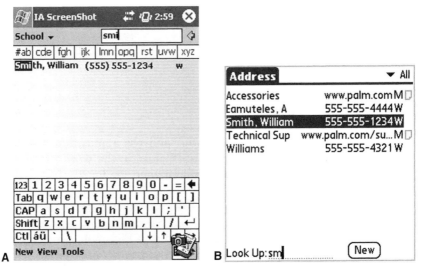

Figure 4.16 **A** Pocket PC Look Up feature. **B** Palm Look Up feature.

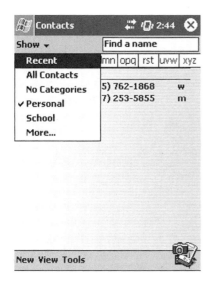

Figure 4.17 Pocket PC view category filters.

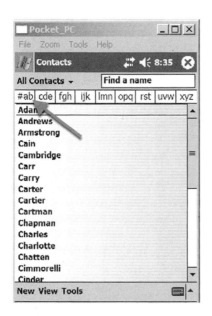

Figure 4.18 ABC tabs navigation.

the two operating systems. In the Palm device the Look Up is located at the bottom of the screen and in the Windows device the Find a Name is at the top of the screen. You need only input a portion (the first few letters) of the last name in the text box to quickly access that contact.

Because both devices allow you to organize your contacts according to categories, you can easily access an important contact by also selecting the specific category you desire.

Pocket PC/Windows CE

For Windows-based devices, when you are in the Contacts area of your PDA, just tap on All Contacts (located on the upper left corner of your screen) to view categories. From this view you can easily access specific contact information that has been filed in a category (see Figure 4.17).

In Pocket PC devices, the ABC tabs are another useful tool that speeds up the process of accessing important contacts. Rather than scrolling through the entire list, you can use the ABC tabs feature by tapping on the letter tabs at the top of the screen (see Figure 4.18). This tool is useful only if you have many contacts in your database. Tapping once on the *cde* tab will take you to the start of the Cs in your contacts. Tapping again will take you to the start of the Ds, and so on.

You can also customize how contacts will be displayed on your screen. In the Windows device, tap on the Tools tab at the bottom of the Contact screen and select Options. From this view you can select how your contacts will be displayed (showing ABC tabs, showing names only, and font size) as well as customize your regional settings, including setting the default area code for your phone numbers (another time-saver!). This item is especially useful, if most of your telephone contacts are within a single area code. Once an area code is entered in this information box, it will automatically default to any new contact telephone number you enter. If the new number entered is in a different area code, you will need to manually modify the entry.

Try modifying the options selected to obtain a screen format that best suits your needs. Displaying contact names only will minimize clutter on the screen, and the large font may be helpful for easy view of specific contact data. You will see that this screen will enable you to select a default area code for telephone contact information.

Test Drive . . . .

Follow these steps to modify contact options:

1. Press the Contacts button.
2. Tap on All Contacts located on the upper left corner of the screen (see Figure 4.19A).
3. From the options view, as shown in Figure 4.19B, select School (a category you created in an earlier activity).
4. You will see that Smith, William is the only contact in that category (see Figure 4.19C).
5. Tap on Tools located on the bottom of the screen (see Figure 4.19D).
6. Select Options to change the way your contacts are displayed. You will notice that the Show ABC tabs option is checked, but Show contact names only is not (see Figure 4.19E).
7. Place a check mark in Show contact names only, as depicted in Figure 4.19F, and change the area code to the one you most frequently use.

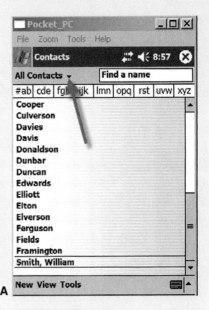

A

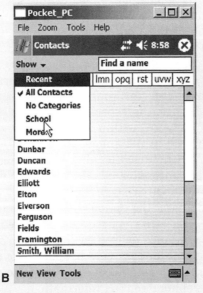

B

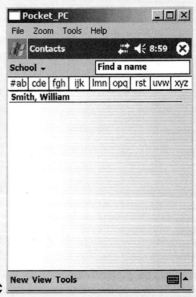

C

Figure 4.19 Test Drive: **A–F** Changing contact view options. **G** Customized contact list view.

(Continued)

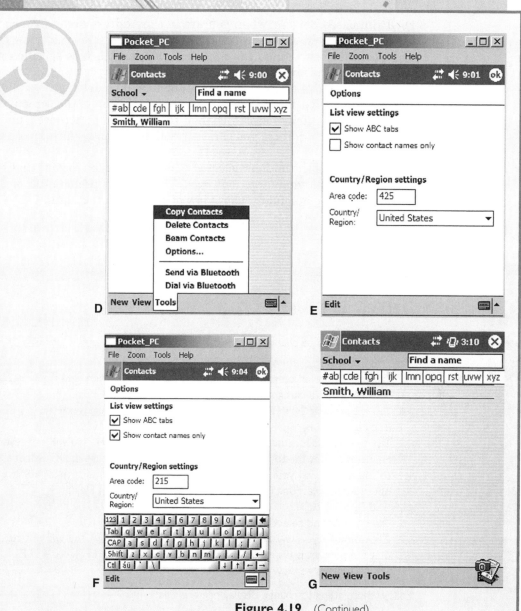

Figure 4.19 (Continued)

8. Be sure the Country/Region is correct for your area.
9. Tap on OK on the upper right side of the screen.

Your screen should look something like the one shown in Figure 4.19G. Keep in mind that the area code will be different. Note that the phone number is no longer visible on this screen.

Palm

For Palm-based devices, when you are in the Address area of your PDA, just tap on All (located on the upper right hand of the screen) to view the list of available categories. From this view you can easily access specific contact information that has been filed in a category.

You can also customize how your contacts will be displayed on your screen. In the Palm device, tap on Address located at the top of the screen and select Options. In this view, you can change the font, set preferences, and rename custom fields. In addition, you can set security options, which are discussed in Chapter 6.

Try modifying the options selected to obtain a screen format that best suits your needs. Displaying large font, modifying display preferences, or customizing fields may be helpful for easy view of specific contact data.

Test Drive . . . .

Follow these steps to change the font:

1. Press the Address button.
2. Tap on All located on the upper right corner of the screen (see Figure 4.20A).
3. Select School (a category you created in an earlier activity).
4. You will see that Smith, William is the only contact in that category (see Figure 4.20B).
5. Tap on Address located at the top right side of the screen. You will see several new tabs across the top of the screen, as depicted in Figure 4.20C. Select Options to change the way your contacts are displayed. You will notice that you have three options available: Font, Preferences, and Rename Custom Fields (see Figure 4.20D).
6. Tap on Font and select the largest font (see Figure 4.20E).
7. Click on OK (you will be taken back to the address view). You will notice that the contact is displayed in a larger font, as depicted in Figure 4.20F.
8. Select Address to view the font changes.

Follow these steps to change display preferences:

1. Repeat steps 1–6 from the previous exercise for changing the font.
2. Select Preferences (see Figure 4.21A).
3. Select Company, Last Name (see Figure 4.21B).
4. Tap on OK.
5. You will see your contact, Mr. Smith, displayed by his company name, CEVA, as depicted in Figure 4.21C.

(Continued)

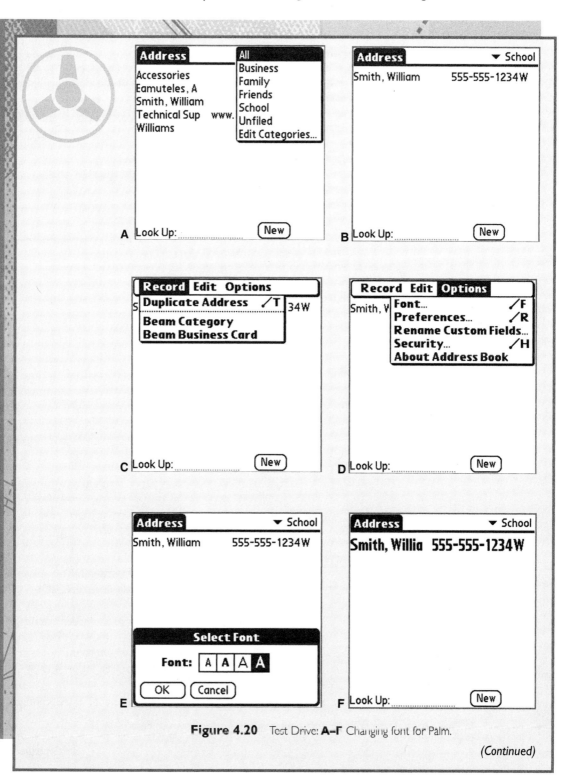

Figure 4.20 Test Drive: **A–F** Changing font for Palm.

(Continued)

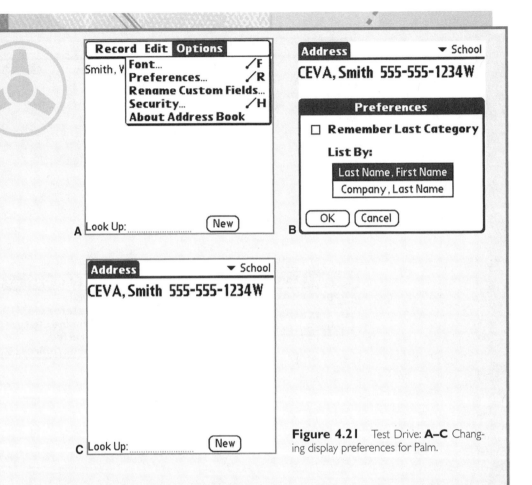

Figure 4.21 Test Drive: **A–C** Changing display preferences for Palm.

Follow these steps to rename custom fields:

1. Repeat steps 1–6 from the first exercise for changing the font.
2. Select Rename Custom Fields (Figure 4.22A).
3. Move your stylus across the word Custom 1 to highlight (Figure 4.22B).
4. Use any input method to enter the following: Spouse's Name (Figure 4.22C).
5. Tap on OK.
6. Tap on CEVA. (Remember, you changed the display options in an earlier activity.)
7. Select Edit.
8. Tap on the small arrow on the lower right hand side to scroll down to the newly created custom field, Spouse's Name, and enter the following: Barbara (Figure 4.22D).
9. Tap on Done to finish.
10. To view your newly configured settings and edited contact, select CETA, Smith....

Your screen should look something like the one shown in Figure 4.22E.

(Continued)

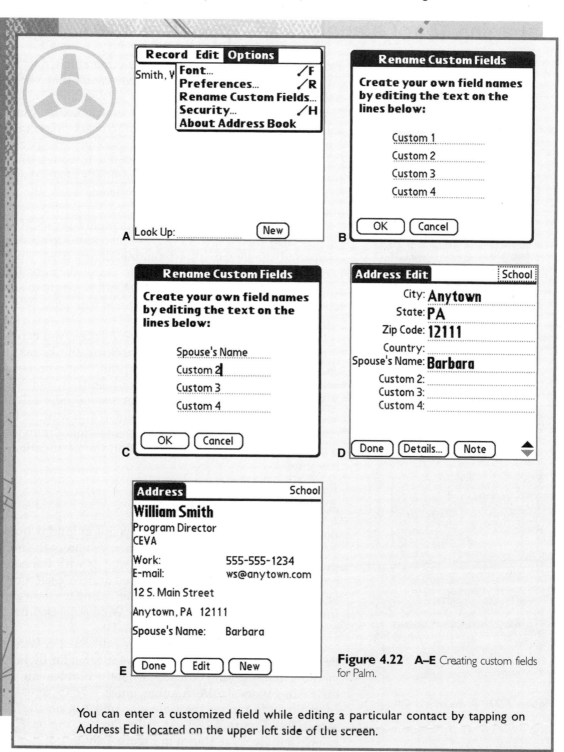

Figure 4.22 A–E Creating custom fields for Palm.

You can enter a customized field while editing a particular contact by tapping on Address Edit located on the upper left side of the screen.

Managing Your Calendar and Appointments

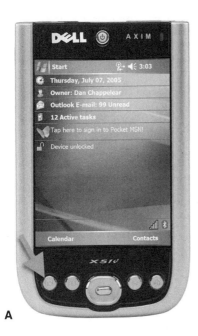

A

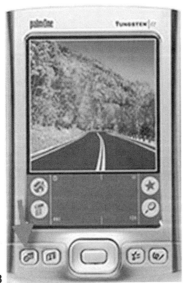

B

Figure 4.23 **A** Pocket PC Calendar button. (2005 Dell, Inc. All rights reserved.) **B** Palm Calendar button (Image courtesy of Palm, Inc.)

Your PDA cannot create more hours in a single day, but it can help you make the most efficient use of that very precious commodity called *time*. The use of standard calendar formats presented here will assist in organizing your appointment calendar. Some manufacturers also include other calendar enhancement programs that are specific to their PDAs, and you are encouraged to check the accompanying product information for details about these enhancements after you become proficient with the basic applications.

Because managing our time is a highly personal task, you are also encouraged to review the options available for setup and display of this valuable information. Just as pocket calendars are available in many formats (daily, weekly, or monthly displays), the PDA can be set up to accommodate your preferences for viewing and managing items on your calendar.

In both Palm and Windows-based devices, you can easily customize your calendar by checking the boxes indicated on the options screen. Be careful, however, because selecting some of these options may clutter your screen and are not necessary for efficient use of your calendar. You can also set the reminder alarm, if you want to be reminded about upcoming appointments. Some individuals really like the reminders; others find the notification distracting.

Accessing the Calendar

Both devices have a time-saving, quick link **calendar button**, as shown in Figure 4.23A and B. When you press the button, the calendar immediately opens. Again, as with the address book in both Palm and Windows-based devices, each time you press this button you will see another calendar view ranging from day, week, month, and, in the Windows-based devices, year (see Figures 4.24A–E and 4.25A–D).

There is another way to access the calendar. For Windows-based devices, you can also access your calendar by tapping on Start and selecting Calendar from the Start menu, as depicted in Figure 4.26A. Another quick way to access your calendar is to tap on the Calendar program on the Today screen (see Figure 4.26B). In Palm devices, tap on 🏠 and select Date Book, as shown in Figure 4.26C.

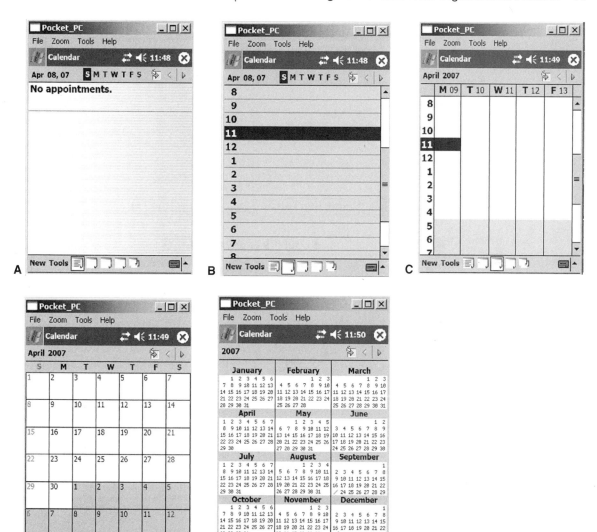

Figure 4.24   A–E Pocket PC Calendar Quick Views.

Using Your Pocket PC/Windows CE Calendar

When in your calendar, you can add a new appointment by tapping on New at the bottom left of the screen. A screen similar to the one in Figure 4.27A will appear. Another way to add an appointment is to tap on New on the bottom left of your Today screen and select Appointment (see Figure 4.27B). This activity will automatically take you to the same screen as before.

As you can see, there are several ways to get to the same place where you can enter your new appointment. Using your preferred input method, you can enter

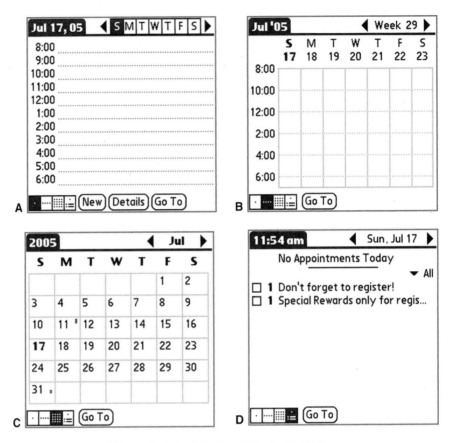

Figure 4.25 **A–D** Palm Calendar Quick Views.

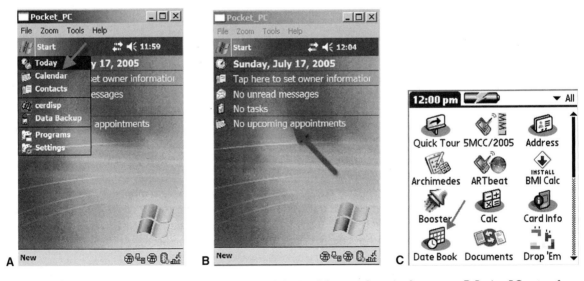

Figure 4.26 Alternative ways to access your calendar: **A** Pocket PC access from the Start menu. **B** Pocket PC access from the Today screen. **C** Palm access from the Home menu.

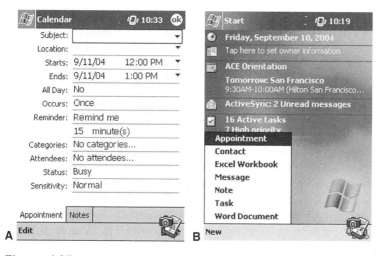

Figure 4.27 Two methods to enter a new appointment: **A** New appointment screen. **B** Selecting new appointment from Today screen.

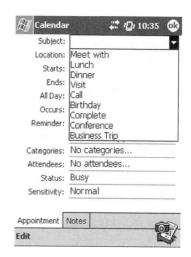

Figure 4.28 Pocket PC: Preset text entry options.

the subject and location of the appointment. You will notice some preset (default) subject topics to help speed up the process for entering information. For example, you can select *Meet with* and then complete your entry more quickly. The same is true for all of the drop-down arrows ▼ you see on any screen. Just click on the ▼, and you will see the drop-down text menu, a list of preset text options available, as depicted in Figure 4.28. The same is true for Location; however, these options in the drop-down menu become available only after you have entered a location for a previous appointment. Because the locations for meetings/appointments are unique for each individual user, having factory set default locations would not make sense. However, having the PDA "remember" your individual meeting places is very convenient and time-saving.

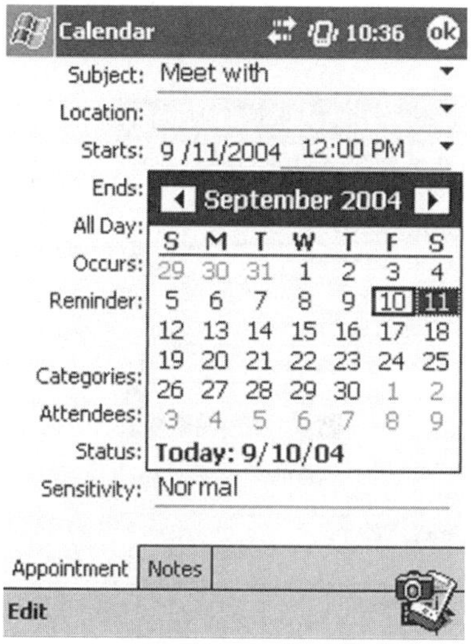

The date of the meeting can be changed by simply placing the stylus on the date. This action will give you a drop-down menu that will enable you to select the month, day, and year for the appointment, as you can see in Figure 4.29. Start time and end time can also be adjusted by using the drop-down menus activated by the arrow next to the times listed. The screen defaults to No when asking you if the meeting is an all-day occurrence. Selecting Yes for this answer will block out a full 24 hours for the event.

Recurring Appointments

The Occurs section allows you the option of setting recurring appointments; the default "once" indicates that it is a one-time appointment. If the appointment recurs in a set pattern, you can tap on Occurs and you will get a drop-down menu of

Figure 4.29 Pocket PC: Modifying the date.

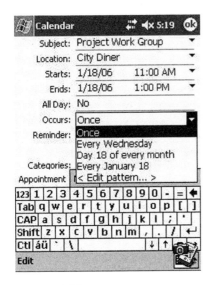

Figure 4.30 Entering a recurring appointment.

choices (see Figure 4.30). Please remember that your PDA has an infinite timeline, so, if you select any of the options that use the term Every, this recurring appointment will be scheduled indefinitely at the indicated interval. For recurring appointments that do have a specific end date, select <Edit pattern . . .> and follow the prompts to complete the process.

Setting Reminders

You can set your PDA to remind you of upcoming meetings by tapping on the Reminder tab and selecting Remind me. You will see 15 minute(s) as the default setting for the time increment allotted, indicating you will receive a reminder of the appointment 15 minutes before the event is due to start. If you would like to change that, tap on 15 to change the numeric value and on minute(s) to change the hours, days, or weeks (see Figure 4.31A and B).

The advantage of this feature is that even if your PDA is turned off when the notification is due, it will automatically turn itself on to activate the reminder. The reminder screen will stay activated even if you miss the initial notification.

Creating Categories

As with Contacts, you can also organize your calendar according to categories such as Business, Holiday, Personal, or even create a new category (see Figure 4.32A). To do so, tap on Categories and either click to place a check mark in one of the existing categories, as shown in Figure 4.32B, or use the Add/Delete tab located on the bottom of the screen to enter a new category. This handy feature allows you to view specific recurring events, such as work or your favorite team's home games.

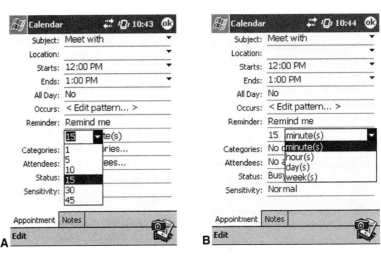

Figure 4.31 **A–B** Setting reminders (alarms).

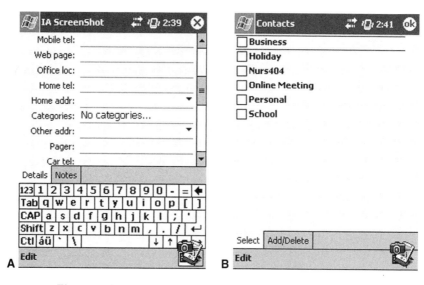

Figure 4.32 **A** Calendar categories. **B** Adding/editing categories.

Test Drive . . . .

Now you try it. Follow these steps to enter a new appointment and organize it by category:

1. Access the calendar program using one of the following methods:
   a. Press the Calendar button on the front of your PDA.
   b. Select the Calendar program from the Start menu.
   c. Tap on the Calendar program on the Today screen.

2. Using the menu located on the top of the screen, select F for Friday. As you can see in Figure 4.33A, the F is now highlighted.
3. Tap on New, located on the lower left hand corner of the screen.
4. Using the preset ▼ options, enter the following (see Figure 4.33B):
   a. Subject: Meet with planning committee
   b. Location: 4th floor conference room

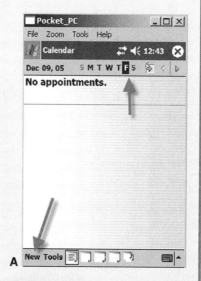

Figure 4.33 Test Drive: **A–C** Entering a recurring appointment/meeting. **D–E** Two calendar views of planning group meeting.

(Continued)

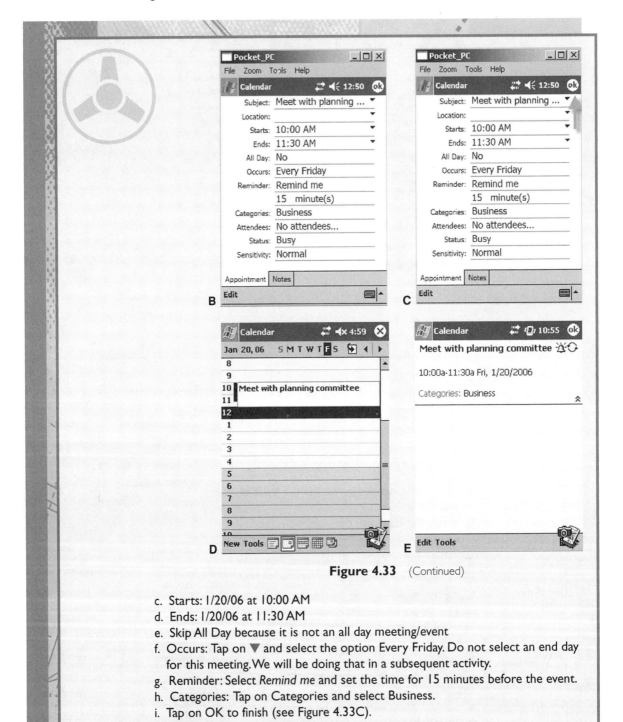

Figure 4.33 (Continued)

c. Starts: 1/20/06 at 10:00 AM

d. Ends: 1/20/06 at 11:30 AM

e. Skip All Day because it is not an all day meeting/event

f. Occurs: Tap on ▼ and select the option Every Friday. Do not select an end day for this meeting. We will be doing that in a subsequent activity.

g. Reminder: Select *Remind me* and set the time for 15 minutes before the event.

h. Categories: Tap on Categories and select Business.

i. Tap on OK to finish (see Figure 4.33C).

Your screen should look something like the one in Figure 4.33D. To see more details, tap on the appointment, as shown in Figure 4.33E.

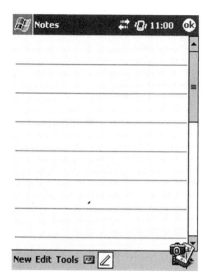

Figure 4.34 Adding notes to a scheduled appointment or meeting.

Notes

Another important feature in setting up an appointment is the Notes tab at the bottom of the Calendar screen. Tapping on the Notes tab will bring you to a blank text screen, where you can enter supplemental information that will allow you to be better prepared for the appointment or meeting (see Figure 4.34). Whenever the appointment is selected for review, the note will also be displayed. Notes can contain text, writing, drawings, or voice recordings. Choose the appropriate input item by selecting from the icons displayed when the Notes option is selected. To make a voice recording of a note, tap on the tape icon and the recording toolbar will appear. Press and hold the Record button. Record your message and tap on the stop icon. A speaker symbol will appear in the Notes section. To hear the message, tap on the speaker icon and play back the recording.

Scheduling a Meeting

The Schedule a Meeting feature is available only if you are using Outlook as your calendar. In reality, a meeting is nothing more than an appointment that involves several people. The steps for creating a meeting are the same as for scheduling an appointment, with the additional step of identifying attendees. To complete this process, create a new appointment as previously described and add participants to the Attendees list (see Figure 4.35A). As soon as you tap on the line item for attendees, you will automatically be directed to a list of individuals whose e-mail addresses are listed in your Contacts information, similar to the list shown in Figure 4.35B. Place a check next to the intended participants and click on OK when finished. When a meeting is

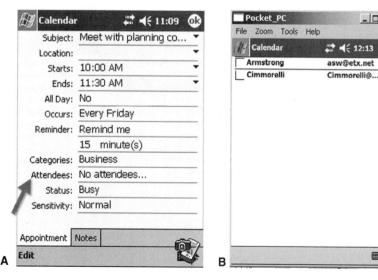

Figure 4.35 **A–B** Inviting attendees to meetings.

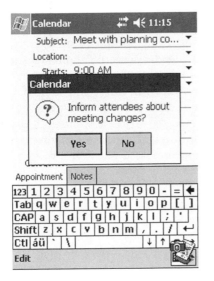

Figure 4.36 Editing a meeting.

created in Calendar, a meeting request can be sent to the intended participants identified in the Attendees field the next time you sync or are connected to the Internet. To send the e-mail, the Inbox must be configured with an e-mail server. Tips for managing e-mail are provided in Chapter 6.

Editing and Deleting Appointments and Meetings

In Windows applications, editing and deleting information in the calendar is easy; open the item and tap on Edit at the bottom left of the screen, make any necessary editorial changes in the appropriate line detail, and click on OK. Adjustments will automatically be made to your calendar as noted. If the item is a meeting, you will be prompted by a dialog box asking whether you want to inform attendees about meeting changes, as illustrated in Figure 4.36.

You can also cut, copy, delete, and beam appointments and meetings by using the drop-down menu that appears when you press and hold the stylus on a scheduled activity (see Figure 4.37A). (Note that you must do this from the contact list view, not the individual contact.) As in any Windows-based product, you can perform a cut-and-paste procedure to move an appointment or to add an additional date but retain the original appointment on your calendar. If you select the option of deleting an appointment, you will be alerted, as shown in Figure 4.37B, that the appointment is scheduled to be deleted and will be asked whether you want to continue and to inform attendees about changes. These confirmation steps afford an additional layer of protection for your data so that you do not delete something in error.

If you are deleting an appointment that is set up as a recurring appointment, you will be asked whether or not you want to delete all appointments in the series, as shown in Figure 4.37C. Selecting No will enable you to delete a

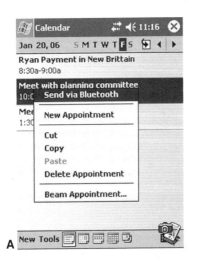
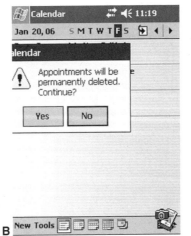
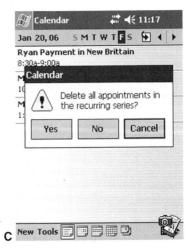

Figure 4.37 **A** Cut, copy, delete, or beam appointment. **B** Confirm choice to delete. **C** Choose to delete recurring series or single occurrence of appointment.

single occurrence in a recurring series without affecting other scheduled meeting dates and times.

Now try something a bit more challenging. Assume that you and your colleagues have decided to meet for lunch every Wednesday from 11:00 A.M. to 1:00 P.M. for the next 6 weeks to discuss an important project. The meeting will be held at the City Diner. While reviewing your calendar, you notice that the boss has scheduled an important conference from 9:00 A.M. to 3:00 P.M. on the third Wednesday of this series of meetings. You discuss the situation with your colleagues, and they decide that the regularly scheduled luncheon meeting for that Wednesday can be canceled without any significant disruption to the project timeline. The remaining luncheon meetings will be held as scheduled. How would you deal with managing your calendar in this situation? If you are unsure, consider following the few easy steps outlined here and illustrated in the following Test Drive.

Test Drive . . . .

1. Open your Calendar and select Wednesday of this week for your first luncheon appointment. Using the menu located on the top of the screen, select W for Wednesday (refer to Figure 4.38 A–J for guidance).
2. Tap on New, located on the lower left corner of the screen (see Figure 4.38A).
3. Enter the following (using the preset ▼ options when possible; see Figure 4.38B–F):
   a. Subject: Meet with Project Work
   b. Location: City Diner
   c. Starts: this week's date at 11:00 A.M.
   d. Ends: this week's date at 1:00 P.M.
   e. Skip All Day because it is not an all day meeting/event

4. Tap on Occurs and schedule the meeting as a recurring appointment as shown in Figures 4.38F–J. (Remember to select <Edit pattern ...> to end the meeting after six sessions and click on OK. [*Tip:* To select six meeting times, you must manually enter the numeral 6.] The luncheon meeting will be listed as a weekly occurrence on your calendar for the next 6 weeks.)
5. Tap on Finish and then OK.

Now that you have the recurring appointment in your calendar, follow the next steps to cancel the meeting on the third Wednesday in the series and to add the conference to your calendar.

(Continued)

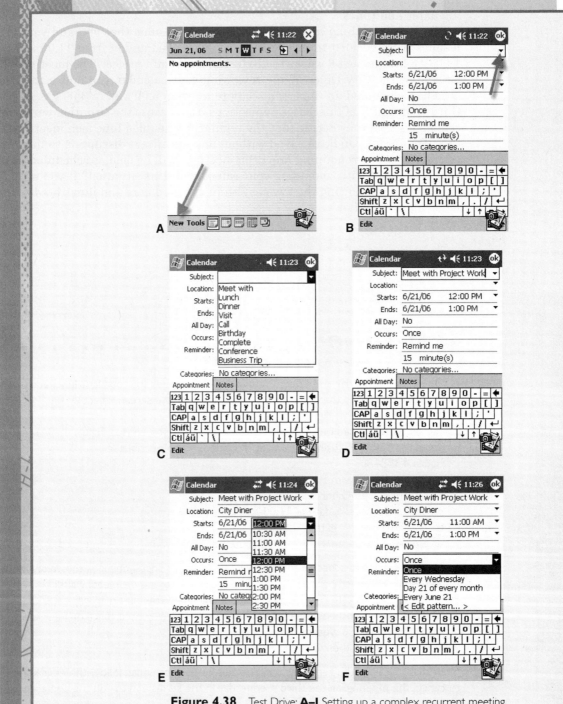

Figure 4.38 Test Drive: **A–J** Setting up a complex recurrent meeting.

(Continued)

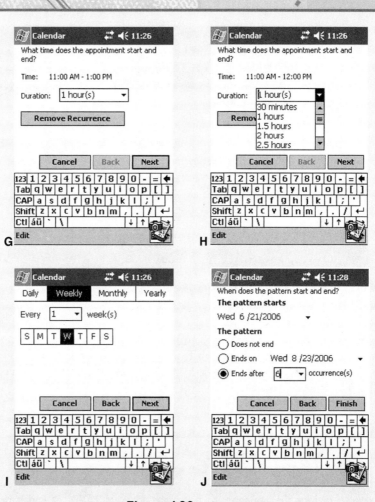

Figure 4.38 (Continued)

6. From the calendar view, move ahead to the third week in the series using the ◀ and ▶, located at the top of the screen. Place and hold your stylus on the appointment until a drop-down menu appears, as shown in Figure 4.39A, and select Delete Appointment.

7. You will be prompted by a message box that asks whether you want to delete all appointments in the recurring series (see Figure 4.39B). In this case, you want to keep the remaining appointments, so select No and only this single occurrence of the luncheon meetings will be deleted.

8. Now you can put the details of the conference that the boss would like you to attend from 9:00 A.M. to 3:00 P.M. on your calendar for that Wednesday.
   a. Select New.
   b. Enter details for Business Conference scheduled for 9:00 A.M. to 3:00 P.M.

(Continued)

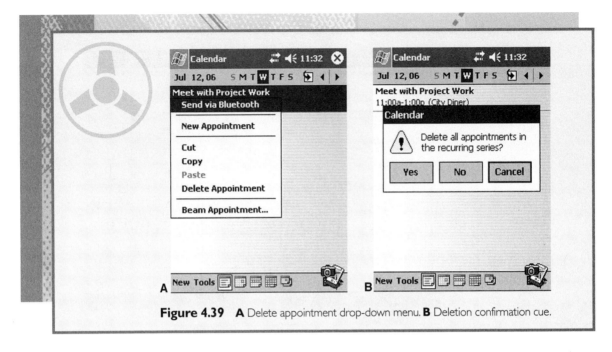

Figure 4.39   **A** Delete appointment drop-down menu. **B** Deletion confirmation cue.

Now, that was not so hard, was it? Give it a try again. Assume that you are scheduled for lab from 8:00 to 10:00 A.M. on Monday mornings for the next 10 weeks. Week 5 is spring break, and you have scheduled a well-deserved vacation.

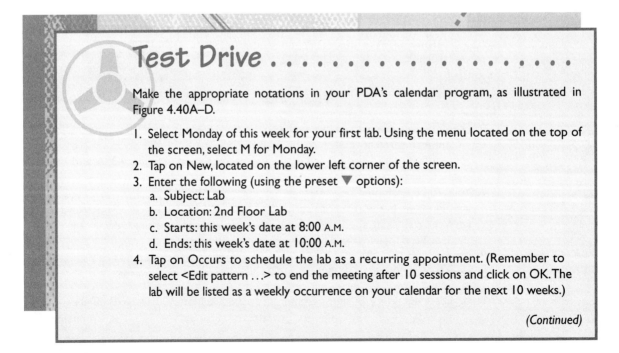

Test Drive . . . .

Make the appropriate notations in your PDA's calendar program, as illustrated in Figure 4.40A–D.

1. Select Monday of this week for your first lab. Using the menu located on the top of the screen, select M for Monday.
2. Tap on New, located on the lower left corner of the screen.
3. Enter the following (using the preset ▼ options):
   a. Subject: Lab
   b. Location: 2nd Floor Lab
   c. Starts: this week's date at 8:00 A.M.
   d. Ends: this week's date at 10:00 A.M.
4. Tap on Occurs to schedule the lab as a recurring appointment. (Remember to select <Edit pattern ...> to end the meeting after 10 sessions and click on OK. The lab will be listed as a weekly occurrence on your calendar for the next 10 weeks.)

(Continued)

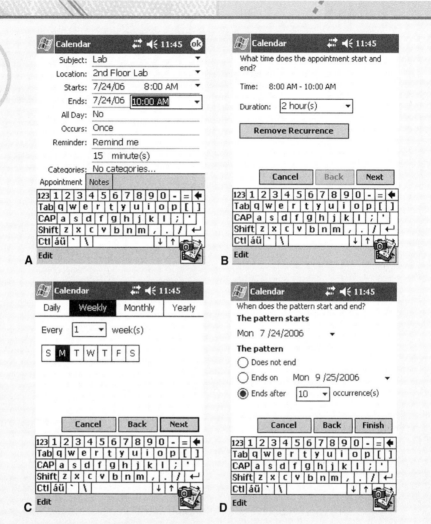

Figure 4.40 Test Drive: **A–D** Scheduling weekly class.

5. Move ahead to the fifth week in the series. Place and hold your stylus on the appointment until a drop-down menu appears and select Delete Appointment (Figure 4.40E).

6. You will be prompted by a message box that asks whether you want to delete all appointments in the recurring series (Figure 4.40F). In this case, you want to keep the remaining appointments, so select No and only this single occurrence of the lab meetings will be deleted.

7. Now you can enter the details of the spring break:
   a. Select New.
   b. Enter details.

(Continued)

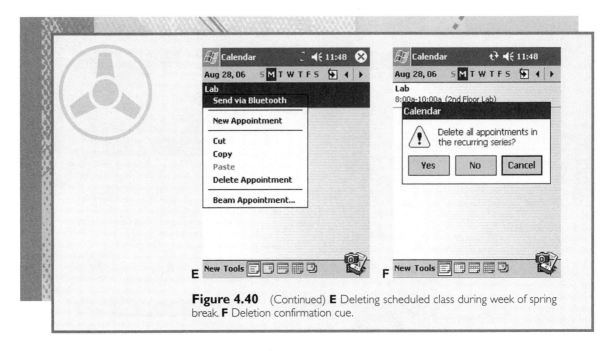

Figure 4.40 (Continued) **E** Deleting scheduled class during week of spring break. **F** Deletion confirmation cue.

The last example will walk you through setting up a calendar event over several days. Assume that you will be attending a 3-day conference and would like to have the event displayed on your calendar.

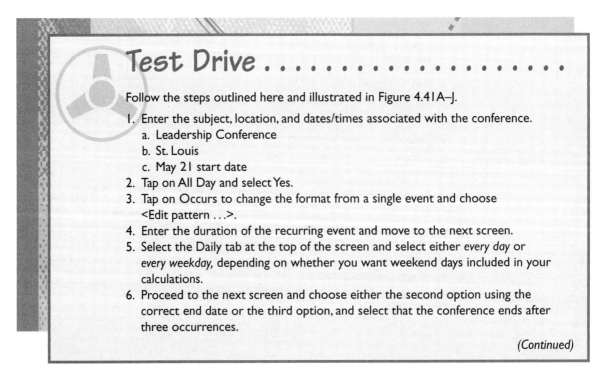

Test Drive . . . .

Follow the steps outlined here and illustrated in Figure 4.41A–J.

1. Enter the subject, location, and dates/times associated with the conference.
   a. Leadership Conference
   b. St. Louis
   c. May 21 start date
2. Tap on All Day and select Yes.
3. Tap on Occurs to change the format from a single event and choose <Edit pattern . . .>.
4. Enter the duration of the recurring event and move to the next screen.
5. Select the Daily tab at the top of the screen and select either *every day* or *every weekday,* depending on whether you want weekend days included in your calculations.
6. Proceed to the next screen and choose either the second option using the correct end date or the third option, and select that the conference ends after three occurrences.

(Continued)

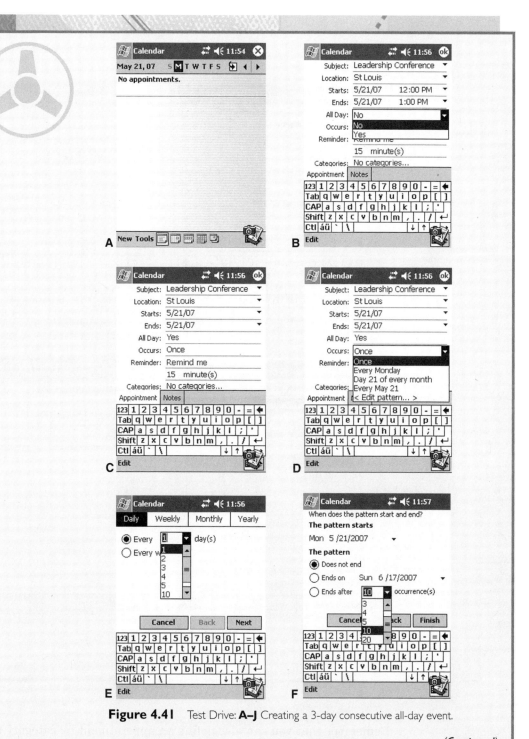

Figure 4.41 Test Drive: **A–J** Creating a 3-day consecutive all-day event.

(Continued)

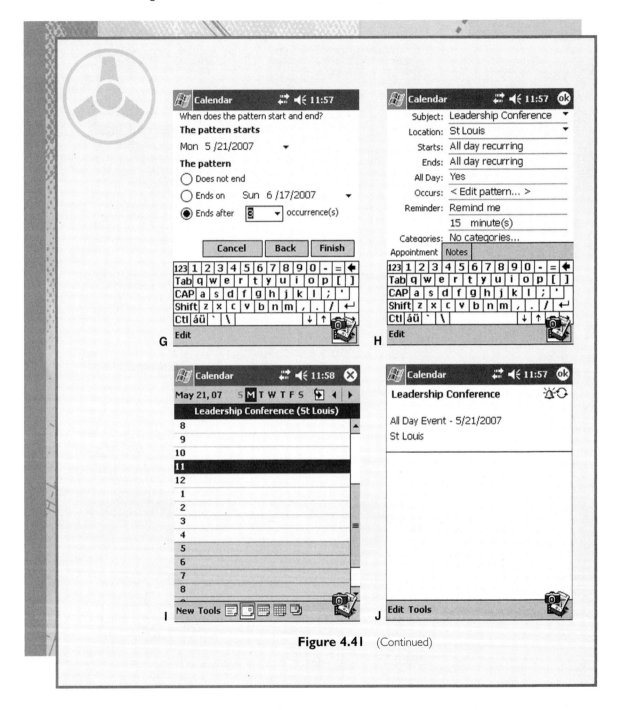

Figure 4.41 (Continued)

Remember that you can also define an appointment by category or identify your availability during an appointment by selecting options in the Categories and Status sections on the calendar screen.

Using Your Palm Calendar

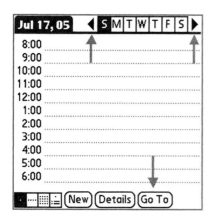

Figure 4.42   Palm: Navigating through the calendar

As stated earlier, you can directly access the calendar program by either pushing the Calendar button on the front of your PDA or selecting the Date Book program from the main menu. Again, as with the Pocket PC, you can see there are several ways to get to the same place where you can enter your new appointment.

When in the Date Book, use the navigation arrows located at the top of the screen to get to the correct date for your new appointment (see Figure 4.42). On the same screen, you can also tap on Go To located on the bottom of the screen. Using these features will enable you to quickly skim through the months and select the appropriate date. You can change your calendar View by tapping on the calendar view icons located at the bottom of the screen. Pressing repeatedly on the Calendar button on the lower left corner of your PDA will also achieve this objective.

When in your calendar, you can add a new appointment by tapping on New at the bottom of the screen. Here you can enter the time of the meeting by selecting the appropriate hour and minute increment from the two columns on the right side of the screen and then tapping on the Start Time text box. The default setting automatically sets the appointment for 1 hour; however, by tapping on the End Time text box, you can easily change the appointment to the appropriate time.

Test Drive . . . .

Now try it out! Refer to Figure 4.43A–D for clarification of the steps involved in this activity.

1. Open your Date Book, using one of the methods described earlier.
2. Using the navigation bar at the top of the screen, select Friday of this week.
3. Tap on New (located on the bottom of the screen).
4. In the Set Time window, enter the following:

   Start Time: 12:00 P.M.
   End Time: 1:30 P.M.

5. Tap on OK.
6. In the calendar view, you will notice that the cursor is flashing at 12:00. Using your preferred input method, enter the following information:

   Planning Committee Lunch Meeting

7. Tap on 🏠 to finish and return to the main screen.   *(Continued)*

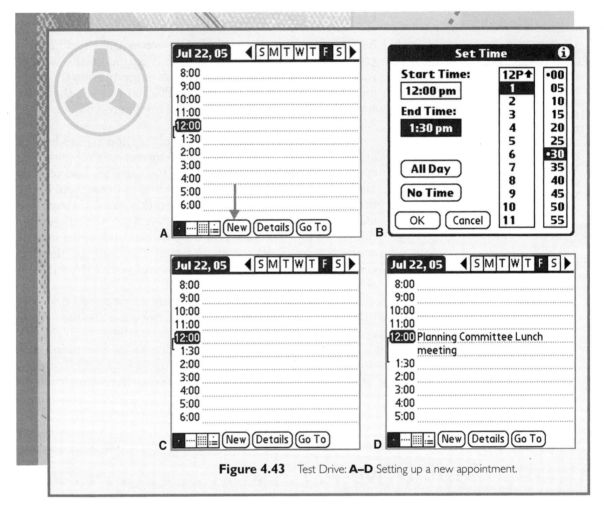

Figure 4.43   Test Drive: **A–D** Setting up a new appointment.

The time or date of the meeting can be changed by placing the stylus on the appointment and selecting Details located on the bottom of the screen. This action will open up the Event Details window in which you may edit the appointment. To change the time of your appointment, tap on the text box next to Time and make the desired adjustments. To change the date, tap on the text box next to Date and select the desired date. For example, suppose that you had a dentist appointment scheduled for August 1. Because of a conflict in your schedule, you must reschedule this appointment. As luck would have it, your appointment has been rescheduled for the same time next week. Using Figure 4.44 as a guide, make the necessary changes on your calendar.

Setting Alarm and Recurring Appointments

From the Event Details window, you can set the alarm to remind you of an upcoming appointment and schedule recurring appointments. To set the alarm, tap to put a check mark in the box next to Alarm (see Figure 4.45A) and then

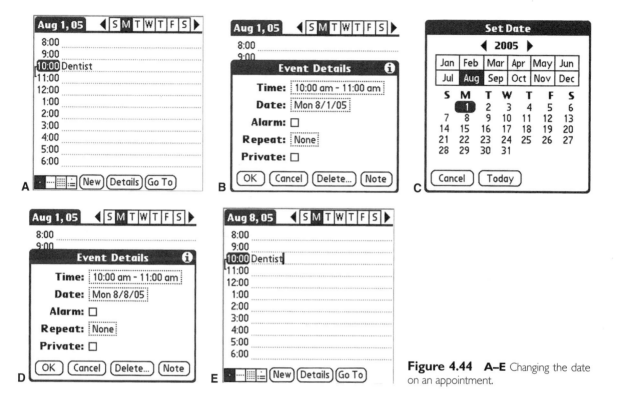

Figure 4.44 A–E Changing the date on an appointment.

choose when you wish to be reminded of the appointment; the default setting is for a reminder of 5 minutes before the appointment, but you can change this by highlighting the numeral 5 and changing it (see Figure 4.45B and C). You can change the interval from minutes to hours or days by tapping on the down arrow next to the numeral. On your calendar, you will see a small alarm clock to the right of the item.

The advantage of the alarm feature is that even if your PDA is turned off when the notification is due, it will automatically turn itself on to activate the

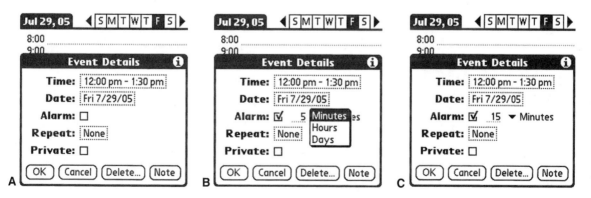

Figure 4.45 A–C Setting an alarm for Palm.

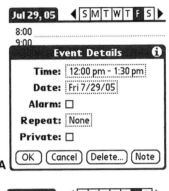

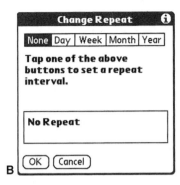

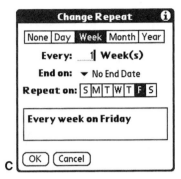

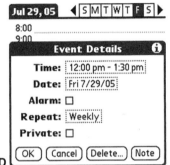

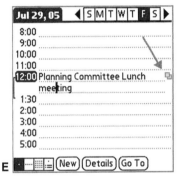

Figure 4.46 **A–D** Setting a recurring appointment. **E** Calendar view of a recurring appointment.

reminder. The reminder screen will stay activated even if you miss the initial notification.

To set a recurring appointment, tap on the text box next to Repeat (see Figure 4.46A). In the Change Repeat window, you can select the repeat interval: day, week, month, or year (see Figure 4.46B). For example, if you wanted to schedule a weekly appointment for the next 3 weeks, select Week and leave the default setting to Every 1 Week (Figure 4.46C). To save your changes, tap on OK and you will return to the Event Details screen (Figure 4.46D). Then tap on OK again to return to the calendar view. The appointment will have a screen on your PDA that should look something like the one in Figure 4.46E. The small icon to the right of the appointment symbolizes that the appointment is recurring.

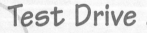

Assume that the luncheon you scheduled in the previous exercise has been rescheduled to next Friday from 1:00 to 2:45 P.M. Make the changes in your Date Book.

1. Open your Date Book.
2. Locate the appointment you entered in the last activity and highlight it by tapping on Planning Committee Lunch Meeting.

(Continued)

3. Tap on Details (located on the bottom of the screen), as shown in Figure 4.47A.
4. In the Event Details window, tap on the text box next to Time to change the meeting time (see Figure 4.47B).
5. Enter the following (see Figure 4.47C), and then tap on OK:

   Start Time: 1:00 P.M.
   End Time: 2:45 p.m.

6. Change the date to the following Friday by tapping on the text box next to Date (Figure 4.47D). Using the Set Date window, select next Friday (Figure 4.47E).
7. Tap on OK to finish (Figure 4.47F). Your rescheduled appointment will appear on your calendar (Figure 4.47G).
8. Tap on 🏠 to finish and return to the main screen.

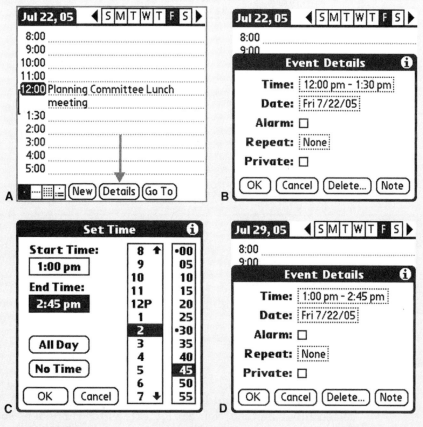

Figure 4.47 Test Drive: **A–G** Editing an appointment on the calendar

(Continued)

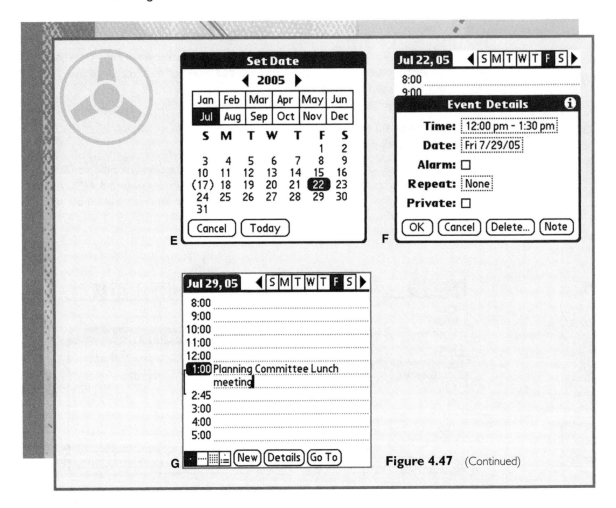

Figure 4.47 (Continued)

Creating Categories

Creating categories within your appointments is not an available feature in Palm devices.

Notes

You can add a note to your appointment by tapping on Details and then on Note while in the Event Details window (see Figure 4.48A–C). Using your preferred input method, you can quickly enter reminders such as "Bring work manual to meeting" or "Bring insurance card." In addition, you can edit or delete notes in the window as well. When you return to the calendar view, you will notice that there is a small icon on the right margin of the screen (see Figure 4.48D); this indicates that there is a note associated with that particular appointment.

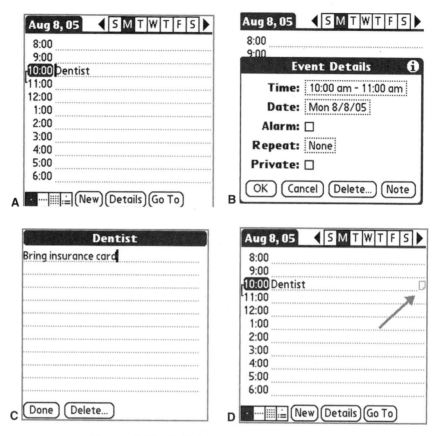

Figure 4.48 **A–D** Adding a note to an appointment.

Editing and Deleting Appointments and Meetings

In Palm applications, editing and deleting information in the calendar is easy; select the item and tap on Details at the bottom of the screen, make any necessary editorial changes in the appropriate line detail, and click on OK (see Figure 4.49A and B). Another way to make changes is to tap on the date in the upper right corner of the screen; this will provide similar options to edit and delete (see Figure 4.49C and D). Adjustments will automatically be made to your calendar as noted.

You can also cut, copy, delete, or paste appointments and meetings by using the Edit drop-down menu that appears when you tap on the date in the upper right corner of the screen (see Figure 4.50). (Note that you must do this while you have an appointment selected.) You can perform a cut-and-paste procedure to move an appointment or to add an additional date, by selecting Copy, while still retaining the original appointment on your calendar. If you select the option of deleting an appointment, you will be alerted, as shown in Figure 4.51, that the appointment is scheduled to be deleted, and asked whether you want to continue and inform attendees about changes. These confirmation steps afford an additional layer of protection for your data so that you do not delete something in error.

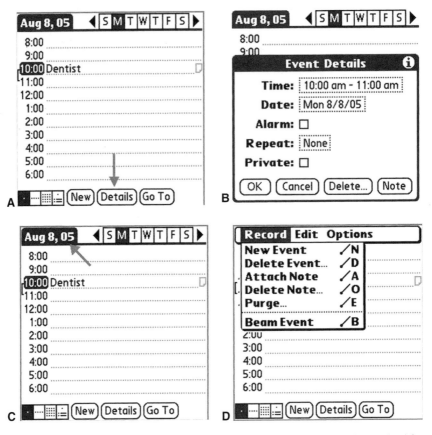

Figure 4.49 **A–B** Editing or deleting an appointment. **C–D** An alternative method for editing or deleting an appointment.

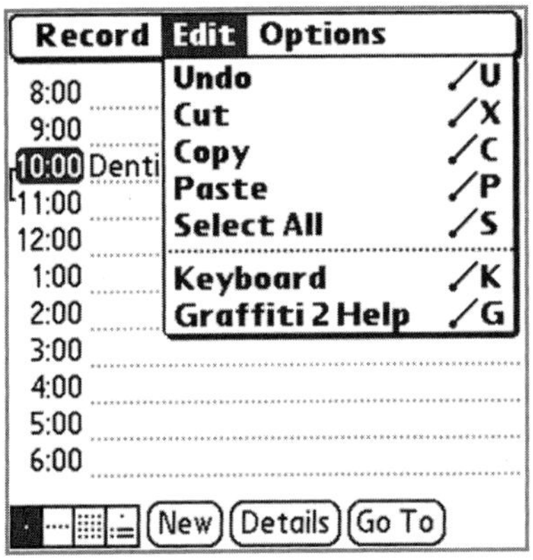

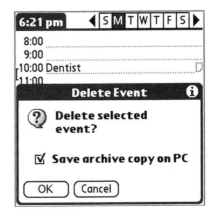

Figure 4.50 Palm: Cut, copy, and paste menu.

Figure 4.51 Palm: Deleting an appointment confirmation.

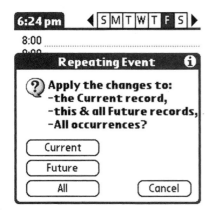

Figure 4.52 Deleting a recurring appointment.

If you are deleting an appointment that is set up as a recurring appointment, you will be asked whether or not you want to delete all appointments in the series. Selecting No will enable you to delete a single occurrence in a recurring series, without affecting other scheduled meeting dates and times (see Figure 4.52).

Now you give it a try. Assume that you and your colleagues have decided to meet for lunch every Wednesday from 11:00 A.M. to 1:00 P.M. for the next 6 weeks to discuss an important project. The meeting will be held at the City Diner. While reviewing your calendar, you notice that the boss has scheduled an important conference from 9:00 A.M. to 3:00 P.M. on the third Wednesday of this series of meetings. You discuss the situation with your colleagues, and they decide that the regularly scheduled luncheon meeting for that Wednesday can be canceled without any significant disruption to the project timeline. The remaining luncheon meetings will be held as scheduled. How would you deal with managing your calendar in this situation? If you are unsure, consider following the few easy steps outlined here and illustrated in Figure 4.53A–K.

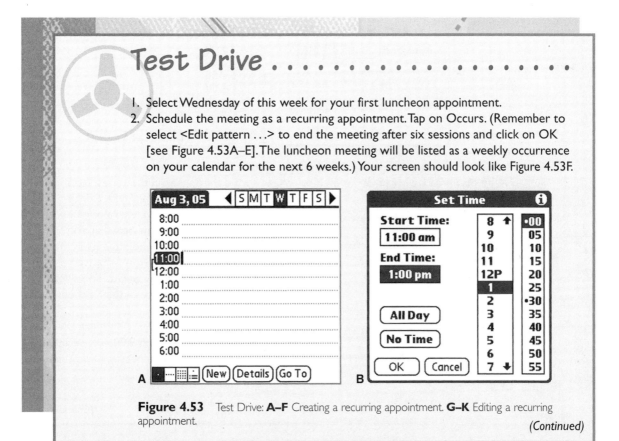

Test Drive . . . .

1. Select Wednesday of this week for your first luncheon appointment.
2. Schedule the meeting as a recurring appointment. Tap on Occurs. (Remember to select <Edit pattern . . .> to end the meeting after six sessions and click on OK [see Figure 4.53A–E]. The luncheon meeting will be listed as a weekly occurrence on your calendar for the next 6 weeks.) Your screen should look like Figure 4.53F.

Figure 4.53 Test Drive: **A–F** Creating a recurring appointment. **G–K** Editing a recurring appointment.

(Continued)

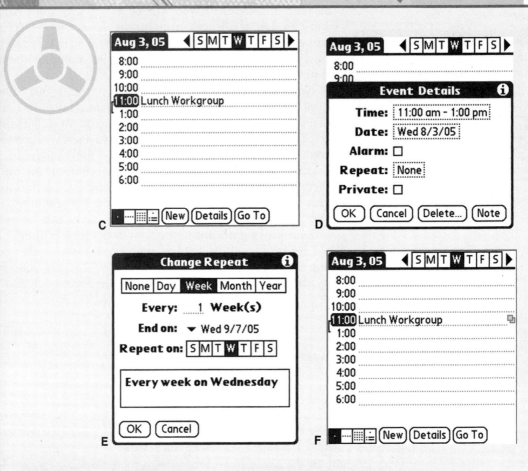

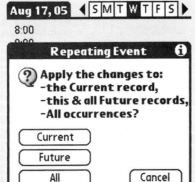

3. Move ahead to the third week in the series. Tap and hold your stylus on the appointment until a drop-down menu appears, and select Delete Appointment.

4. You will be prompted by a message box that asks whether you want to delete all appointments in the recurring series (see Figure 4.53G). In this case, you want to keep the remaining appointments so select No and only this single occurrence of the luncheon meetings will be deleted.

5. Now you can put the details of the conference the boss would like you to attend from 9:00 A.M. to 3:00 P.M. on your calendar for that Wednesday. To do this,

Figure 4.53 (Continued)

(Continued)

stay on the same date, tap on New (located at the bottom left) and create an appointment that starts at 9:00 A.M. and ends at 3:00 P.M. (see Figure 4.53H–K).

6. Tap on OK to finish.

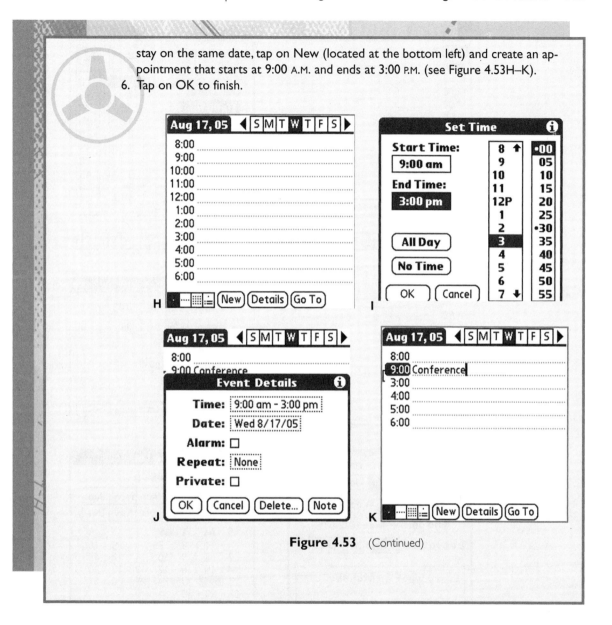

Figure 4.53 (Continued)

Now that was not so hard, was it? Give it a try again. Assume that you are scheduled for lab from 8:00 to 10:00 A.M. on Monday mornings for the next 10 weeks. Week 5 is spring break, and you have scheduled a well-deserved vacation. Make the appropriate notations in your PDA's calendar program. Refer to Figure 4.54A–L for guidance.

The last example will walk you through setting up a calendar event over several days. Assume that you will be attending a 3-day evidence-based practice conference and would like to have the event displayed on your calendar. Refer to Figure 4.55 as a guide for this activity.

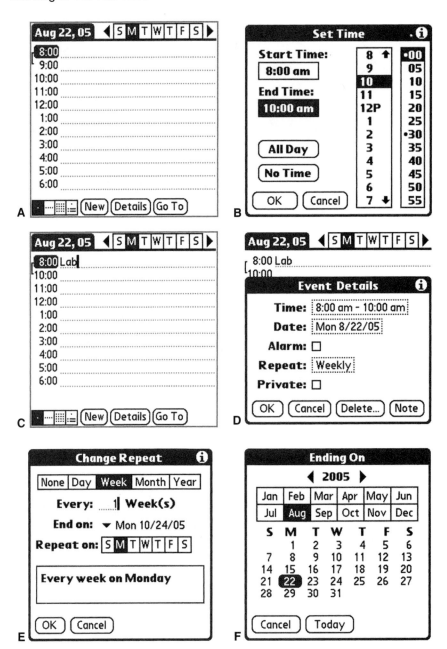

Figure 4.54   A–H Scheduling lab as a recurring event. **I–L** Deleting scheduled lab during week of spring break.

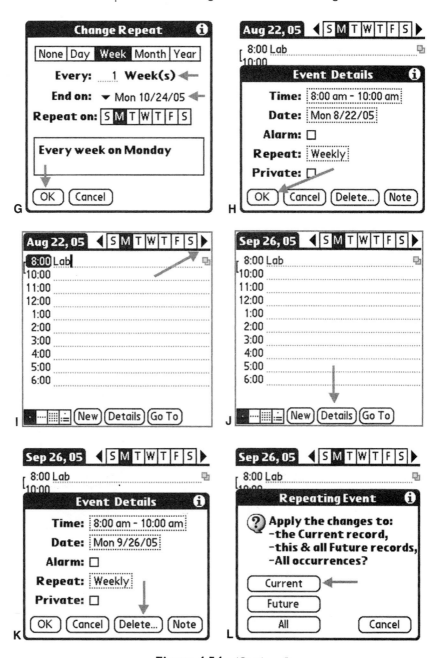

Figure 4.54 (Continued)

Test Drive . . . .

1. Open your Date Book.
2. Locate the date that the conference starts, May 21, and tap on New, located at the bottom of your screen (see Figure 4.55A).
3. Tap on All Day, select Yes, and tap on OK (see Figure 4.55B).
4. Enter: Evidence Based Practice Conference (see Figure 4.55C).
5. Select Details, located at the bottom of the screen (see Figure 4.55D).

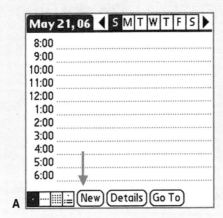
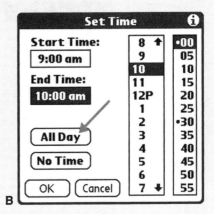

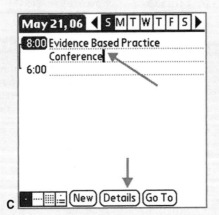
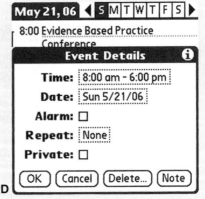

Figure 4.55   A–G Creating a daily recurring event.

(Continued)

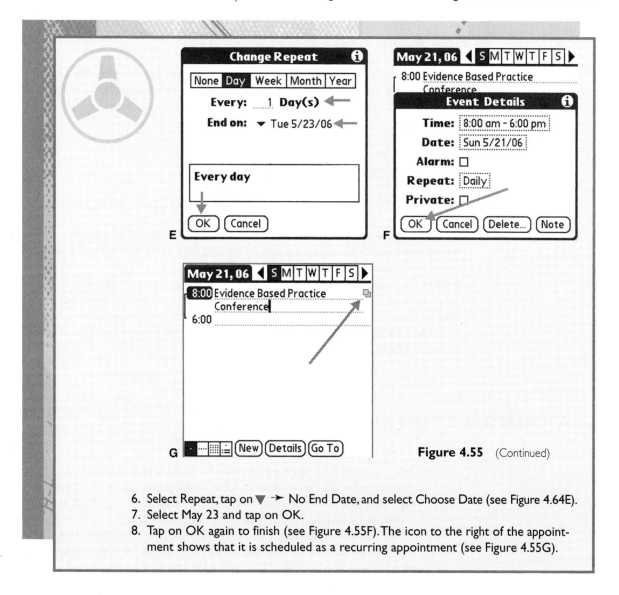

Figure 4.55 (Continued)

6. Select Repeat, tap on ▼ → No End Date, and select Choose Date (see Figure 4.64E).
7. Select May 23 and tap on OK.
8. Tap on OK again to finish (see Figure 4.55F). The icon to the right of the appointment shows that it is scheduled as a recurring appointment (see Figure 4.55G).

Summary

You have now been introduced to the basic organizational features available on your PDA. As with all new things, these tools take time to become second nature; however, given time, you will likely find these features essential for managing your personal information *and*, more importantly, saving you time.

Tips From the Experts

- Palm users can quickly locate an appointment or contact by using the Look Up feature by tapping on the small magnifying glass icon located on the Palm writing area to initiate the search (see Figure 4.56).

Figure 4.56   Palm Look Up feature.

- Palm users can speed up text entry in the Memo Pad and To Do list. You do not have to tap New to create a new record; just start writing and a new record will be automatically created.
- Pocket PC users can organize and manage multiple calendars (for example, your work schedule, your kid's soccer schedule, and his or her class schedule) by assigning categories to the appointments. To view a particular calendar/schedule, select that category from your calendar Tools menu. (Unselect the category to go back to the full calendar view.)

LEARNING ACTIVITIES

1. Schedule a recurring meeting:
   a. You are asked by your supervisor to chair a policy committee that is charged with the task to review and update all current policies. You are asked to meet weekly and complete this task in 3 months. Enter this recurring event in your PDA.
   b. After the first meeting, two of the members inform you that they will not be able to attend the sixth meeting. After some discussion, it was determined that this meeting will be cancelled and the committee will resume work the following week. Remove the meeting from your calendar.
2. Add new contacts: You have three other people who have volunteered to be on your policy committee. Add the following individuals to your PDA:

   Sylvia Stone
   sylvia.stone@anyone.com
   555-555-2626

Mary Loven
mary.loven@anyone.com
555-555-2826

Andrew Bace
andrew.bace@anyone.com
555-555-2999

3. Create a new contact category: Create a new category called Policy Committee, and place the contacts you entered in the previous activity into this category.

Visit http://thePoint.LWW.com/cornelius for supplemental information and activities.

5

Downloading Applications

Mary Gallagher Gordon

Key Terms

Applications • Software or programs that run on your PDA or PC

Default install directory • The location of memory in the handheld device that is automatically selected for the download of programs

Download • The process of transferring data or applications from a server to a computer or handheld device

Drag and Drop • The process of right-clicking on an application, dragging it into another area, and "dropping" it for downloading

Freeware • Software that is developed, usually by individuals or small companies, and distributed at no cost to the user, usually via the Internet. Individuals can freely use this software, and the developer/owner retains the copyright

Shareware • Software that is distributed for free on a trial or limited basis, with the understanding that the user may need or want to pay for it later. Sometimes shareware has a built-in expiration date so the software stops working; other shareware is distributed in a "lite" version of the application with some key functionality becoming operational only after the product is purchased. This strategy often entices users to purchase the full version of the program

Zip file • A folder that contains multiple files that have been compressed or "zipped" to take up less space

Many **applications** are available that can extend the functionality of your PDA. Applications range from those that can support your professional practice, enhance your personal life, or just give you an opportunity to relax a moment by playing a game. Available PDA applications for the health care provider are extensive and include:

- Diagnostic Tools (identification and classification of disease)
- Health and Fitness (lifestyle modification and alternative medicine)
- Interventions (procedural and treatment protocols)
- Investigations (lab tests and other diagnostic tools)
- Record Tracking (databases for tracking health care)
- References (grab-bag of medical knowledge base)
- Research Tools (critical appraisal tools)

Downloading and installing applications (also called *software*) onto your PDA is a fairly simple process. Usually, you will download the application without any problem, but, occasionally, you will run into a snag or two! So, we will review the basic process of downloading and installing applications.

What are applications? Applications are software that you would usually purchase in addition to the computer hardware. Application software is usually a program that is independent of the operating system yet has been adapted to the operating system. You will find applications on the Internet, and they may be **shareware**, a "try before you buy" type of software, usually found on the Internet. An example of shareware would be Pocket Informant, a tool to assist with daily personal information management (PIM). Another type of application is **freeware**, free software applications are also usually found on the Internet. An example of freeware would be the American Cancer Society C-Tools. You can locate available resources by doing an Internet search using a search engine. When selecting programs for your PDA, make sure you are getting the correct version for your specific handheld device.

Now that you know the wealth of resources available, you will want to "load up" your PDA. Before you do this, consider the amount of available memory on your PDA. Where do you want to store these new and wonderful applications? To review information about memory, refer to Chapter 1. When you have decided where you will store the application, you are ready to begin the downloading and installation process.

When you have decided on the application and you begin the "download now" process, sometimes installation goes smoothly, and other times you are struggling to get the application across to the PDA. Why is that? This chapter should assist you in the processes of installing an application from the Web or from your computer onto your PDA, deleting unwanted applications, and backing up your PDA to protect your settings and applications.

Basic Downloads and Installation

When preparing to install/download programs to your PDA, you must begin with your PDA in its cradle and synchronized to your computer. The two primary ways to install programs onto your PDA are (1) directly from the Internet or (2) using a CD that contains the application or program. When completing the installation, the installation wizard will launch and assist you with the step-by-step instructions for the installation. Depending on the amount of memory that you have available on your PDA, you may choose to install your programs on a storage card rather than in the main memory; you will be able to select this option during the process of the installation wizard. Some programs, such as Norton Antivirus for the Windows PDA, require that they be installed on the main memory of the PDA to function properly.

Installation for Windows CE/Pocket PC

Basic Download and Installation From the Internet

To download and install an application from the Internet into your Windows CE/Pocket PC device, start with your handheld device in the cradle. Locate on the Internet the program you want to install. Make sure to select the correct version of the program that matches the format of your handheld. You will be asked whether you want to save or run the file; if this is an application you will be putting on various PDAs, then save it to the desktop; if this application will be used on this PDA only, you may want to select run.

During the download process, you will be asked where the program should be installed (main memory or storage card, for example). Usually, the message you will see is "Install using default install directory?" (see Figure 5.1). The default install directory is the main memory of the PDA. If you have a storage card, you can select No, and in the next screen, you will have the option of instead selecting where you wish to install the application. From the drop-down menu, you can select Main (default) or a memory card if you have one on your PDA (see Figure 5.2). The rule of thumb is that all programs be installed to the storage card to save space on your main memory, unless the application specifically states that it must be stored on the main memory. Two exceptions would be when you are installing an antivirus program or an external keyboard driver. Many of these programs will not function properly if not installed on the main memory.

When the program is downloaded, you will see a notice on your computer to check your handheld device for any further instructions (e.g., "Please check

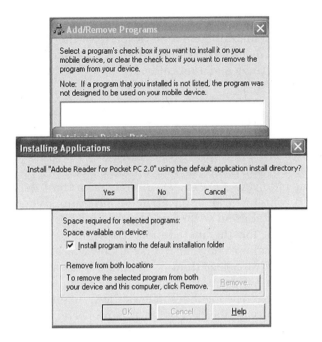

Figure 5.1 Download process and direction regarding installing using the default application install directory.

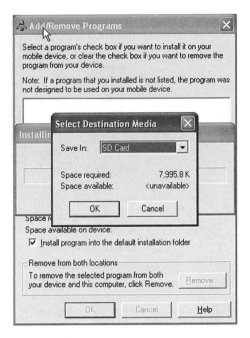

Figure 5.2 Changing where to place the application, using the storage card as the final destination.

your mobile device screen to see if additional steps are necessary to complete this installation"). If available, follow those specific instructions; otherwise, the download of the program is now complete. To access the new program, click on Start, Programs, and then tap on the desired application icon to open the program.

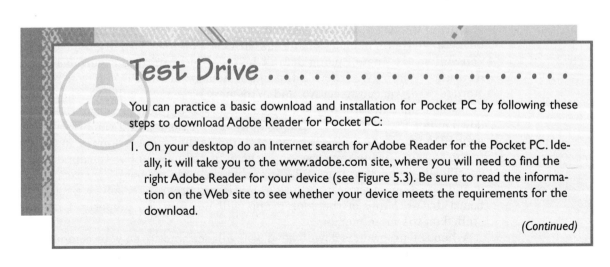

Test Drive . . . .

You can practice a basic download and installation for Pocket PC by following these steps to download Adobe Reader for Pocket PC:

1. On your desktop do an Internet search for Adobe Reader for the Pocket PC. Ideally, it will take you to the www.adobe.com site, where you will need to find the right Adobe Reader for your device (see Figure 5.3). Be sure to read the information on the Web site to see whether your device meets the requirements for the download.

(Continued)

2. If it does meet requirements, continue to the section where you are given directions to download Adobe Reader. It will ask you the operating system that you are using on your device. You will need to identify the language that you wish to use for the download process (e.g., English). When asked whether you want to run or save the program, select run (see Figure 5.4A and B).

3. Press No when you get to the screen that shows "Install Adobe Reader 2.0 for Pocket PC using the default application install directory?"

4. The next screen will ask you where you want the application to be placed. Again, it defaults to the main memory. You will need to use the drop-down bar to place the application in the storage card and press OK (see Figure 5.2).

5. The program will complete the process and prompt you that the files are being transferred to the PDA. Look onto the PDA and see whether the process is moving forward, as shown in Figure 5.5.

6. To verify that you have placed the application on your PDA, tap on Start, Programs, and then look for Adobe Reader. Because programs are listed alphabetically, Adobe should be at the top of the screen.

Adobe **Reader**

Download Adobe Reader for mobile devices

Select your operating system:

↓ Pocket PC
↓ Palm OS for Windows
↓ Palm OS for Macintosh
↓ Symbian OS

Pocket PC Version 2.0
Pocket PC 2002 and Windows Mobile 2003 with update 2

English Pocket PC v2.0 13.5MB
French Pocket PC v2.0 14.3MB
German Pocket PC v2.0 14MB
Italian Pocket PC v2.0 14MB
Japanese Pocket PC v2.0 14MB
Spanish Pocket PC v2.0 14MB

Pocket PC 2002
All models - ARM, X-Scale

English Pocket PC 2002 8.4MB
French Pocket PC 2002 8.4MB
German Pocket PC 2002 8.3MB
Italian Pocket PC 2002 8.3MB
Japanese Pocket PC 2002 10.1MB
Spanish Pocket PC 2002 8.3MB

Adobe® Reader® updates
Get the latest updates available for your version of Adobe Reader.

Distribute Adobe Reader
Find out how to distribute Adobe Reader software on an intranet, CD, or other media, or place an "Includes Adobe Reader" logo on your printed material.

More info
Adobe Reader
Adobe Reader for Symbian OS™
Adobe Reader for Pocket PC
Adobe Reader for Palm OS®
What is Adobe PDF?

Figure 5.3 Using the Adobe Reader for installation requirements for your device. (Adobe product screen shot reprinted with permission from Adobe Systems, Inc.)

(Continued)

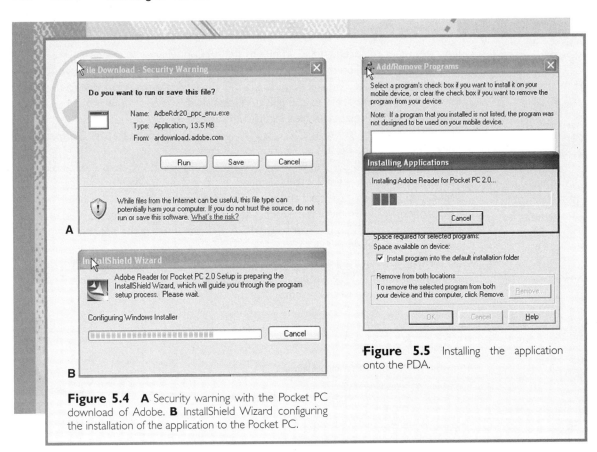

Figure 5.5 Installing the application onto the PDA.

Figure 5.4 A Security warning with the Pocket PC download of Adobe. **B** InstallShield Wizard configuring the installation of the application to the Pocket PC.

Basic Installation From a CD

If you are installing an application from a CD onto your Windows CE/Pocket PC device, you can follow these steps:

1. Place your handheld device into the cradle and make sure it is connected (synchronized).
2. Insert the desktop CD-ROM into your computer's CD-ROM drive.
3. The installation program will automatically launch with on-screen instructions that will guide you through the installation process.
4. You will be prompted during the installation process to identify where you would like the program installed: the main memory (default install directory) or on a storage card (if available).
5. Follow the on-screen instructions and enter your registration information.

A Word About Zip Files

You may come across a **zip file** when downloading an application. A zip file is a folder that contains multiple files that have been compressed or zipped to take up less space. A zipped file is frequently used for sending multiple files via e-mail or with applications. If you would like more information on zip files, tutorials and information can be found online using a search engine.

Drag and Drop

You may need to install an application for which the developer did not include an installer, so the installation onto the PDA must be performed manually. In many cases, this application will be provided to you in a zipped folder. After unzipping the folder, you can install the program manually through a simple process called **drag and drop**, using the explorer function on your PDA. To drag and drop an application, follow these steps:

1. Find the application you want to install.
2. Follow the directions and save the zipped application to the desktop. Unzip the application using WinZip or a similar program. Then find the ARM.CAB file you would like to install, as shown in Figure 5.6. (Some applications are also distributed as MIPS.CAB and SH3.CAB files. ARM, MIPS, and SH3 describe the different types of processors that are used in Pocket PC-based PDAs; the early processors had a combination of all three, but, lately, most are of the Intel processor type, based on the ARM version.)
3. Open ActiveSync on your desktop.
4. Select Explore, located on the top toolbar (see Figure 5.7A and B).
5. While Explore is open, drag the ARM.CAB folder into a white spot in the explore section of your mobile device, as shown in Figure 5.8.
6. A message will appear, stating it will need to convert files to the PDA format (see Figure 5.9A). After you click on OK, it will copy and convert the files (see Figure 5.9B).

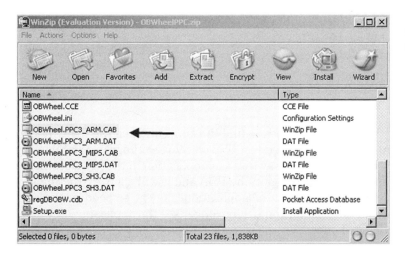

Figure 5.6 Selecting program to install after unzipping the downloaded application file.

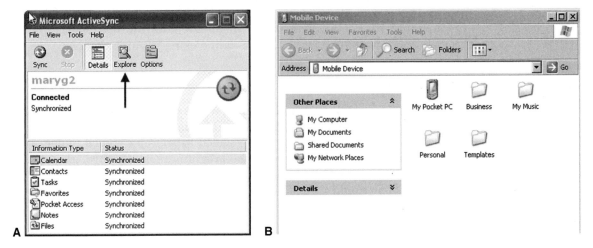

A   B

Figure 5.7   Using the Explore feature in Microsoft ActiveSync to install an ARM.CAB file: **A** Click on Explore tab. **B** Open Explore window.

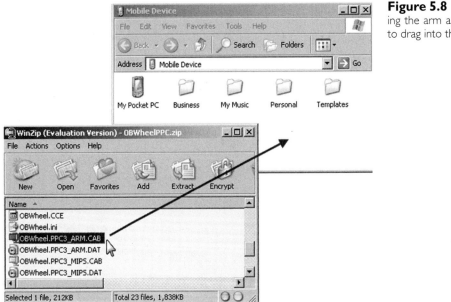

Figure 5.8   Opening the file and finding the arm application; selecting the file to drag into the Explore window.

7. Now the tricky part; you need to find the application on the PDA. To do this, go to your PDA Today screen. Tap on Start → Programs → File Explorer. Frequently, you may find the application in the My Documents folder. Tap on the application in the PDA and it will open, extracting itself onto your PDA. Some of the applications may be embedded; therefore, once you open them, you will no longer see the application in the My Documents folder.

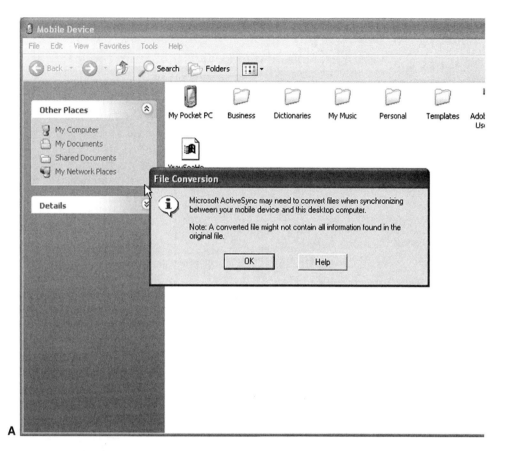

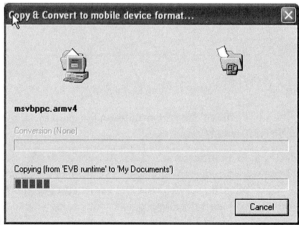

Figure 5.9 **A** File conversion message with the option to click on OK or read the Help message. **B** Copying and converting files to the Mobile Device format.

Installation for Palm

Basic Download and Installation From the Internet

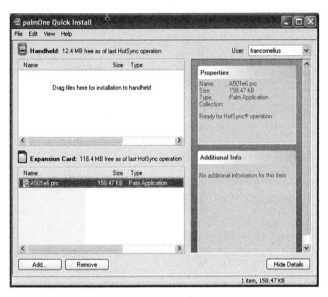

Figure 5.10 Quick Install window in Palm.

To install an application from the Internet onto your Palm handheld, start with your handheld device in its cradle. Locate the program that you want to install on the Internet, and make sure to select the correct version of the program that matches the format of your handheld.

The Palm handheld provides you with various choices when downloading programs or applications. A process called *Quick Install* will allow you to drag and drop files onto the Palm Quick Install icon on your Windows desktop. To take advantage of Quick Install, you can drag and drop files onto the Palm Quick Install Window seen in Figure 5.10, use the commands or buttons on the Quick Install Window, or right-click on a file and send it to the Palm Quick Install.

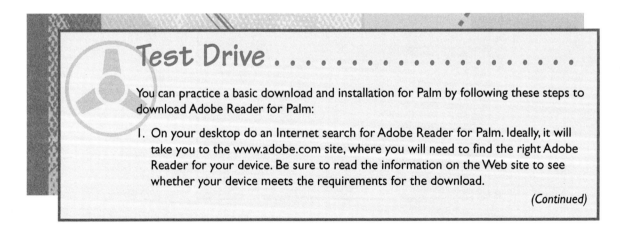

Test Drive

You can practice a basic download and installation for Palm by following these steps to download Adobe Reader for Palm:

1. On your desktop do an Internet search for Adobe Reader for Palm. Ideally, it will take you to the www.adobe.com site, where you will need to find the right Adobe Reader for your device. Be sure to read the information on the Web site to see whether your device meets the requirements for the download.

(Continued)

2. If it does meet requirements, continue to the section where you are given directions to download Adobe Reader. When you choose the language version of the application, it will then ask you whether you want to run or save. If this is an application that you will be putting on various PDAs, then save to the desktop. If this application will be used on this PDA only, press run (see Figure 5.11A). The process will ask you to verify if you want to run the program. If it is a trusted site, press run (see Figure 5.11B).

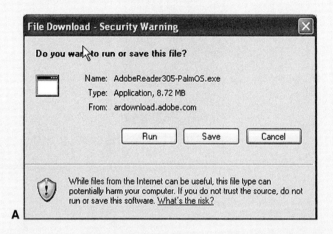

A

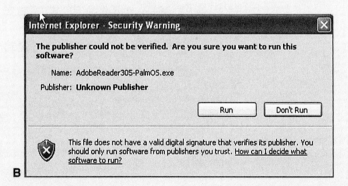

B

Figure 5.11   A Selecting whether to run or save the application. **B** Microsoft security warning verifying information that is being downloaded.

(Continued)

3. The installation process begins, and you need to respond to each question in a positive tone, usually a *yes, accept,* or *continue* response, as shown in Figure 5.12.

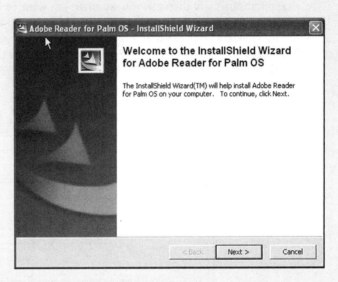

Figure 5.12   InstallShield Wizard for Palm OS: Following the directions for the process.

4. Once the process is completed on the desktop, you will then install on the device (see Figure 5.13). Be sure to sync after the transfer of information has occurred.

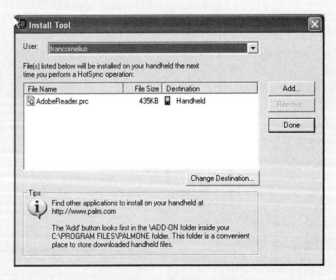

Figure 5.13   Installing onto Palm device: Files to be installed upon syncing.

(Continued)

5. Downloading applications from a zip file will require you to have a desktop program to unzip the files. Now you will have to decide which file to use (see Figure 5.14). Figure 5.15A shows the application being moved into the main memory; you

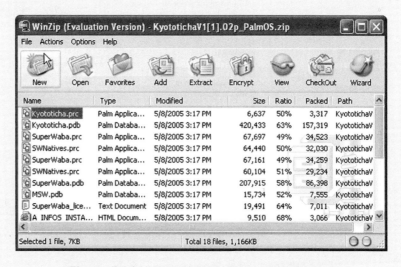

Figure 5.14   Selecting a file to unzip and place in Palm.

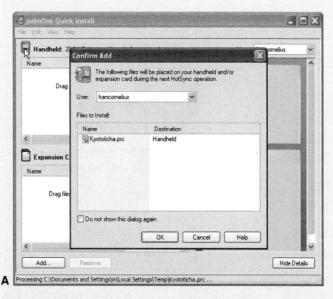

Figure 5.15   A Confirming files to be placed onto the Palm with the next HotSync operation.

(Continued)

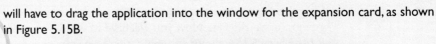

will have to drag the application into the window for the expansion card, as shown in Figure 5.15B.

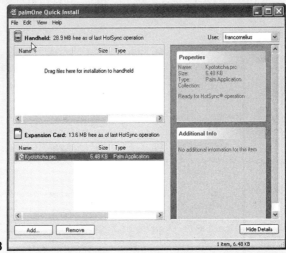

B

Figure 5.15 (Continued) **B** Dragging an application into the expansion card.

6. After you receive a message that installation is complete (see Figure 5.16), click on Finish, and then perform a HotSync on the Palm.

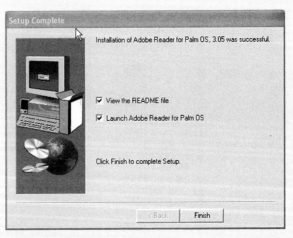

Figure 5.16 Completed installation with the completion of HotSync.

7. To find the application, you will need to recall where you directed it during the application process. In this case, the program is on the SD card. Now the fun begins. Open the application and enjoy!

Basic Download From a CD

If you are installing an application from a CD onto your Palm device, you can follow these steps. This process is the same as for a Windows CE/Pocket PC device.

1. Insert the desktop CD-ROM into your computer's CD-ROM.
2. The installation program will automatically launch with on-screen instructions that will guide you through the installation process.
3. You will be prompted during the installation process to identify where you would like the program installed: the main memory or on a memory card (if available).
4. Follow the on-screen instructions and enter your registration information.

Deleting Applications From Your PDA

Sometimes you may wish to delete programs or tools from your PDA. Deleting applications is a simple process. To delete applications from a Windows CE/Pocket PC device, follow these steps:

1. From your PDA Today screen, tap on Start.
2. Select Settings from the drop-down menu.
3. Select the System tab located at the bottom of the screen.
4. Locate and select the Remove Programs icon.
5. Locate the program you wish to remove, highlight it, and then tap on Remove.

To delete applications from a Palm device, follow these steps:

1. On your Palm, tap on the time display located at the upper left corner of the screen.
2. Choose Delete from the options.
3. Highlight the application you would like to delete.
4. Tap on Delete.
5. When you have deleted the applications you will no longer be using, press Done.

Backing Up Your PDA

A backup is a mirror image or snapshot of all of the programs and data you have on your PDA at the time the backup is created. You can back up the main memory, the storage card, or a compact flash, if available. In some instances, if space is limited, you may perform a partial backup, saving only the most important data. Save yourself some grief by doing a backup of your device routinely before you install any new applications. That way, if you really do not like the new application or the application does not function properly, you can do a "restore" from your backup and not have to worry whether you got the entire program off your PDA. Restoring in this situation is a real time-saver, especially if you have spent considerable time setting up your PDA according to your personal preferences. It is recommended that you create a new backup whenever you install new applications or make modifications on your PDA.

Backing Up Windows CE/Pocket PC

You can back up your Pocket PC device from your PDA or from your computer. To do a backup on your PDA, follow these steps:

1. Press Start in the top left corner.
2. Scroll down and press Programs.
3. In Programs find Data Backup or whatever your device calls the backing up process.
4. Be sure to select the option to back up all information or all data.
5. If you do not have a storage card, back up the information to the main memory.
6. If you have a storage card, open up the drop-down bar, where the backup to main memory is located and tap on storage card.
7. If there is an option to name the file, it is suggested that you give it a meaningful name, such as the date. That way you will know the last time you backed up your PDA.
8. If you need to restore your information, you would go to the same site and look for the restore key.
9. On some devices you may see a message indicating that it is preferable, but not essential, to be hooked up to power when doing a backup. You can tap on OK and continue the process.

To back up your Windows CE/Pocket PC PDA from the desktop, perform an ActiveSync, and then open the Tools option at the top of the ActiveSync section. Go down to *backup/restore* and do either a full backup or an incremental backup. An incremental backup will back up only the information that has changed since the last backup. You will then press the *backup now* button. Once the process is completed, you may close the application on the desktop.

Backing Up Palm

You do not have an option in your Palm menu to do a quick backup, so you will need to follow these steps:

1. Create a new folder on your desktop and give it a meaningful name.
2. Open the Palm desktop on your desktop computer.
3. Press on the Save All icon in the top left corner of the desktop application.

4. Go to the Start icon on your desktop in the bottom left corner.
5. Go to My Computer.
6. Go to the C drive or local file.
7. Go to program files.
8. Go to Palm One.
9. Open the folder that is labeled with the name of your Palm.
10. Right-click in the white area in the folder and click on paste; all of the information that is in your Palm will now be in this folder.
11. Depending on how often you use your PDA, you should do a backup when you load new applications or files.

Summary

You have learned how to download and install applications onto your PDA using various methods depending upon the delivery method provided by the application designers; how to install applications that use automatic installation wizards as well as those that require the manual "drag and drop" technique; how to direct the installation either to the main memory or to the memory card (CF or SD) of your PDA; and how to provide a layer of security (and peace of mind) by performing a device backup, which will allow you to restore your PDA to optimal functioning status quickly and easily.

Tips From the Experts

- Occasionally, you may see the following message after you have downloaded an application: "The program you have installed may not display properly because it was designed for a previous version of Windows Mobile software." When you see this message, you will need to press OK. The reasons for this message vary; you may have a PDA with a newer version of the operating system than that for which the application was built.
- Once you have the settings on your PDA the way you like them, you should do a backup of your PDA.
- Conduct a backup before you download an application that you are not sure you really want on your PDA. Then, if you decide you want to remove the application, you can do a restore on your PDA, and all parts of that application will be removed.
- Palm: If you write the first letter of the program you are looking for in the Graffiti area, it will scroll to that program.

LEARNING ACTIVITIES

1. Using the skills discussed in this chapter, locate an article of interest regarding health promotion at the Centers for Disease Control and Prevention (CDC) Web page (http://www.cdc.gov) and save it as a PDF file on your PDA. Use Adobe Reader, which you installed earlier, to view the article on your PDA. This can be done on either a Palm or a Pocket PC device.

2. Perform a backup on your device. Be sure to date the backup, as well as back it up to the memory card (SD or CF) to conserve memory on your PDA.

 WebLink. | Visit http://thePoint.LWW.com/cornelius for supplemental information and activities.

References

Adobe Systems Incorporated. (2005). Retrieved October 26, 2005, from http://www.adobe.com.

Department of Health and Human Services, Centers for Disease Control and Prevention. (2005). Retrieved October 26, 2005, from http://www.cdc.gov.

6

Connectivity

Linda Wilson • H. Lynn Kane

Key Terms

Hotspot • A connection point for a Wi-Fi network, supported by a small box (hub) that is hardwired into the Internet

Infrared (IR) • An invisible radiation wavelength used to transmit data

Modem • A device that allows digital data to be transmitted over a phone line (The term is an abbreviation of the words *modulator-demodulator*)

Wireless • A feature that allows you to read, transmit, or receive information via the Internet without your PDA or PC being physically connected by a cable

Depending on the type of handheld device that you purchase, you will have various connectivity options, which include infrared (IR), wireless, modem, and Bluetooth. These options can greatly increase the functionality of your device and enhance your ability to perform various tasks in a mobile environment. This expanded functionality can help the busy professional work more efficiently by streamlining workflow and information sharing. For example, shift report information can be beamed via infrared to a coworker, or library databases can be accessed via wireless to locate current literature to guide practice.

Although every type of PDA does not have all of the connectivity options previously listed, most have infrared. Many devices that do not have those features built-in can usually be upgraded with add-on accessories that can be purchased. These accessories are discussed in more detail in Chapter 18. In this chapter we will review the various connectivity options listed previously and provide step-by-step instructions for using each.

Infrared

Most PDAs have an IR port that uses IR light to transmit information to a PC or to another PDA. Depending on the type of handheld device that you select, you may have many options for the use of IR. Usually, IR ports are located on the top of your device, as depicted in Figure 6.1. The benefit of IR capability is the opportunity to share files and information through the use of a simple beaming process. Beaming is the process of sending an item from one device to another. You can beam documents (i.e., Word or Excel files), notes, contact information, appointments on your calendar, themes, and images. Infrared technology has also become useful for importing literature search results to your handheld device while at the library. Many libraries are currently offering this service. Limitations of IR devices include the proximity needed for the beaming process to function (maximum of only a few feet) and the amount of battery power used during the process. Beaming can be accomplished between any two devices that have IR capabilities; Figure 6.2 demonstrates beaming between two handheld devices. The basic steps involved in the beaming process are explained in the following section.

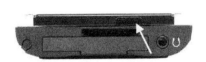

Figure 6.1 Typical infrared port. (Image courtesy of Dell, Inc.)

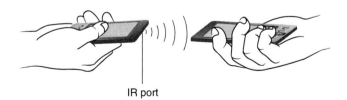

IR port

Figure 6.2 Beaming between two handheld devices. (Redrawn with permission from Palm, Inc.)

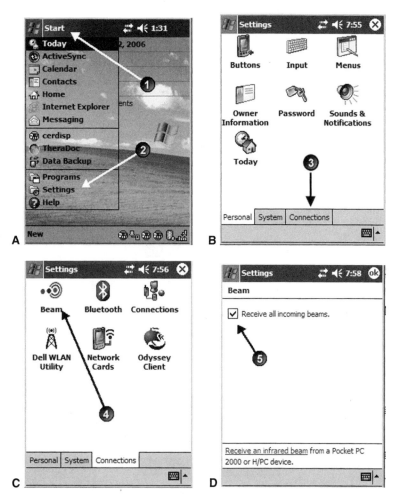

Figure 6.3 Enabling beam function on Pocket PC.

Beaming for Windows CE/Pocket PC

Before you start, make sure your beam function is enabled. To enable it, refer to Figure 6.3 and follow these steps:

1. Locate Start on the Today screen.
2. From the drop-down menu, select Settings (Figure 6.3A).
3. Select Connections (Figure 6.3B).
4. Select Beam (Figure 6.3C).
5. Put a check mark in the box labeled *Receive all incoming beams* (Figure 6.3D).

Now that your IR port is enabled, you are ready to beam.

Test Drive . . . .

For the purposes of this Test Drive, you can use the calendar appointment you created in Chapter 4 and refer to Figure 6.4 as you follow these steps:

1. On your handheld device, select Start and then select Calendar.
2. Locate and select the appointment that you want to beam (Figure 6.4A).
3. Press and hold your stylus on the appointment and from the drop-down menu, select Beam Appointment (Figure 6.4B).

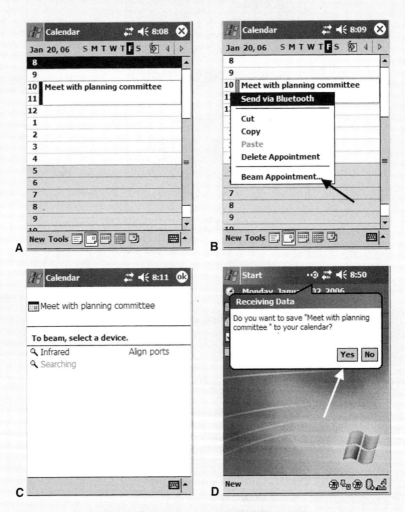

Figure 6.4 Beaming an appointment on Pocket PC.

(Continued)

4. Locate the IR site on your device and line up the IR port on your handheld device with the IR port on the device that will be receiving the file (Figure 6.4C). Remember that the handheld devices can be up to a maximum of a few feet apart for the IR beaming to work effectively. Please note that if the device is low on battery power, beaming may not be possible.

5. The handheld device receiving the beam will give a notification upon receipt of the file, and the owner will have to accept the appointment for it to be incorporated into the calendar (Figure 6.4D).

Beaming for Palm

The process of beaming an appointment from a Palm PDA is similar to that for a Pocket PC. Before you start, make sure your beam function is enabled. To enable it, refer to Figure 6.5 and follow these steps:

1. On your Palm screen, select Prefs (Preferences) (Figure 6.5A).
2. Tap on Power (Figure 6.5B).
3. Be sure that the beam function is turned on, and tap on Done to finish (Figure 6.5C).

Now that you are certain that the beam function is enabled, try it out in the following activity.

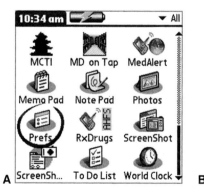
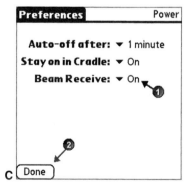

Figure 6.5   Enabling beam function on Palm.

Test Drive . . . .

For beaming with a Palm device, refer to Figure 6.6 and follow these steps:

1. Locate the IR site on your device.
2. On your handheld device, open the Date Book and locate the appointment you created earlier (Figure 6.6A).
3. Tap to select the appointment.
4. From the drop-down menu on the upper left corner of the screen, select Beam Event (Figure 6.6B).
5. Line up IR port on your handheld device with the IR port on the device that will be receiving the document. The handheld devices can be a maximum of a few feet apart for the IR beaming to work effectively.
6. The handheld device receiving the beam will have a notification or beam dialog box upon receipt of the document, and you will have to either accept or reject the document by tapping on Yes or No (Figure 6.6C).

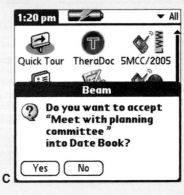

Figure 6.6　Beaming an appointment on a Palm device.

Wireless

Many handheld devices today have wireless capability, which allows you to communicate via voice or Internet depending on your specific device. A clear benefit of wireless capability is the availability of communication at any time in almost any location, provided that there is wireless access available. A major limitation of wireless is the varying strength of signal you receive in different locations from your service provider, which may cause you to be "out of range" and therefore not be able to connect to the Internet.

If you purchase a handheld device with wireless capability, you will also need to sign up for a wireless service or locate and access an ever-growing network of wireless hotspots. Many Wi-Fi hotspots are now available in public places, for instance, restaurants, hotels, libraries, and airports. Some hotspots provide users free access to the Internet while others require membership. A wireless service can be used for Internet access only or for both Internet access and voice/phone service. The options that you have depend on the handheld device that you select and the wireless services that are available in your geographic area.

Wireless for Windows CE/Pocket PC

Setting up your wireless is a simple process. You can set up your wireless connectivity on a Windows CE/Pocket PC device by following the steps illustrated in Figure 6.7.

1. On the Today screen, select Start and then select Settings (Figure 6.7A).
2. Select Connections (Figure 6.7B).
3. Select Add a new connection (Figure 6.7C).

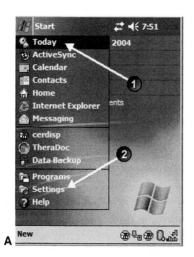
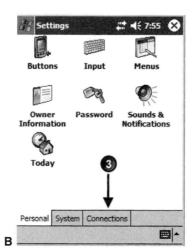
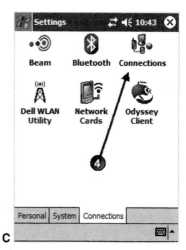

Figure 6.7 Setting up wireless connectivity for Pocket PC.

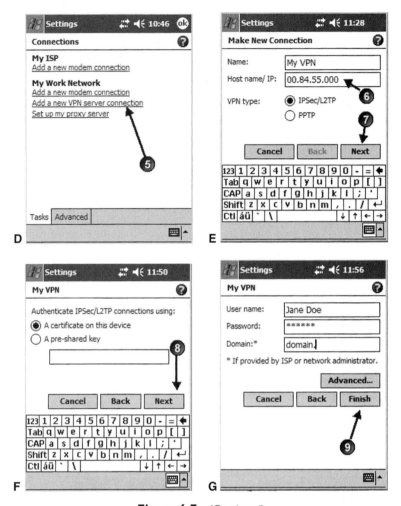

Figure 6.7 (Continued)

4. Select Add a new VPN server connection (Figure 6.7D).
5. Identify the name for the connection and the IP address and select Next (Figure 6.7E).
6. Select to authenticate the device and select Next (Figure 6.7F).
7. Enter a user name and password and select Finish (Figure 6.7G).

Now that you have set up the wireless connection, return to the Today screen and check to make sure your connection functions properly. Select Programs from the Start menu (see Figure 6.8A), and then select Internet Explorer (see Figure 6.8B). Type Web address http://www.google.com/pda into the URL bar and tap on the green Go arrow on the upper right corner (see Figure 6.8C). If you were successful in setting up your Internet access, you should see the Google search engine screen (see Figure 6.8D). Once you are able to verify that you are connected to the Internet, you can enter any Web address you want and surf to your heart's content. Bear in mind that some Web sites do

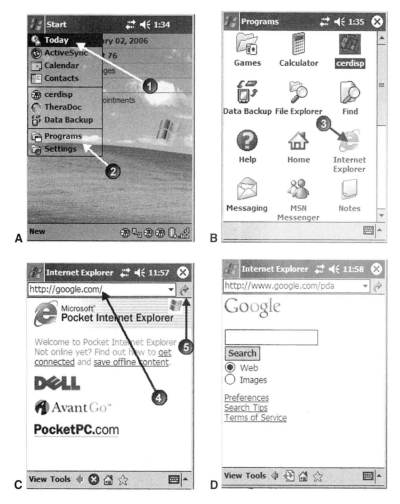

Figure 6.8 Checking wireless connection for Pocket PC. (Part D used with permission from Google, Inc.)

not display well on the smaller PDA screen, but many other Web sites are more "PDA-friendly."

Wireless for Palm

For Palm devices that have Wi-Fi capabilities, it is very easy to get connected. To set up your wireless connection, tap on Home on your Palm device and scroll down to Wi-Fi Setup. Tap on Wi-Fi Setup and select Next, as depicted in Figure 6.9. In the next screen, you should select LAN Setup. This action will take you through screens that will detect and display available wireless access points. All you need to do is select the access point you want; in this example, Pico is selected. Once you have set up your wireless connection, you can surf the Internet by pressing on your Wireless button (see Figure 6.10).

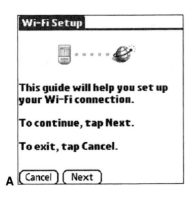

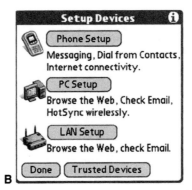

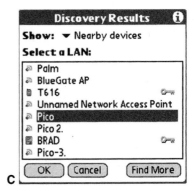

Figure 6.9   Palm Wi-Fi setup.

If your Palm device does not have Wi-Fi capabilities, you can use the IR wireless capabilities or a direct cable connection to connect to the Internet using a cellular phone, as shown in Figure 6.11. To use the wireless feature of your handheld device, follow the instructions listed in the Infrared section of this chapter.

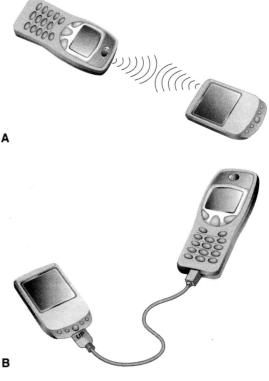

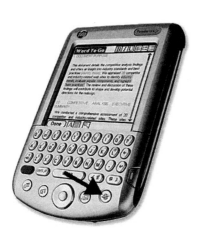

Figure 6.10 Palm wireless button. (Image courtesy of Palm, Inc.)

Figure 6.11 Palm connecting to the Internet using a cellular phone via: **A** Infrared. **B** Cable. (Redrawn with permission from Palm, Inc.)

Add-On Modems

Add-on modems are available and either clip into or on your handheld device. The other end of the modem device can be plugged into your phone jack using the standard phone cable. Once again, the type and capability of your handheld device will determine the options you have for add-on modems. These add-on accessories are discussed in more detail in Chapter 18.

Connecting to a Modem With Windows CE/Pocket PC

To connect your Windows CE/Pocket PC handheld device to either a 56K or LAN modem, follow the steps outlined here and illustrated in Figure 6.12.

1. Connect the modem to your handheld device, following the modem manufacturer instructions. You may need to install a driver for the modem before you proceed.
2. Connect the cable from your modem into the jack (phone line or LAN).
3. On your PDA, tap on Start on the Today screen and select Settings (Figure 6.12A).
4. Select the Connections tab at the bottom of the screen (Figure 6.12B).
5. Select Connections (Figure 6.12C).
6. Select Add a new modem connection (Figure 6.12D).
7. Identify the name for the connection, select a modem, and tap on Next (Figure 6.12E).
8. If you are using a phone line, you will receive a cue to enter the phone number and tap on Next (Figure 6.12F). (If you are using a LAN modem, you will not see this screen.)
9. Enter a user name and password and tap on Finish (Figure 6.12G).

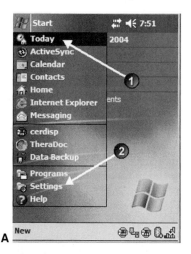
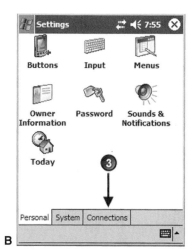
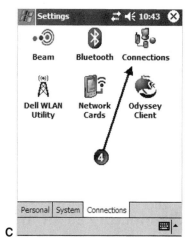

Figure 6.12 Pocket PC connecting to the Internet using an external modem (56K or LAN).

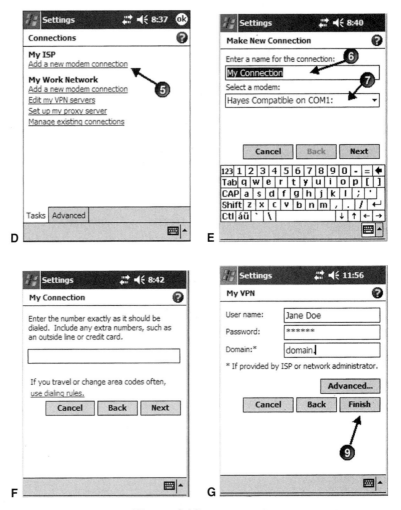

Figure 6.12   (Continued)

Now that you have set up your modem connection, return to the Today screen and check to see that your connection is functioning properly. Select Programs from the Start menu (Figure 6.13A), and then select Internet Explorer (Figure 6.13B). Type Web address http://www.google.com/pda into the URL bar and tap on the green Go arrow on the upper right corner (Figure 6.13C). If you were successful in setting up your modem Internet access, you should see the Google search engine screen (Figure 6.13D).

Connecting to a Modem With Palm

To connect your Palm handheld device to either a 56K or LAN modem, follow the steps outlined here and illustrated in Figure 6.14.

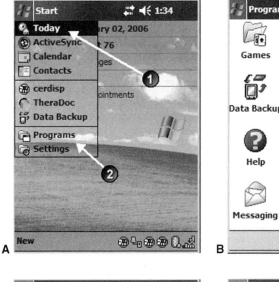
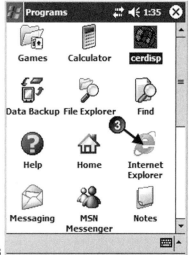
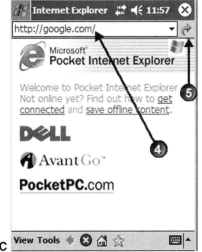
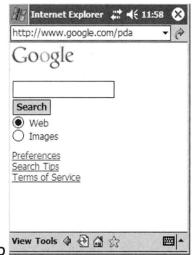

Figure 6.13 Checking external modem connection for Pocket PC. (Part D used with permission from Google, Inc.)

1. Connect the modem to your handheld device following the modem manufacturer instructions. You may need to install a driver for the modem before you proceed.
2. Connect the cable from your modem into the jack (phone line or LAN).
3. On your Palm device, tap on Home and locate and select Preferences (Figure 6.14A).
4. Select Connection (Figure 6.14B).
5. Select Palm Modem US/Canada and tap on New (Figure 6.14C).

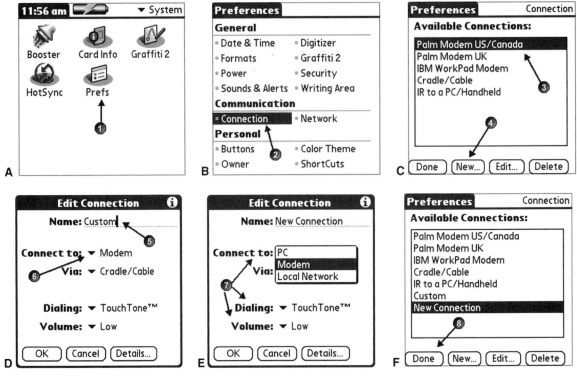

Figure 6.14   Palm connecting to the Internet using an external modem (56K or LAN).

6. Give this new connection a name (Figure 6.14D).
7. Begin configuration of the connection by making selections from the drop-down menus (Figure 6.14E).
8. Select Done to finish setup (Figure 6.14F).

Another useful function of an add-on modem is that it enables you to perform a HotSync to your home PC while at a remote setting, for example, out of town on a business trip. This can be easily set up, but you will need to have two modems—one for your Palm device and one for your PC. Any modem will do for your PC, but it will need to be connected to its own private line. Your handheld will need a modem specifically designed for the device. These accessories will be discussed in more detail in Chapter 18. To set up your device for a modem HotSync, you will need to follow the steps outlined here and illustrated in Figure 6.15.

1. On your Palm device, tap on Home and locate and select HotSync (Figure 6.15A).
2. Select Modem and then tap on Enter phone # (Figure 6.15B).

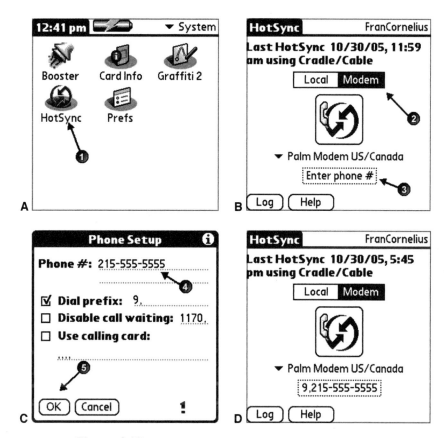

Figure 6.15 Setting up a modem HotSync on a Palm device.

3. Enter the phone number that is connected to your computer and tap on OK to save settings (Figure 6.15C).
4. In the next screen, you will see that the phone number is now stored for performing a HotSync remotely (Figure 6.15D).

Bluetooth

As described in Chapter 1, many handheld devices today have Bluetooth capability. The biggest benefit of Bluetooth is the ability to network within one's own work environment. Bluetooth can allow your handheld device to "communicate" with other devices in your home or office, such as compatible keyboards, printers, and fax machines, without being connected by cables. The Bluetooth capability will enable you to send documents to the printer or fax machine without having to connect your handheld to any additional device. Also, Bluetooth will permit you to share files with other PDA users. Generally, Bluetooth has a range of about 30 feet. Limitations of Bluetooth capability include the proximity needed to complete the wireless process and not all other devices, such as printers and fax machines, are Bluetooth enabled. It is also important to be aware that many Bluetooth enabled devices may need installation of specific drivers to enable the communication between your handheld and the other device.

Bluetooth for Windows CE/Pocket PC

To set up Bluetooth capability on your Windows CE/Pocket PC handheld device, follow the steps depicted in Figure 6.16 and outlined here:

1. From the Today screen, select the Bluetooth icon at the bottom right-hand corner of the screen (Figure 6.16A). You can also access Bluetooth via the pathway Start → Settings → Connections.
2. Select Bluetooth Manager (Figure 6.16B).
3. Select New on the bottom left-hand corner of the screen (Figure 6.16C).
4. You will see the Bluetooth wizard that will give you choices that you can access via Bluetooth, such as (a) creating a connection with another Bluetooth device; (b) connecting to the Internet; (c) joining a personal network; (d) connecting to the Internet via cell phone; (e) using ActiveSync via Bluetooth; (f) browsing a file on a remote device; or (g) connecting to a headset.
5. To proceed, tap on your selection. For this example, we will select the option to Connect to Internet via phone (Figure 6.16D).
6. Select the phone type and tap on Next (Figure 6.16E).
7. Select Next to finish (Figure 6.16F).
8. Once you are finished using the Bluetooth, return to the Today screen and tap on the Bluetooth icon at the bottom right corner to turn off Bluetooth (Figure 6.16G). Remember, leaving Bluetooth enabled when you are not using it will drain your battery.

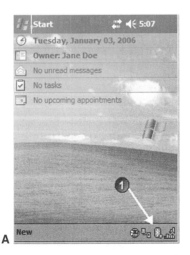 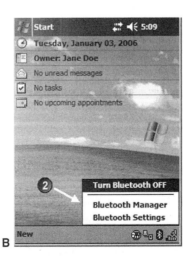 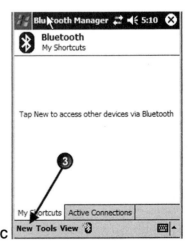

Figure 6.16   Setting up Bluetooth on Pocket PC.

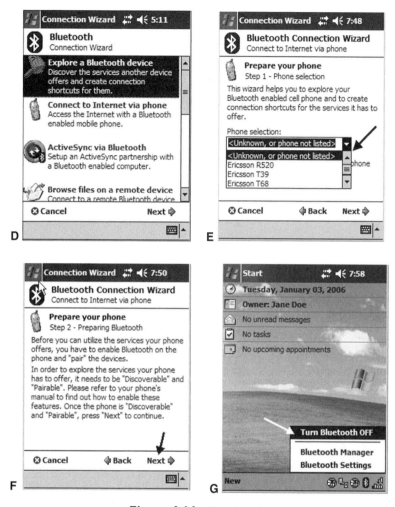

Figure 6.16 (Continued)

Bluetooth for Palm

To set up Bluetooth capability for your Palm handheld device, follow the steps depicted in Figure 6.17 and outlined here.

1. Pair your handheld device with the other device you plan to use Bluetooth (for this example, we will use a phone).
2. Select to power on the Bluetooth (Figure 6.17A).
3. Tap on Setup Devices.
4. Select the type of phone service and tap on Next (Figure 6.17B).
5. Your device will locate all the Bluetooth enabled phones within range. Select the particular phone that you want to connect with and tap on OK to finish (Figure 6.17C).
6. Once you are finished using the Bluetooth, turn it off.

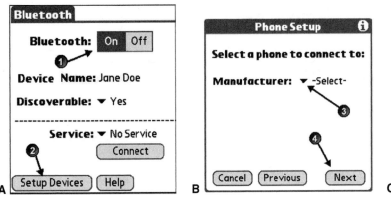
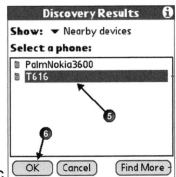

Figure 6.17 Setting up Bluetooth on Palm.

Summary

You have learned about the various connectivity options available for the PDA that expand your ability to work more effectively and efficiently in a mobile environment. These options—IR, Bluetooth, wireless, and modems—enhance your ability to locate and share information with others as well as provide a means for you to stay connected via e-mail. Such functionality clearly helps the busy practitioner bring relevant and current information to the care setting—when and where it is needed—not only saving time but also improving the quality of care provided.

Tips From the Experts

- Take your time when selecting the handheld device that you are going to purchase to ensure that it has all of the features that you need.
- Investigate the specific additional requirements needed to use the wireless, IR, and Bluetooth capabilities of your handheld device.
- Beaming, Bluetooth, and wireless use a lot of battery power, so consider keeping your handheld device plugged into power if you are using these functionalities extensively.

LEARNING ACTIVITIES

1. Beam a document to another person's handheld device.
2. Beam a contact to another person's handheld device.
3. Beam a Today screen theme to another person's handheld device.

4. Set up the wireless capabilities of your handheld device.

5. Connect to the Internet and search for your favorite Web site. Save that Web site as a "favorite."

6. If you have a Bluetooth enabled printer, set up a connection between your handheld device and the printer, and attempt to print a document.

 Visit http://thePoint.LWW.com/cornelius for supplemental information and activities.

Unit 2

CASE SCENARIOS AND LEARNING ACTIVITIES

Introduction

The following section of this book contains case scenarios and learning activities designed to build competency in using the PDA to access information at the point-of-care/point-of-need when a question arises. Each chapter consists of two types of case studies: general and advanced. The General Case Studies provide you with an opportunity to practice accessing information, using the trial references indicated before each case presentation.

The Advanced Case Studies are more in-depth and give you the opportunity to use PDA software you may choose to buy for your PDA. Purchasing the references indicated at the beginning of each case presentation is necessary to complete the case studies. Each advanced case study contains both cross-discipline and discipline-specific learning activities. In this portion you are guided step-by-step in the process of accessing required information residing in the PDA and correlating assessment information as well as findings to plan for short-term and long-term patient care needs. Specific questions are provided to guide your discipline-specific interventions.

The Answers to Case Studies section at the end of each chapter provides you with the PDA references to use and the pathways to follow to find the specific answers to the case study questions. Note that, for some questions, more than one reference could be used to find the same information.

Visit thePoint at **http://thePoint.LWW.com/cornelius** to access the trial versions of the references or to purchase the full versions for the PDA.

7

Medical Surgical
Case Studies

Magdeleine Vasso • Francine Gelo

The case studies in this chapter focus on adult clients with complex medical health care needs. As stated in the unit introduction, the exercises in each case study offer opportunities to practice using your PDA as a resource in the clinical setting. The General Case Studies section will provide you with an opportunity to practice accessing information on your PDA, using the trial references indicated before each case presentation. The Advanced Case Studies section is more in-depth and will require that you purchase the references indicated at the beginning of each case presentation. Both types of case studies explore the acute and chronic health issues that arise when dealing with this population. To maximize health and to restore an independent lifestyle for the adult with complex medical issues, an interdisciplinary team approach is needed. This team approach is vital within the acute care setting, as is the ability to access community services outside the specific institution.

➤ General Case Studies

For the following three case studies, you will need to download the trial versions of the following references:

- Griffith's 5-Minute Clinical Consult (5MCC)
- Lippincott's Nursing Drug Guide (LNDG)
- Physician's Drug Handbook (PDH)

- Stedman's Medical Dictionary for the Health Professions and Nursing (HPND)
- Manual of Psychiatric Therapeutics (PsychThrp)
- Nurse's Quick Check: Diseases (NDisCheck)

CASE STUDY 1 • *Mr. Volartez*

Mr. Volartez is a 55-year-old electrician, who, in a routine annual physical exam, presented with the following: anemia, occult blood in his stool, and a mass (3 cm) in the right lower quadrant. He denies pain but does report that, on occasion, his stools "look funny." His diagnosis is colorectal malignancy.

1. What is colorectal malignancy?
2. What are the signs and symptoms associated with this disease?
3. What are the causes associated with this disease?
4. What are the available treatments for this disease?

Mr. Volartez has surgery. During his postoperative recovery, Mr. Volartez is started on medication.

5. What are the drugs of choice?
6. What are steroids?

After a few weeks, Mr. Volartez is seen and cleared by the surgeon; he begins chemotherapy.

7. What are the side effects of fluorouracil?
8. What should the patient and his family be taught about this medication?
9. What is the prognosis for this patient?

CASE STUDY 2 • *Mr. Bergey*

Mr. Bergey is a 32-year-old firefighter who went to see his doctor with complaints of persistent fever, malaise, very itchy irritated skin, nausea, and vomiting. Upon examination, the doctor notices that Mr. Bergey's scleras are jaundiced and that he has hepatomegaly. Following a series of tests, the following diagnosis is made: acute hepatitis B virus and acute dermatitis. Mr. Bergey has many questions about his diagnosis.

1. What is a virus?
2. Specifically, what is hepatitis B?
3. Is there a genetic link associated with hepatitis B?
4. What are the symptoms of hepatitis B?
5. What are the risk factors associated with hepatitis B?
6. How can one minimize his or her risk of getting hepatitis B? How can he protect his family?

The doctor prescribed a topical corticosteroid to help relieve Mr. Bergey's discomfort related to the skin irritation.

7. What is dermatitis?
8. What is the action of hydrocortisone?
9. What instruction should Mr. Bergey receive regarding this medication?
10. What are the specific instructions regarding application of this ointment?

CASE STUDY 3 • *Ms. Hardy*

Ms. Hardy is a 47-year-old single woman with a history of alcohol abuse. She presents in the emergency room with significant abdominal distension and discomfort. She does not appear intoxicated but has a blood alcohol level of 200 mg/dL. The attending physician tells you that Ms. Hardy has abdominal ascites caused by cirrhosis (liver damage) associated with her alcoholism.

1. What is ascites?
2. When treating ascites, what are the dietary restrictions?
3. What is alcohol abuse?
4. How does alcohol affect the body?
5. What is the incidence of alcoholism in the United States?
6. What are the risk factors associated with alcohol abuse?

The attending physician uses the CAGE questionnaire for additional assessment.

7. What is the CAGE questionnaire?

Ms. Hardy is admitted to the hospital. Given her history of alcoholism, she is to be monitored for signs and symptoms (s/s) of alcohol withdrawal.

8. What signs and symtoms of alcohol withdrawal should you watch for?
9. You decide to use an assessment scale to facilitate monitoring your patient. What questions are on the Clinical Institute Withdrawal Assessment Scale for Alcohol?

➤ Advanced Case Studies

For the following three case studies, you will need to download full versions of these references:

- Griffith's 5-Minute Clinical Consult (5MCC)
- Stedman's Medical Dictionary for the Health Professions and Nursing (HPND)
- Nurse's Quick Check: Diseases (NDisCheck)
- Lippincott's Nursing Drug Guide (LNDG) *or* Physician's Drug Handbook (PDH)
- Nursing Procedures (NurProc)
- Nurses' Handbook of Health Assessment (HlthAssess)
- Handbook of Diagnostic Tests (HbDxTests)
- Manual of Psychiatric Therapeutics (PsychThrp)
- Physical Medicine and Rehabilitation Pocketpedia (PMRRx)

CASE STUDY 1 • *Mrs. Nazardo*

Mrs. Nazardo is a 28-year-old Caucasian woman who weighs 128 pounds and is 5 feet, 6½ inches tall. Approximately 2 years ago, she presented to the clinic with complaints of fatigue, generalized weakness, numbness, and loss of balance. She reported that she "constantly dropped objects" and would "stumble and fall." She reports occasional or transient diplopia. Extensive diagnostic studies were done and, eventually, the patient was diagnosed with multiple sclerosis. The patient was started on prednisone 30 mg orally daily and baclofen 5 mg orally t.i.d. The patient's condition seemed to stabilize.

Six months ago the patient's husband was killed in a work-related accident. Since that time, Mrs. Nazardo has noticed an increase in her fatigue and muscle weakness, and her balance and gait have been extremely unsteady. The patient reports that she constantly falls and is unable to hold objects in her hand. Although she was not totally dependent on her husband for her daily activities of self-care and dressing, she was dependent on him to complete the household chores, including food shopping and the preparation of meals. Although her family lives nearby, it has been difficult for them to be a consistent support to help Mrs. Nazardo. Additionally, it has been increasingly difficult for her to report to work and to perform her duties as an administrative secretary. Her employer has asked her to resign and apply for permanent disability.

Today, the patient is being admitted to the hospital with an exacerbation of her multiple sclerosis. She presents with spastic weakness of the extremities, urinary incontinence, tremors, and dysphagia. She is extremely weak and is unable to hold a glass of water without spilling the contents. She complains of severe muscle spasms of the lower extremities. Mrs. Nazardo has a flat affect and cries frequently. On admission to the unit her vital signs were as follows: blood pressure, 112/80; heart rate, 78; respiratory rate, 22 breaths per minute; and oral body temperature, 98.6°F.

Cross-Discipline Learning Activities

1. What is multiple sclerosis?
2. What physical signs and symptoms did Mrs. Nazardo display that are consistent with the diagnosis of multiple sclerosis?
3. Identify three different clinical courses of multiple sclerosis.

Discipline-Specific Learning Activities

Nursing

As the nurse caring for Mrs. Nazardo, you are responsible for ensuring the patient's safety and monitoring her response to treatment.

1. What are the adverse effects of baclofen on the central nervous system (CNS)?
2. What measures should be taken to ensure that it is safe for this patient to take in food orally and to prevent aspiration?

3. What are three techniques to evaluate the nutritional status of this client?
4. Identify the equipment needed to promote proper body alignment and to prevent complications in patients needing prolonged bed rest.

Medicine/PA/NP

1. What tests would you expect to be ordered to confirm the diagnosis of exacerbation of multiple sclerosis?
2. What precautions should be taken to address Mrs. Nazardo's complaints of dysphagia?
3. The drug prednisone (prednisolone/Predalone) may be beneficial to this client; what is the intravenous dosage of prednisone given to adults experiencing an exacerbation of multiple sclerosis?
4. Depression is often present in patients suffering with a chronic disease; what medication has been associated with depression in patients with multiple sclerosis?

Physical and Occupational Therapy

Mrs. Nazardo needs to start a comprehensive rehabilitation program at the bedside and continue at a rehabilitation center until her condition stabilizes.

1. What are the goals of a comprehensive physical and occupational therapy program for patients with multiple sclerosis?
2. What are the indications for treatment for spasticity?
3. Multiple sclerosis patients cannot tolerate high temperatures. What education regarding this problem should be provided to the patient to help her avoid exacerbations in her condition?

Behavioral Health

1. Mrs. Nazardo is grieving the loss of her husband. Describe the mourning process.
2. What community referrals should be considered as part of the patient's discharge planning?

Critical Thinking—Correlating Patient Data/Assessment Findings to Plan Care

Mrs. Nazardo wishes to be discharged home. What needs to be included as part of the discharge teaching plans regarding her medication regimen as well as safety issues within the home?

What additional information specific to this case would be beneficial to facilitate a plan of care for this patient and to promote an independent lifestyle? What resources are available to this client to promote an independent lifestyle within the community?

What assessments regarding the patient's home environment, community, and support systems would need to be assessed to promote an independent lifestyle?

CASE STUDY 2   •   *Mr. Victor*

Mr. Victor is a 59-year-old man who is the vice president of a major communications company. He works extremely long hours, is rarely at home, and travels often for work. He has a history of hypertension, coronary artery disease, and unstable angina. Two years prior he was diagnosed with an acute myocardial infarction (AMI) and underwent interventional cardiac procedures with stent placement in his proximal and medial left anterior descending (LAD) artery. In addition to the LAD, Mr. Victor had a stent placed proximally in his right coronary artery.

After the initial myocardial infarction, Mr. Victor was dedicated to altering his lifestyle; however, in the past year he has been less compliant with his cardiac regimen and changes in lifestyle. Mr. Victor has resumed his long working hours. He has regained all of the initial weight loss and is currently 20 pounds heavier than he was at the time of his AMI. He leads a sedentary lifestyle because he is always at work on the computer. He continues to smoke two packs of cigarettes per day. His diet consists mostly of "fast foods," and a diet recall reveals that he primarily eats foods high in fat and sodium. His medications regimen includes ASA, Lopressor, and furosemide.

On this hospital admission, Mr. Victor presented to the emergency room with complaints of shortness of breath (SOB), dyspnea with exertion, and a productive cough of frothy, blood-tinged sputum. Before coming to the emergency room, he called the cardiologist to see if he could take "more of his water pill" because he felt short of breath, extremely bloated, and lower extremity edema. He started to cough frothy mucus just prior to his arrival to the emergency room.

The client was admitted to the hospital for treatment of acute pulmonary edema secondary to congestive heart failure (CHF).

Cross-Discipline Learning Activities

1. What is the definition of CHF?
2. Identify the clinical manifestations of left- versus right-sided ventricular heart failure.
3. What is the definition of pulmonary edema?
4. What are the classic clinical manifestations of pulmonary edema? With which of these signs and symptoms did this client present on admission?
5. What are the treatment goals, including medication, for pulmonary edema?

Discipline-Specific Learning Activities

Nursing

1. What tests are usually ordered to support the diagnosis of pulmonary edema?
2. What are two risk factors of intravenous potassium?
3. What are the cardiovascular effects of administering furosemide intravenously?

4. What nursing measures should be used on a daily basis to evaluate the progress of Mr. Victor's medical regimen?
5. What dietary restrictions are important for this patient?

Medicine/PA/NP

On day 2 of admission, the client complains of tingling and numbness of his fingers, muscle weakness, and cardiac palpitations. He appears confused and restless. An arterial blood gas is drawn and reveals the following: pH, 7.56; $PaCO_2$, 45; PaO_2, 69; HCO_3, 33; and SaO_2 saturation, 92%. An electrolyte panel reveals a potassium level of 2.8 mEq/L. The patient's electrocardiogram (ECG) reveals that he is having frequent premature ventricular contractions (PVCs).

1. What is the patient's acid base imbalance, and what are the most likely causes of this imbalance?
2. What medications should be considered as part of this patient's regimen on admission?
3. What diet should be ordered for this patient?
4. What are the normal potassium parameters?
5. What are the signs and symptoms of hypokalemia?

Physical and Occupational Therapy

1. What elements should be included for a comprehensive cardiac rehabilitation program for this client?
2. What exercises should be emphasized in Mr. Victor's rehabilitation plan?
3. During your initial evaluation of Mr. Victor, you note that he becomes short of breath with exertion. What should be included in the patient's teaching plan regarding energy conservation?

Behavioral Health

1. Before discharge, what other services should be consulted to help Mr. Victor with his change in lifestyle, including smoking cessation and physical activity?
2. Mr. Victor is concerned about returning to his usual daily activities. What type of information is needed to assist Mr. Victor?
3. Included in Mr. Victor's discharge-teaching plan should be information regarding resumption of sexual activity. List the information that should be shared with this patient.

Critical Thinking—Correlating Patient Data/Assessment Findings to Plan Care

Mr. Victor is scheduled to be discharged home. What teaching will need to be included in his discharge plan? What additional information specific to Mr. Victor, including physical assessment, diagnostic testing, medications, and cardiac rehabilitation, would the team need to include in his plan of care to prevent his recurrent admission to the hospital with CHF? What education does this patient need regarding diet and exercise before being discharged?

CASE STUDY 3 • *Mr. Malvinado*

Mr. Malvinado is a 45-year-old Hispanic man with a history of uncontrolled diabetes mellitus and hypertension. He was involved in a work-related accident, in which a piece of equipment fell on his lower extremities. He was trapped under the heavy equipment for 90 minutes. After he was finally extricated, he was taken to the hospital and diagnosed with crush injuries to his lower extremities—bilateral femur, right tibia, and right fibula fractures.

He was taken to the operating room for an open reduction of the fractures and was admitted to the orthopedic unit. His postoperative phase was unremarkable until day 2, when the patient's urine became scant and dark amber. The patient was evaluated and diagnosed with acute renal failure (ARF).

Cross-Discipline Learning Activities

1. What is the definition of ARF?
2. What is the definition of rhabdomyolysis?
3. What is the treatment for this patient's ARF?
4. What diagnostic and laboratory tests should be performed both to aid in the diagnoses of ARF and direct the management of this patient?

Discipline-Specific Learning Activities

Nursing

1. What are the priority nursing diagnoses for this patient?
2. What are the causes of hypocalcemia and hyperphosphatemia?
3. What is a positive Trousseau's sign? Identify the steps to assess for a positive Trousseau's sign.
4. An indwelling urinary catheter must be inserted to monitor this patient's urinary output. What are the possible complications of this type of monitoring device?

Medicine/PA/NP

1. What is the significance of an elevated serum creatinine level?
2. What are the goals in the management of ARF?
3. Explain the differences between hemodialysis and peritoneal dialysis to the patient, in terms easily understood.
4. This patient is given Procrit to treat his anemia. What is the pharmacological drug class of Procrit, and what is its mechanism of action to prevent anemia?

Physical and Occupational Therapy

1. What is the functional independence measure?
2. What types of exercises should be initiated during the early phase of the patient's hospitalization?

Behavioral Health

1. The patient with traumatic injury as well as ARF may suffer from stress and anxiety related to the injuries and complications. What are the five Rs of stress and anxiety reduction?
2. Relaxation techniques may be beneficial for this patient. What instruction would be helpful for this patient?

Critical Thinking—Correlating Patient Data/Assessment Findings to Plan Care

The patient would like to be discharged home. What assessments of Mr. Malvinado's home environment need to occur for him to be discharged? Discuss an interdisciplinary plan to meet this patient's discharge needs. What community resources are available to this patient so that he can continue to receive physical and occupational therapy? What resources are available to facilitate an independent lifestyle at home?

Chapter Summary—Tying It All Together

This chapter has challenged the participant to explore patient care issues that are typical of an adult population in the acute care setting. When dealing with complex medical issues that face this group, health care providers must resolve the acute health care issues of clients as well as address the needs that clients face when they return to their normal environment. A multidisciplinary approach using the resources that are available both in the acute care setting and in the community may reduce the length of stay in the hospital. Additionally, if health care providers address the challenges that face this population in their homes, the number of readmissions to acute care settings will be decreased.

 Visit http://thePoint.LWW.com/cornelius for supplemental information and activities.

ANSWERS TO CASE STUDY QUESTIONS

➤ General Case Studies

CASE STUDY 1 • *Mr. Volartez*

1. What is colorectal malignancy?

    5MCC → Colorectal Malignancy → Basics

2. What are the signs and symptoms associated with this disease?

    5MCC → Colorectal Malignancy → Basics → scroll down to Signs and Symptoms

3. What are the causes associated with this disease?

    5MCC → Colorectal Malignancy → Basics → scroll down to Causes

4. What are the available treatments for this disease?

    5MCC → Colorectal Malignancy → Treatment

5. What are the drugs of choice?

    5MCC → Colorectal Malignancy → Medications → Drugs of Choice

6. What are steroids?

    HPND → Steroids

7. What are the side effects of fluorouracil?

    LNDG → Fluorouracil → Adverse Effects

8. What should the patient and his family be taught about this medication?

    LNDG → Fluorouracil → Nursing Considerations → scroll down to Teaching Points

9. What is the prognosis for this patient?

    5MCC → Colorectal Malignancy → Follow-up → scroll down to Expected Course/Prognosis

CASE STUDY 2 • *Mr. Bergey*

1. What is a virus?

    HPND → Virus

2. Specifically, what is hepatitis B?

    HPND → Virus → scroll down to Hepatitis B Virus

3. Is there a genetic link associated with hepatitis B?

    5MCC → Hepatitis B → Basics → scroll down to Genetics

4. What are the symptoms of hepatitis B?

    5MCC → Hepatitis B → Basics → scroll down to Signs and Symptoms

5. What are the risk factors associated with hepatitis B?

    5MCC → Hepatitis B → Basics → scroll down to Risk Factors

6. How can one minimize his or her risk of getting hepatitis B? How can he protect his family?

    5MCC → Hepatitis B → Follow-up → scroll down to Prevention/Avoidance

7. What is dermatitis?

    HPND → Dermatitis

8. What is the action of hydrocortisone?

    PDH → Hydrocortisone (topical) → Pharmacodynamics

9. What instruction should Mr. Bergey receive regarding this medication?

    PDH → Hydrocortisone (topical) → Patient Education

10. What are the specific instructions regarding application of this ointment?

    PDH → Hydrocortisone (topical) → Special Considerations

CASE STUDY 3 • *Ms. Hardy*

1. What is ascites?

    5MCC → Ascites → Basics

2. When treating ascites, what are the dietary restrictions?

    5MCC → Ascites → Treatment → scroll down to Diet

3. What is alcohol abuse?

    5MCC → Alcohol Use Disorders → Basics

4. How does alcohol affect the body?

    NDisCheck → Alcoholism → Overview → scroll down to Pathophysiology

5. What is the incidence of alcoholism in the United States?

    NDisCheck → Alcoholism → Overview → scroll down to Incidence

6. What are the risk factors associated with alcohol abuse?

    5MCC → Alcohol Use Disorders → Basics → scroll down to Risk Factors

7. What is the CAGE questionnaire?

    5MCC → Alcohol Use Disorders → Basics → scroll down to Pathophysiology

8. What signs and symptoms of alcohol withdrawal should you watch for?

    PsychThrp → Alcohol Withdrawal → scroll down to Signs and Symptoms

9. You decide to use an assessment scale to facilitate monitoring your patient. What questions are on the Clinical Institute Withdrawal Assessment Scale for Alcohol?

    PsychThrp → Alcohol Withdrawal → scroll down to Assessment Scale

---

➤ Advanced Case Studies

CASE STUDY 1 • *Mrs. Nazardo*

Cross-Discipline Learning Activities

1. What is multiple sclerosis?

    NDisCheck → Main Index → Multiple Sclerosis → Description
    5MCC → Main Index → Multiple Sclerosis → Basics

2. What physical signs and symptoms did Mrs. Nazardo display that are consistent with the diagnosis of multiple sclerosis?

    NDisCheck → Main Index → Multiple Sclerosis → on right of screen select A for Assessment → scroll down to Physical Findings
    5MCC → Main Index → Multiple Sclerosis → Basics → scroll down to Signs and Symptoms

3. Identify three different clinical courses of multiple sclerosis.

    PMRRx → Main Index → Multiple Sclerosis → Clinical Categories and Tx

Discipline-Specific Learning Activities

Nursing

1. What are the adverse effects of baclofen on the central nervous system (CNS)?

    LNDG → Medication Index → Baclofen → on right of screen select AE for Adverse Effects → CNS
    PDH → Baclofen → Adverse Effects

2. What measures should be taken to ensure that it is safe for this patient to take in food orally and to prevent aspiration?

   PMRRx ➛ Main Index ➛ scroll down to Dysphagia Treatment ➛ on right of screen select O for Outline ➛ Suboptimal Cognitive Status

3. What are three techniques to evaluate the nutritional status of this client?

   HlthAssess ➛ Table of Contents ➛ scroll down to #18 Nutritional Assessment ➛ Adult Assessment ➛ on right of screen select O for Outline ➛ Objective Data Assessment Techniques

4. Identify the equipment needed to promote proper body alignment and to prevent complications in patients needing prolonged bed rest.

   NurProc ➛ Procedure Index ➛ scroll down to Alignment and Pressure Reducing Devices ➛ on right of screen select EQ for Equipment

Medicine/PA/NP

1. What tests would you expect to be ordered to confirm the diagnosis of exacerbation of multiple sclerosis?

   HbDxTests ➛ Main Index ➛ Multiple Sclerosis ➛ Information

2. What precautions should be taken to address Mrs. Nazardo's complaints of dysphagia?

   PMRRx ➛ Main Index ➛ scroll down to Dysphagia ➛ on right of screen select O for Outline ➛ select Oral Phase Dysphagia

3. The drug prednisone (prednisolone/Predalone) may be beneficial to this client; what is the intravenous dosage of prednisone given to adults experiencing an exacerbation of multiple sclerosis?

   LNDG ➛ Main Index ➛ Drug Index ➛ Predalone ➛ on right of screen select D for Dosage ➛ scroll down to Adults
   PDH ➛ Prednisolone (systemic) ➛ Indications and Dosage ➛ scroll down to Acute Exacerbation of Multiple Sclerosis

4. Depression is often present in patients suffering from a chronic disease; what medication has been associated with depression in patients with multiple sclerosis?

   PsychThrp ➛ Main Index ➛ enter Multiple Sclerosis ➛ Medical Conditions ➛ scroll down to fourth bullet point

Physical and Occupational Therapy

1. What are the goals of a comprehensive physical and occupational therapy program for clients with multiple sclerosis?

   PMRRx ➛ Main Index ➛ Multiple Sclerosis ➛ Clinical Categories and Tx ➛ scroll down to fourth bullet ➛ Rehabilitation Management

2. What are the indications for treatment for spasticity?

PMRRx → Main Index → Spasticity → scroll down to Topic Outline → select Tx

3. Multiple sclerosis patients cannot tolerate high temperatures. What education regarding this problem should be provided to the patient to help her avoid exacerbations in her condition?

NDisCheck → Main Index → Heat Syndrome → on right of screen select P for Patient Teaching

Behavioral Health

1. Mrs. Nazardo is grieving for the loss of her husband. Describe the mourning process.

PsychThrp → Table of Contents → scroll down to #16, Bereavement Reactions and Grief → Mourning Period

2. What community referrals should be considered as part of the patient's discharge planning?

NDisCheck → Main Index → Multiple Sclerosis → on right of screen select P for Patient Teaching, → scroll down to Discharge Planning

CASE STUDY 2 • *Mr. Victor*

Cross-Discipline Learning Activities

1. What is the definition of CHF?

HPND → Main Index → Congestive Heart Failure → Definition → select SYN Heart Failure
5MCC → Congestive Heart Failure → Basics
NDisCheck → Main Index → Heart Failure → Description

2. Identify the clinical manifestations of left- versus right-sided ventricular heart failure.

HPND → Main Index → Congestive Heart Failure → Definition → select SYN Heart Failure → select Right Ventricular Failure and Left Ventricular Failure
NDisCheck → Main Index → Heart Failure → Pathophysiology (left- and right-sided heart failure)
5MCC → Congestive Heart Failure → Diagnosis → Differential Diagnosis (third and fourth bullets)

3. What is the definition of pulmonary edema?

HPND → Main Index → scroll down to Pulmonary Edema
5MCC → Pulmonary Edema → Basics
NDisCheck → Main Index → Pulmonary Edema → Overview → Description

4. What are the classic clinical manifestations of pulmonary edema? With which of these signs and symptoms did this client present on admission?

   HPND ➔ Main Index ➔ scroll down to Pulmonary Edema ➔ at top of screen select Link ➔ HbDxTests
   NDisCheck ➔ Main Index ➔ Pulmonary Edema ➔ Assessment ➔ scroll down to Physical Findings
   5MCC ➔ Pulmonary Edema ➔ Basics ➔ scroll down to Signs and Symptoms

5. What are the treatment goals, including medication, for pulmonary edema?

   NDisCheck ➔ Main Index ➔ Pulmonary Edema ➔ on right of screen tap on T for Treatment
   5MCC ➔ Pulmonary Edema ➔ Treatment and 5MCC ➔ Pulmonary Edema ➔ Medications

Discipline-Specific Learning Activities

Nursing

1. What tests are usually ordered that support the findings of pulmonary edema?

   HbDxTests ➔ Main Index ➔ Pulmonary Edema ➔ Information
   NDisCheck ➔ Pulmonary Edema ➔ Assessment ➔ Test Results (special tests and imaging)

2. What are two risk factors of intravenous potassium?

   Nurproc ➔ Main Index ➔ Medication Index ➔ Potassium Chloride ➔ Risk of Peripheral IV Therapy

3. What are the cardiovascular side effects of administering furosemide intravenously?

   LNDG ➔ Drug Index ➔ Furosemide ➔ on right of screen select AE for Adverse Effects ➔ scroll down to CV
   PDH ➔ Furosemide ➔ Adverse Effects ➔ CV

4. What nursing measures should be used on a daily basis to evaluate the progress of Mr. Victor's medical regimen?

   NDisCheck ➔ Disease Index ➔ Pulmonary Edema ➔ Nursing Considerations ➔ Nursing Interventions
   5MCC ➔ Pulmonary Edema ➔ Follow-up ➔ scroll down to Patient Monitoring

5. What dietary restrictions are important for this patient?

   NDisCheck ➔ Disease Index ➔ Pulmonary Edema ➔ on right of screen select T for Treatment ➔ General Outline
   5MCC ➔ Pulmonary Edema ➔ Treatment ➔ scroll down to Diet and Patient Education

Medicine/PA/NP

1. What is the patient's acid base imbalance, and what are the most likely causes of this imbalance?

   HbDxTests → Main Index → Arterial Blood Gas Analysis → on right of screen select AF for Abnormal Findings → scroll to bottom and tap on Acid-Base Disorders → Metabolic Alkalosis → Possible Causes → #2 bullet

2. What medications should be considered as part of this patient's regimen on admission?

   NDisCheck → Disease Index → Pulmonary Edema → on right of screen select T for Treatment → scroll down to Medications
   5MCC → Pulmonary Edema → Medications

3. What diet should be ordered for this patient?

   NDisCheck → Disease Index → Pulmonary Edema → on right of screen select T for Treatment → scroll down to General Outline
   5MCC → Pulmonary Edema → Treatment → scroll down to Diet

4. What are the normal potassium parameters?

   HbDxTests → Main Index → Potassium → on right of screen select NF for Normal Findings

5. What are the signs and symptoms of hypokalemia?

   HbDxTests → Main Index → Potassium → on right of screen select AF for Abnormal Findings
   5MCC → Hypokalemia → Basics → scroll down to Signs and Symptoms
   NDisCheck → Hypokalemia → Assessment → History and Physical Findings

Physical and Occupational Therapy

1. What elements should be included for a comprehensive cardiac rehabilitation program for this client?

   PMRRx → scroll down to Cardiac Rehabilitation → select Introduction

2. What exercises should be emphasized in Mr. Victor's rehabilitation plan?

   PMRRx → scroll down to Cardiac Rehabilitation → select Exercise Rx

3. During your initial evaluation of Mr. Victor you note that he becomes short of breath with exertion. What should be included in the patient's teaching plan regarding energy conservation?

   HPND → Main Index → Energy Conservation Techniques

Behavioral Health

1. Before discharge, what other services should be consulted to help Mr. Victor with his change in lifestyle, including smoking cessation and physical activity?

    NDisCheck → Main Index → Pulmonary Edema → on right of screen select P for Patient Teaching → scroll down to Discharge Planning

2. Mr. Victor is concerned about returning to his usual daily activities. What type of information is needed to assist Mr. Victor?

    HlthAssess → Main Index → Activity Exercise Pattern → Outline → Subjective and Objective Data

3. Included in Mr. Victor's discharge-teaching plan should be information regarding resumption of sexual activity. List the information that should be shared with this patient.

    PMRRx → Table of Contents → scroll down to #11 Cardiac Rehabilitation → Post-Cardiac Event Sexual Counseling

CASE STUDY 3 • *Mr. Malvinado*

Cross-Discipline Learning Activities

1. What is the definition of ARF?

    NDisCheck → Main Index → Renal Failure → Acute → Overview → Description
    5MCC → Acute Renal Failure → Basics

2. What is the definition of rhabdomyolysis?

    NDisCheck → Main Index → Rhabdomyolysis → Overview → Description
    5MCC → Rhabdomyolysis → Basics → Description

3. What is the treatment for this patient's ARF?

    NDisCheck → Main Index → Acute Renal Failure → on right of screen select T for Treatment
    5MCC → Acute Renal Failure → Treatment

4. What diagnostic and laboratory tests should be performed to both aid in the diagnoses of ARF and direct the management of this patient?

    HbDxTests → Main Index → Acute Renal Failure
    5MCC → Acute Renal Failure → Diagnosis → scroll down to Laboratory
    NDisCheck → Acute Renal Failure → Diagnosis → scroll down to Laboratory

Discipline-Specific Learning Activities

Nursing

1. What are the priority nursing diagnoses for this patient?

   HlthAssess → Main Index → Acute Renal Failure → Nursing Diagnosis → Risk Diagnosis

2. What are the causes of hypocalcemia and hyperphosphatemia?

   HbDxTests → Main Index → Calcium → on right of screen select AF for Abnormal Findings
   5MCC → Hypokalemia → Basics → scroll down to Causes

3. What is a positive Trousseau's sign? Identify the steps to assess for a positive Trousseau's sign.

   NDisCheck → Main Index → Trousseau's sign → Outline

4. An indwelling urinary catheter must be inserted to monitor this patient's urinary output. What are the possible complications with this type of monitoring device?

   NurProc → Table of Contents → scroll down to Renal and Urologic Care → Catheter (indwelling) → on right of screen select CO for Complications

Medicine/PA/NP

1. What is the significance of an elevated serum creatinine level?

   HbDxTests → Main Index → Creatinine, Serum → on right of screen select AF for Abnormal Findings

2. What are the goals in the management of ARF?

   NDisCheck → Main Index → Acute Renal Failure → on right of screen select O for Outline and NC for Nursing Considerations

3. Explain the differences between hemodialysis and peritoneal dialysis to the patient, in terms easily understood.

   HPND → Main Index → Hemodialysis → return to Main Index → Peritoneal Dialysis

4. This patient is given Procrit to treat his anemia. What is the pharmacological drug class of Procrit, and what is its mechanism of action to prevent anemia?

   LNDG → Main Index → Procrit → on right of screen select G for General → scroll down to Drug Class → Therapeutic Actions
   PDH → Procrit → Classification and PDH10 → Procrit → Pharmacodynamics

Physical and Occupational Therapy

1. What is the functional independence measure?

   PMRRx ➤ Table of Contents ➤ scroll down to #8 Disability ➤ select Functional Independence Measure

2. What types of exercises should be initiated during the early phase of the patient's hospitalization?

   PMRRx ➤ Table of Contents ➤ scroll down to #10 Therapeutic Exercise ➤ Strength Training ➤ Isometric Exercise

Behavioral Health

1. The patient with traumatic injury as well as ARF may suffer from stress and anxiety related to the injuries and complications. What are the five Rs of stress and anxiety reduction?

   PsychThrp ➤ Main Index ➤ Stress ➤ Anxiety ➤ Five Rs

2. Relaxation techniques may be beneficial to this patient. What instruction would be helpful for this patient?

   PsychThrp ➤ Main Index ➤ Relaxation Techniques ➤ scroll down to Instructions

8

Rehabilitation Case Studies

Judith L. Draper

T
he case studies in this chapter focus on the care of clients with rehabilitation needs. As with the previous case studies, these clients are complex and have additional concerns and needs beyond the primary rehabilitation issues. The goal of health care providers working with clients with rehabilitation needs is to provide comprehensive care to enhance the quality of life for those affected by disability and chronic illness. It requires a multidisciplinary approach to achieve success.

➤ General Case Studies

For the following three case studies, you will need to download the trial versions of the following references:

- The 5-Minute Orthopaedic Consult (5MOrtho)
- Physician's Drug Handbook (PDH)
- Stedman's Medical Dictionary for the Health Professions and Nursing (HPND)
- Nurse's Quick Check: Diseases (NDisCheck)
- Lippincott's Nursing Drug Guide (LNDG)

CASE STUDY 1 • *John Simpson*

John Simpson is an athletic 18-year-old college student who plays on the school tennis team. He comes into the clinic complaining of severe left knee pain. He reports that he has had intermittent aching and swelling below his kneecap in the past, but he says it is much worse. John states that he is not able to walk up stairs using his left leg. Inspection finds that the knee is swollen. John states he does not recall injuring his knee while playing tennis yesterday. He says that his knee was a bit puffy today when he woke and became more swollen throughout the day. John is also complaining of severe seasonal allergies (itchy eyes, sneezing, and runny nose) and is requesting medication to relieve these symptoms.

1. What could be the cause of John's knee pain?
2. What are some of the signs and symptoms associated with knee pain?

The physician on call orders a magnetic resonance imaging (MRI) of the left knee. While John is having the MRI done, his mother arrives at the emergency room and tells you that he has a history of Osgood-Schlatter disease.

3. What is an MRI?
4. What is Osgood-Schlatter disease?
5. What are the causes of this disease?
6. Who is at risk for this disease?
7. What is the usual treatment for pain associated with Osgood-Schlatter disease?

The physician reviews the MRI results and gives the diagnosis of meniscal tear. He explains to John and his mother that this is an injury that can occur without a traumatic injury, but it is likely that the tear occurred over time due to repeated twisting movements characteristic of tennis. John is discharged with a leg brace, prescriptions for acetaminophen with codeine for pain and diphenhydramine hydrochloride, and a physical therapist (PT) referral.

8. What are the trade names of diphenhydramine hydrochloride?
9. For what is diphenhydramine hydrochloride prescribed?
10. What instructions should you give John regarding this medication?

CASE STUDY 2 • *Mr. Johnstone*

Mr. Johnstone is a 54-year-old gentleman who is brought to the emergency room via ambulance after falling down a flight of stairs in his home. He denies hitting his head or losing consciousness and complains of severe pain in his right arm. The right forearm is deformed, bruised, and swollen, and he cannot move his wrist. Mr. Johnstone is diabetic and has been on insulin for 10 years to control his diabetes (IDDM). He is legally blind due to diabetic retinopathy and has osteoarthritis.

1. What is the standard management of a forearm fracture?
2. What should Mr. Johnstone be taught about this kind of injury?

3. What is diabetic retinopathy?
4. What is diabetes?
5. The ID in IDDM stands for "insulin dependent." What does DM stand for?

The physician suspects a fracture of the forearm and orders an x-ray. The x-ray confirms multiple fractures of the ulna and radius. Mr. Johnstone is scheduled for surgery and is given fentanyl citrate 75 mg IM.

6. Why was fentanyl citrate administered?
7. What are the side effects of fentanyl citrate?
8. What are the special considerations associated with fentanyl citrate?

CASE STUDY 3 • *Mrs. Palu*

Mrs. Palu is a 47-year-old, married woman who is brought to the clinic by her husband. She is complaining of a severe and debilitating headache for the past several days. Past medical history includes a diagnosis of uncontrolled hypertension that has responded poorly to treatment. Mrs. Palu has osteoporosis, and the admitting physician writes the following on her chart: "osteoporosis with kyphosis." The physician on call gives a diagnosis of pheochromocytoma and orders verapamil hydrochloride 80 mg three times a day (t.i.d.). Mr. and Mrs. Palu have many questions about this new diagnosis.

1. What is pheochromocytoma?
2. What patient education is indicated for pheochromocytoma?
3. What is kyphosis?
4. Mrs. Palu asks, "What causes kyphosis?" What answer can you give her?
5. What are the risk factors associated with kyphosis?
6. The physician makes a referral for physical therapy. What kind of physical therapy exercises might be prescribed for Mrs. Palu?
7. For what is verapamil hydrochloride prescribed?
8. What are the side effects of verapamil hydrochloride?
9. What should you include in your ongoing assessment of Mrs. Palu?

The physician on duty also orders ibuprofen for Mrs. Palu's headache.

10. What is ibuprofen prescribed for in this instance?
11. What are the side effects of ibuprofen?
12. How will ibuprofen affect lab test results?

► Advanced Case Studies

For the following three case studies, you will need to download the full versions of the following references:

* Nursing Procedures (NurProc)
* Handbook of Diagnostic Tests (HbDxTests)

- Physical Medicine and Rehabilitation Pocketpedia (PMRRx)
- Stedman's Medical Dictionary for the Health Professions and Nursing (HPND)
- Nurse's Quick Check: Diseases (NDisCheck)
- Griffith's 5-Minute Clinical Consult (5MCC)
- Lippincott's Nursing Drug Guide (LNDG) *or* Physician's Drug Handbook (PDH)

CASE STUDY 1 • *Mrs. Sharp*

Mrs. Roberta Sharp is a 78-year-old, white, non-Hispanic woman. She lives with her spouse in a multistory home with 10 steps leading up to the outside door. She was diagnosed with osteoarthritis over 20 years ago and has experienced chronic pain with decreasing physical function over the past 10 years, primarily affecting the right hip.

Two years ago, Mrs. Sharp injured her right hip further in a motor vehicle accident. Medical treatment after the accident included Buck traction and physical therapy during the hospitalization. She returned home with a rolling walker to assist with ambulation and a prescription for celecoxib (Celebrex) 200 mg every day.

Within the past 6 months, she has received intra-articular corticosteroid injections with minimal improvement in physical function or pain relief. Three days ago, Mrs. Sharp underwent a total right hip replacement surgery for degenerative joint disease at the acute care hospital. Her postoperative course was uneventful, and she is transferred to the rehabilitation hospital today.

The physician's orders read:

Total hip precautions
Physical therapy daily
Out of bed with assistance only
Nonweight-bearing right lower extremity
Anticoagulation with Coumadin daily per prothrombin time/international normalized ratio (INR)

Cross-Discipline Learning Activities

You want to be sure that you understand the history and recent course of events for this patient, so you consult your PDA to answer the following questions:

1. What is Buck traction?
2. What is intra-articular?
3. What is a total hip arthroplasty?
4. What is osteoarthritis?
5. What are hip precautions?
6. What is anticoagulation?

Discipline-Specific Learning Activities

Nursing

1. What are the nursing considerations associated with warfarin (Coumadin)?
2. What is a prothrombin time? What is an INR?
3. Because of concerns for Mrs. Sharp's new hip, you will need to take certain precautions in her care. What are the nursing interventions for arthroplasty care following total hip replacement?
4. What is the potentially fatal complication to assess the patient for after arthroplasty surgery?

Medicine/PA/NP

The physician has ordered Coumadin daily per prothrombin time/INR.

1. What is prothrombin time? What is an INR?
2. What is the therapeutic INR level that should be achieved for this patient?
3. How much warfarin (Coumadin) should the patient be prescribed initially?
4. What is the potentially fatal complication to assess the patient for after arthroplasty surgery?

Physical and Occupational Therapy

1. What nonsurgical physical therapy interventions are used for osteoarthritis?
2. After arthroplasty surgery, what kinds of equipment might be used to aid in ambulation, transfers, and bed mobility?
3. After arthroplasty surgery, what kinds of interventions would the therapist be doing?

Behavioral Health

1. What are the potential psychosocial needs of this patient?
2. What kinds of interventions might this patient need after discharge to home?

Critical Thinking—Correlating Patient Data/Assessment Findings to Plan Care

What additional information specific to this case (physical assessment, diagnostic testing, and medications) would you need to know to further your assessment of the patient's needs and to guide your interventions? What is your plan of care for this patient (what should you do next)?

CASE STUDY 2 • *Mr. Diaz*

Mr. Thomas Diaz is a 39-year-old Hispanic man who is admitted to the acute care hospital following a fall off of his roof while repairing shingles. The fall results in an incomplete spinal cord injury at the C4 level of the spine. The patient is stabilized at the acute care hospital. He has an intracranial computed tomography (CT) scan and spinal x-rays to determine his injuries. He is monitored in the intensive care unit and assessed using the Glasgow Coma Scale frequently during the first few days in the hospital. He undergoes surgery to have a halo-vest traction attached to stabilize his cervical spine, and complications during the hospitalization include autonomic dysreflexia.

Mr. Diaz is a partner in a law firm and has three children ages 18, 14, and 7. His wife does not work outside the home. He lives in a multistory home with two steps to enter the first level and a powder room on the first floor.

The physician's orders read:

> Halo-vest traction care daily
> Antiembolism stockings
> Physical and occupational therapy daily
> Bowel and bladder program
> • Catheterize patient three times a day for urine
> • Dulcolax suppository one per rectum every other day
> Case management regarding discharge arrangements before going home

Cross-Discipline Learning Activities

You want to be sure that you understand the history and recent course of events for this patient, so you consult your PDA to answer the following questions:

1. What is a spinal injury?
2. What is an intracranial CT scan?
3. What are spinal x-rays (vertebral radiography)?
4. What is halo-vest traction?
5. What is the Glasgow Coma Scale?
6. What are the types of classifications used to describe spinal cord injuries?

Discipline-Specific Learning Activities

Nursing

1. What are the nursing considerations/key outcomes for a patient with a spinal cord injury?
2. List two topics about what the nurse would need to teach the patient with a spinal cord injury.
3. What is autonomic dysreflexia?
4. What are some precipitating factors for autonomic dysreflexia that the nurse can watch for during assessments?

5. Why are antiembolism stockings ordered for this patient?
6. Why is the use of antiembolism stockings important for this patient?

Medicine/PA/NP

1. What is autonomic dysreflexia?
2. What are some precipitating factors for autonomic dysreflexia to watch for during assessments?
3. Why are antiembolism stockings ordered for this patient?
4. Why is the use of antiembolism stockings important for this patient?
5. What are the three classifications of medications often ordered for a patient with spinal cord injury?

Physical and Occupational Therapy

1. Why are antiembolism stockings ordered for this patient?
2. Why is the use of antiembolism stockings important for this patient?
3. What are the goals of physical and occupational therapies to be reached before discharge?

Behavioral Health

1. Why is a psychosocial assessment important to conduct for this patient?
2. What guidelines need to be met by this patient before discharge to home?

Critical Thinking—Correlating Patient Data/Assessment Findings to Plan Care

What additional information specific to this case (physical assessment, diagnostic testing, and medications) would you need to know to further your assessment of the patient's needs and to guide your interventions? What is your plan of care for this patient (what should you do next)?

CASE STUDY 3 • *Ms. Tomlinson*

Ms. Rebecca Tomlinson is a 19-year-old African American woman who is admitted to the acute care hospital after a skiing accident that resulted in head trauma and a broken left lower extremity. She is airlifted from the mountainside to the closest regional trauma center for evaluation and care. The patient has a CT scan of the brain and skull, cervical spine, and femoral x-rays to determine the injuries. She is found to have an intracerebral hemorrhage, and a craniotomy is performed to evacuate the blood that is accumulating in her brain. Ms. Tomlinson requires close monitoring in the intensive care unit, including intracranial pressure monitoring and neurologic assessments. During her first night in the hospital, she develops seizures and requires anticonvulsant therapy. She also has a displaced fracture of the left femur that requires an external fixation device for repair. Initially, she is intubated with an endotracheal tube and has arterial blood gas (ABG) monitoring several times a day. As she begins to recover and regain consciousness, she is noted having cognitive changes, including disorientation and confusion at times, along with diminished abilities to follow directions, word finding difficulties, and a slowed speech pattern.

Ms. Tomlinson is a college student majoring in the sciences at a university in New England, where the accident occurred. She lives at school in a dormitory. Her parents, two sisters, and one brother live in a ranch-style house in California. Her mother has flown to the East Coast to be with her daughter and is staying at a local hotel. She will remain as long as she is needed to assist her daughter.

Ms. Tomlinson does not smoke or drink alcohol and enjoys bike riding, skiing, and tennis. She is being admitted to the rehabilitation hospital today.

The physician's orders read:

Local pin care daily to external fixation device on lower left extremity
Dilantin 150 mg p.o. b.i.d.
OOB with assistance only
Nonweight-bearing left lower extremity
Physical/occupational/speech therapy daily
Dilantin level in 1 week

Cross-Discipline Learning Activities

You want to be sure that you understand the history and recent course of events for this patient, so you consult your PDA to answer the following questions:

1. What does femoral mean?
2. What is an intracranial hemorrhage?
3. What is a craniotomy?
4. What is intracranial pressure monitoring?
5. What are seizures?
6. What is anticonvulsant therapy?
7. What is an external fixation device?
8. What is an endotracheal tube?
9. What does *intubated* mean?
10. What is an ABG?
11. What is the purpose of doing an ABG?

Discipline-Specific Learning Activities

Nursing

1. What is local pin care to external fixation device?
2. What equipment is needed for local pin care?
3. In what drug class is Dilantin?
4. What is important to teach a patient who is taking Dilantin?

5. What is the clinically effective serum (therapeutic) level for Dilantin?
6. What needs to be monitored for a patient with a seizure disorder?

Medicine/NP/PA

The patient is exhibiting signs of slowed brain patterns.

1. What is a neurologic vital sign assessment?
2. What is the adult dosage range for Dilantin?
3. What is the clinically effective serum (therapeutic) level for Dilantin?
4. What symptoms occur when Dilantin levels fall above or below the therapeutic range?
5. What are possible complications after a traumatic brain injury?
6. What general treatment measures are instituted after a traumatic brain injury?

Physical and Occupational Therapy

1. What patient monitoring of physical capabilities should be done in the posttraumatic brain injury patient?
2. What documentation of physical and occupational therapies should occur for a patient with an external fixation device on the lower extremity?
3. What prevention teaching should be done to avoid head trauma in the future?

Behavioral Health

1. What are the potential psychosocial needs of this patient?
2. What kinds of interventions might this patient need after discharge to home?

Critical Thinking—Correlating Patient Data/Assessment Findings to Plan Care

What additional information specific to this case (physical assessment, diagnostic testing, and medications) would you need to know to further your assessment of the patient's needs and to guide your interventions? What is your plan of care for this patient (what should you do next)?

Chapter Summary—Tying It All Together

You have explored several patient scenarios typical for the rehabilitation setting. In each case, the patient presented with an acute or chronic diagnosis requiring multiple diagnostic studies like CT scans and x-rays followed by some type of surgery requiring implantable metal devices (halo traction, external fixation device, and so on).

In the second and third advanced cases, there were medical complications (autonomic dysreflexia, seizure disorder) related to the initial diagnosis that required the attention and care of various health care providers. As with all rehabilitation patients, there needs to be a multidisciplinary approach (physicians, nurses, physical/occupational therapists, and case management) to the patient's care because of the many issues related to a successful course of treatment and return of the patient to the home environment. Remember, the primary goal is to enhance the quality of life for those affected by disability and chronic illness.

 WebLink. | Visit http://thePoint.LWW.com/cornelius for supplemental information and activities.

ANSWERS TO CASE STUDY QUESTIONS

➤ General Case Studies

CASE STUDY I • *John Simpson*

1. What could be the cause of John's knee pain?

   5MOrtho ➙ Knee Pain ➙ Basics (scroll down to Causes)

2. What are some of the signs and symptoms associated with knee pain?

   5MOrtho ➙ Knee Pain ➙ Diagnosis ➙ Signs and Symptoms

3. What is an MRI?

   HPND ➙ MRI ➙ Imaging ➙ scroll down to Magnetic Resonance Imaging

4. What is Osgood-Schlatter disease?

   NDisCheck ➙ Osgood-Schlatter Disease ➙ Overview

5. What are the causes of this disease?

   NDisCheck ➙ Osgood-Schlatter Disease ➙ Overview (scroll down to Causes)

6. Who is at risk for this disease?

   NDisCheck ➙ Osgood-Schlatter Disease ➙ Overview (scroll down to Risk Factors)

7. What is the usual treatment for pain associated with Osgood-Schlatter disease?

   NDisCheck ➤ Osgood-Schlatter Disease ➤ Treatment ➤ General

8. What are the trade names of diphenhydramine hydrochloride?

   PDH ➤ Diphenhydramine Hydrochloride ➤ Trade Names

9. For what is diphenhydramine hydrochloride prescribed?

   PDH ➤ Diphenhydramine Hydrochloride ➤ Indications and Dosages

10. What instructions should you give John regarding this medication?

    PDH ➤ Diphenhydramine Hydrochloride ➤ Patient Education

CASE STUDY 2 • *Mr. Johnstone*

1. What is the standard management of a forearm fracture?

   5MOrtho ➤ Forearm Fractures ➤ Management ➤ General

2. What should Mr. Johnstone be taught about this kind of injury?

   5MOrtho ➤ Forearm Fractures ➤ Management ➤ General (scroll down to Patient Education)

3. What is diabetic retinopathy?

   HPND ➤ Retinopathy ➤ scroll down to Diabetic Retinopathy

4. What is diabetes?

   HPND ➤ Diabetes

5. The ID in IDDM stands for "insulin dependent." What does DM stand for?

   HPND ➤ Diabetes ➤ scroll down to Insulin Dependent

6. Why was fentanyl citrate administered?

   PDH ➤ Fentanyl Citrate ➤ Indications and Dosages

7. What are the side effects of fentanyl citrate?

   PDH ➤ Fentanyl Citrate ➤ Adverse Reactions

8. What are the special considerations associated with fentanyl citrate?

   PDH ➤ Fentanyl Citrate ➤ Special Considerations

CASE STUDY 3 • *Mrs. Palu*

1. What is pheochromocytoma?

   NDisCheck ➤ Pheochromocytoma ➤ Overview

2. What patient education is indicated for pheochromocytoma?

   NDisCheck ➤ Pheochromocytoma ➤ Nursing Considerations (scroll down to Teaching Points)

3. What is kyphosis?

   5MOrtho ➤ Kyphosis ➤ Basics

4. Mrs. Palu asks, "What causes kyphosis?" What answer can you give her?

   5MOrtho ➤ Kyphosis ➤ Basics ➤ scroll down to Causes

5. What are the risk factors associated with kyphosis?

   5MOrtho ➤ Kyphosis ➤ Basics ➤ scroll down to Risk Factors

6. The physician makes a referral for physical therapy. What kind of physical therapy exercises might be prescribed for Mrs. Palu?

   5MOrtho ➤ Kyphosis ➤ Management ➤ scroll down to Physical Therapy

7. For what is verapamil hydrochloride prescribed?

   LNDG ➤ Verapamil ➤ Verapamil [Appendix S] ➤ Verapamil ➤ Indications

8. What are the side effects of verapamil hydrochloride?

   LNDG ➤ Verapamil ➤ Verapamil [Appendix S] ➤ Verapamil ➤ Adverse Effects

9. What should you include in your ongoing assessment of Mrs. Palu?

   LNDG ➤ Verapamil ➤ Verapamil [Appendix S] ➤ Verapamil ➤ Indications ➤ Nursing Considerations (scroll down to Interventions)

10. What is ibuprofen prescribed for in this instance?

    LNDG ➤ Ibuprofen ➤ Indications and Dosages (second bullet)

11. What are the side effects of ibuprofen?

    LNDG ➤ Ibuprofen ➤ Adverse Reactions

12. How will ibuprofen affect lab test results?

    LNDG ➤ Ibuprofen ➤ Effects on Lab Test Results

➤ Advanced Case Studies

CASE STUDY 1 • *Mrs. Sharp*

Cross-Discipline Learning Activities

1. What is Buck traction?

   HPND ➤ Traction ➤ scroll down to Buck Traction

2. What is intra-articular?

   HPND → Intra-articular

3. What is a total hip arthroplasty?

   PMRRx → Hip Arthroplasty

4. What is osteoarthritis?

   NDisCheck → Osteoarthritis → Overview

5. What are hip precautions?

   PMRRx → Hip Precautions

6. What is anticoagulation?

   HPND → Anticoagulant Therapy → scroll down to Anticoagulant Therapy

Discipline-Specific Learning Activities

Nursing

1. What are the nursing considerations associated with warfarin (Coumadin)?

   LNDG → Coumadin → Nursing Considerations

2. What is prothrombin time? What is an INR?

   HbDxTests → Prothrombin Time → International Normalized Ratio

3. Because of concerns for Mrs. Sharp's new hip, you will need to take certain precautions in her care. What are the nursing interventions for arthroplasty care following total hip arthroplasty?

   NurProc → Arthroplasty Care → Implementation → After Hip Arthroplasty

4. What is the potentially fatal complication to assess the patient for after arthroplasty surgery?

   NurProc → Arthroplasty Care → Complications → scroll down to Fat Embolism

Medicine/PA/NP

1. What is prothrombin time? What is an INR?

   HbDxTests → Prothrombin Time → International Normalized Ratio

2. What is the therapeutic INR level that should be achieved for this patient?

   LNDG → Coumadin → Dosages
   (This information is not found in PDH.)

3. How much warfarin (Coumadin) should the patient be prescribed initially?

LNDG → Coumadin → Dosages
PDH → Coumadin → Indications and Dosages

4. What is the potentially fatal complication to assess the patient for after arthroplasty surgery?

NurProc → Arthroplasty Care → Complications → scroll down to Fat Embolism

Physical and Occupational Therapy

1. What nonsurgical physical therapy interventions are used for osteoarthritis?

NDisCheck → Osteoarthritis → Treatment

2. After arthroplasty surgery, what kinds of equipment might be used to aid in ambulation, transfers, and bed mobility?

NurProc → Arthroplasty Care → Equipment and Preparation of Equipment

3. After arthroplasty surgery, what kinds of interventions would the therapist be doing?

NurProc → Arthroplasty Care → Implementation → scroll down to bullets 14 and on

Behavioral Health

1. What are the potential psychosocial needs of this patient?

NDisCheck → Osteoarthritis → Nursing Considerations

2. What kinds of interventions might this patient need after discharge to home?

NDisCheck → Osteoarthritis → Patient Teaching

CASE STUDY 2 • *Mr. Diaz*

Cross-Discipline Learning Activities

1. What is a spinal injury?

NDisCheck → Spinal Injury → Overview

2. What is an intracranial CT scan?

HbDxTests → Intracranial CT → Introduction

3. What are spinal x-rays (vertebral radiography)?

HbDxTests → Vertebral Radiography → Introduction

4. What is halo-vest traction?

NurProc → Halo-vest Traction → Introduction

5. What is the Glasgow Coma Scale?

   HPND ➤ Glasgow Coma Scale ➤ Coma Scale

6. What are the types of classifications used to describe spinal cord injuries?

   PMRRx ➤ Spinal Cord Injury ➤ Classification of SCI ➤ scroll down to #4 and 5

Discipline-Specific Learning Activities

Nursing

1. What are the nursing considerations/key outcomes for a patient with a spinal cord injury?

   NDisCheck ➤ Spinal Cord Injury ➤ Nursing Considerations ➤ Key Outcomes

2. List two topics that the nurse would need to teach the patient with a spinal cord injury.

   NDisCheck ➤ Spinal Cord Injury ➤ Patient Teaching

3. What is autonomic dysreflexia?

   PMRRx ➤ Autonomic Dysreflexia ➤ Info ➤ scroll down to second bullet

4. What are some precipitating factors for autonomic dysreflexia that the nurse can watch for during assessments?

   PMRRx ➤ Autonomic Dysreflexia ➤ Management of Acute Autonomic Dysreflexia (AD) ➤ scroll down through #4

5. Why are antiembolism stockings ordered for this patient?

   NurProc ➤ Antiembolism Stockings ➤ Introduction

6. Why is the use of antiembolism stockings important for this patient?

   NurProc ➤ Antiembolism Stockings ➤ Introduction

Medicine/PA/NP

1. What is autonomic dysreflexia?

   PMRRx ➤ Autonomic Dysreflexia ➤ Info ➤ scroll down to second bullet

2. What are some precipitating factors for autonomic dysreflexia to watch for during assessments?

   PMRRx ➤ Autonomic Dysreflexia ➤ Management of Acute Autonomic Dysreflexia (AD) ➤ scroll down through #4

3. Why are antiembolism stockings ordered for this patient?

   NurProc ➤ Antiembolism Stockings ➤ Introduction

4. Why is the use of antiembolism stockings important for this patient?

NurProc → Antiembolism Stockings → Introduction

5. What are the three classifications of medications often ordered for a patient with spinal cord injury?

NDisCheck → Spinal Injury → Treatment → scroll down to Medication

Physical and Occupational Therapy

1. Why are antiembolism stockings ordered for this patient?

NurProc → Antiembolism Stockings → Introduction

2. Why is the use of antiembolism stockings important for this patient?

NurProc → Antiembolism Stockings → Introduction

3. What are the expected functional levels after discharge based on the injury level of the spinal cord?

PMRRx → Spinal Cord Injury → Expected Functional Levels

Behavioral Health

1. Why is a psychosocial assessment important to conduct for this patient?

NDisCheck → Spinal Injury → Nursing Considerations → Key Outcomes

2. What guidelines need to be met by this patient before discharge to home?

NDisCheck → Spinal Injury → Patient Teaching

CASE STUDY 3 • *Ms. Tomlinson*

Cross-Discipline Learning Activities

1. What does femoral mean?

HPND → Femoral

2. What is an intracranial hemorrhage?

HPND → Intracranial Hemorrhage → scroll down to Intracranial Hemorrhage

3. What is a craniotomy?

HPND → Craniotomy

4. What is intracranial pressure monitoring?

NurProc → Intracranial Pressure Monitoring → Introduction

5. What are seizures?

NDisCheck → Seizure Disorder → Epilepsy → Overview

6. What is anticonvulsant therapy?

   HPND ➤ Anticonvulsant

7. What is an external fixation device?

   NurProc ➤ External Fixation ➤ Introduction

8. What is an endotracheal tube?

   HPND ➤ Endotracheal tube ➤ scroll down to Endotracheal Tube

9. What does *intubated* mean?

   HPND ➤ Intubate

10. What is an ABG?

    HbDxTests ➤ Arterial Blood Gas Analysis ➤ Introduction

11. What is the purpose of doing an ABG?

    HbDxTests ➤ Arterial Blood Gas Analysis ➤ Purpose

Discipline-Specific Learning Activities

Nursing

1. What is local pin care to external fixation device?

   NurProc ➤ External Fixation ➤ Implementation

2. What equipment is needed for local pin care?

   NurProc ➤ External Fixation ➤ Implementation

3. In what drug class is Dilantin?

   LNDG ➤ Dilantin ➤ Phenytoin ➤ General ➤ scroll down to Drug Class
   PDH ➤ Dilantin ➤ Phenytoin ➤ Classification

4. What is important to teach a patient who is taking Dilantin?

   LNDG ➤ Dilantin ➤ Phenytoin ➤ Nursing Considerations ➤ scroll down to Teaching Points
   PDH ➤ Dilantin ➤ Phenytoin ➤ Patient Education

5. What is the clinically effective serum (therapeutic) level for Dilantin?

   LNDG ➤ Dilantin ➤ Phenytoin ➤ Dosages ➤ scroll down to Individualize Dosage

6. What needs to be monitored for a patient with a seizure disorder?

   NDisCheck ➤ Seizure Disorder ➤ Epilepsy ➤ Nursing Considerations ➤ Monitoring

Medicine/NP/PA

1. What is a neurologic vital sign assessment?

   NurProc ➙ Neurologic Vital Sign Assessment ➙ Introduction

2. What is the adult dosage range for Dilantin?

   LNDG ➙ Dilantin ➙ Phenytoin ➙ Dosages
   PDH ➙ Dilantin ➙ Phenytoin ➙ Indications and Dosages

3. What is the clinically effective serum (therapeutic) level for Dilantin?

   LNDG ➙ Dilantin ➙ Phenytoin ➙ Dosages

4. What symptoms occur when Dilantin levels fall above or below the therapeutic range?

   LNDG ➙ Dilantin ➙ Phenytoin ➙ Adverse Effects
   PDH ➙ Dilantin ➙ Phenytoin ➙ Adverse Effects

5. What are possible complications after a traumatic brain injury?

   5MCC ➙ Brain Injury, Traumatic ➙ Follow-Up ➙ scroll down to Possible Complications

6. What general treatment measures are instituted after a traumatic brain injury?

   5MCC ➙ Brain Injury, Traumatic ➙ Treatment ➙ scroll down to General Measures

Physical and Occupational Therapy

1. What patient monitoring of physical capabilities should be done in the posttraumatic brain injury patient?

   5MCC ➙ Brain Injury—Post Acute Care Issues ➙ Follow-Up ➙ Patient Monitoring

2. What documentation of physical and occupational therapies should occur for a patient with an external fixation device on the lower extremity?

   NurProc ➙ External Fixation ➙ Documentation

3. What prevention teaching should be done to avoid head trauma in the future?

   5MCC ➙ Brain Injury, Traumatic ➙ Follow-Up ➙ scroll down to Prevention/Avoidance

Behavioral Health

1. What are the potential psychosocial needs of this patient?

   5MCC ➤ Brain Injury, Traumatic ➤ Follow-Up ➤ scroll down to Patient
   Monitoring and Expected Course/Prognosis

2. What kinds of interventions might this patient need after discharge to
   home?

   5MCC ➤ Brain Injury, Traumatic ➤ Follow-Up ➤ scroll down to Patient
   Monitoring and Expected Course/Prognosis

9

Pediatric
Case Studies

Mary Gallagher Gordon

Pediatric nursing is a profession that cares for children and is intimately involved with children and their families at all levels of growth and development. The major goal of pediatric nursing care is to enable the family and child to actively participate in their care, with the intent that both family and child can return to their community. Ready access to accurate information on a PDA, literally at one's fingertips, is empowering for the pediatric nurse and has clear benefits for pediatric patients and their families.

➤ General Case Studies

For the next three case studies, you will need to download and install the trial versions of the following references:

- Griffith's 5-Minute Clinical Consult (5MCC)
- Taylor's Clinical Nursing Skills (ClinSkills)
- Nurses' Handbook of Health Assessment (HlthAssess)
- Lippincott Manual of Nursing Practice: Procedures (LMNPPr)
- Lippincott's Nursing Drug Guide (LNDG)
- Nelson's Pocket Book of Pediatric Antimicrobial Therapy (Nelson ABX)
- Nurse's Quick Check: Diseases (NDisCheck)
- Handbook of Signs and Symptoms (SignsSx)

- Stedman's Medical Dictionary for the Health Professions and Nursing (HPND)
- The Washington Manual Pediatrics Survival Guide (WUSPeds)

Each case study presented describes a situation that you may encounter in a pediatric setting. Use the trial versions of the software you have downloaded to find answers to the questions presented in each case study.

CASE STUDY 1 • *James*

James is an 11-year-old boy who presents to the pediatric office complaining of abdominal pain. He has had nausea, vomiting, fever, and pain for 2 days. He has become irritable and has a decreased energy level, according to his mother, rebound tenderness, and abdominal rigidity, noted on physical exam. He is sent to the emergency room (ER) with a diagnosis of appendicitis.

1. What is McBurney's sign?
2. Where is McBurney's incision?
3. When does perforation commonly occur?
4. When does anorexia usually occur with appendicitis?
5. The practitioner is giving a medication via ampule. What are some unexpected situations that he or she may encounter?
6. Before starting an IV, the practitioner places EMLA cream over the potential insertion site. What is the total maximum dose that may be given?
7. James may be started on ampicillin before surgery. What are the IV facts to recall when giving this medication?

CASE STUDY 2 • *Ms. Behr and Evan*

Ms. Behr gave birth to her first child, a son Evan, yesterday. He is a product of a normal vaginal delivery with a birth weight of 8 pounds 4 ounces.

1. Ms. Behr is concerned with the pearly white papules in Evan's mouth. What is this form of milia called?
2. Ms. Behr is also questioning the acne on the baby's face. What would you tell her about the acne?
3. Baby Evan needs some oxygen by mask. What equipment would you need on hand?
4. Ms. Behr breaks out in her first episode of genital herpes within 24 hours of birthing Evan. If Evan needed to receive acyclovir, what would the route and dosing be for him?
5. You are teaching Evan's mother about administration of acetaminophen. What is the dose for a newborn?
6. Evan is noted to have a murmur. What is the definition of a murmur?
7. While in the hospital recovering from the birth of Evan, Ms. Behr's 18-month-old child is diagnosed with laryngotracheobronchitis. What are the common characteristics of laryngotracheobronchitis or croup?
8. What parent teaching should be given to Ms. Behr regarding caring for her child with laryngotracheobronchitis or croup?

CASE STUDY 3 • *Patti*

Patti, age 12, has come to the ER complaining of severe abdominal pain, fever, nausea, and vomiting. She ate her last meal 4 hours ago. She is diagnosed with *Staphylococcus aureus* bacterial food poisoning.

1. What laboratory diagnosis tools are used to assist with this diagnosis?
2. What are the medications used with this diagnosis?
3. What is the follow-up with Patti's care?
4. Patti had a bout of emesis and now needs mouth care. What would you assess during this procedure?
5. What are the 10 most common floor calls for fever in a pediatric facility?
6. When performing a pediatric abdominal assessment, what focus questions should you ask Patti?
7. What is the definition of *food fever*?

➤ Advanced Case Studies

You will have the opportunity to further research pediatric cases using the references described. For the next three case studies, you will need to download the full versions of the following references:

- Griffith's 5-Minute Clinical Consult (5MCC)
- The 5-Minute Pediatric Consult (5MPed)
- Handbook of Diagnostic Tests (HbDxTests)
- Lippincott's Nursing Drug Guide (LNDG) *or* Physician's Drug Handbook (PDH)
- Manual of Psychiatric Therapeutics (PsychThrp)
- Nursing Procedures (NurProc)
- Nurse's Quick Check: Diseases (NDisCheck) *or* 5MCC
- Physical Medicine and Rehabilitation Pocketpedia (PMRRx)
- Stedman's Medical Dictionary for the Health Professions and Nursing (HPND)

CASE STUDY 1 • *Suzie*

Suzie is a 6-year-old girl who has been admitted to the pediatric unit following a 2-day stay in the Pediatric Intensive Care Unit (PICU) for a life-threatening asthma attack. She has a history of reactive airway disease and presents to the emergency department with an increase in cough, wheezing, shortness of breath, chest tightness, restlessness, and apprehension. This is her second PICU admission and is ventilated for 1 day and weaned to mask and oxygen within 24 hours of admission. Her pulse oximeter ranges from 89–96%.

Past medical history: Suzie lives in a public housing complex built in the 1950s with her mother, two younger siblings, and an aunt, as well as two small cousins. She is up-to-date on her immunizations. Her present weight is 48 pounds; she has environmental allergies to dust, smoke and a positive skin test for cockroaches; and she has a history of eczema. Her medications at home are albuterol MDI with spacer for wheezing and Advair 100/50 one inhale bid.

Her mom states that Suzie has had a chronic nighttime cough, which worsens as she lies down to sleep at night. Her mom also states that she ran out of Suzie's medications 4 days ago. Neither her mom nor she has done a peak expiratory flow rate to see Suzie's baseline.

On admission to the pediatric floor, Suzie was on O_2 at 1 L via mask with a continuous albuterol nebulizer; she is also on methylprednisolone IV for severe exacerbation and Intal bid in nebulizer for maintenance. Suzie is on a cardiac monitor as well as a continuous pulse oximeter, which has been ranging from 93–97%. Her vital signs are monitored every hour while on the continuous nebulizer. Her heart rate has ranged from 70–100 and with an increase in respiratory rate; her cardiac monitor strips (EKG) show no abnormal rhythm, and no murmur has been noted. Her color is pale pink, mucous membranes are moist, and she has allergic shiners under each eye; her eyes do not appear watery and she has no complaints of itching. Capillary filling time is 2 seconds, chest shape is normal, and she has no nasal flaring. She does have slight sternal, intercostal, and supraclavicular retractions. On auscultation breath sounds are present in all lobes on auscultation, and they are decreased in bilateral bases, with wheezing throughout. Expiration is greater than inspiration on auscultation with an involuntary cough at the end.

Suzie is on a clear diet at present. Her labs and diagnostic tests include CBC, pulmonary function test (PFT), CXR, serum electrolytes, and blood gas. She appears more comfortable in a high Fowler's position. Her skin shows some evidence of eczema on arms and thighs. Her mom is not able to be at the bedside due to her work schedule and younger children at home. According to her mom, Suzie is a pleasant and easy child and able to play alone as easily as she can with others. She is to begin kindergarten in the fall.

Cross-Discipline Learning Activities

1. What are the three components that characterize asthma?
2. What is skin testing?
3. What are common questions that parents may ask when they have a child who has asthma?
4. Why is her heart rate elevated when on prednisone (prednisolone)?

Discipline-Specific Learning Activities

Nursing

1. When discussing patient teaching with Suzie and her family, what should you be sure to cover?
2. When hanging a bag of IV fluid ordered, what steps should be implemented for the pediatric client?
3. Suzie is scheduled for PFTs before discharge to home. What patient prep would you give her?
4. What are the special considerations when giving medication to a child?
5. What is the rationale for cardiac monitoring?
6. What would be a life-threatening reaction to prednisone?

Medicine/NP/PA

1. When looking at the interview of a child diagnosed with reactive airway, the practitioner should address the environmental history. What is included in this history?
2. What is the drug class for methylprednisolone?
3. What is the proper oral dosage for this child?
4. When drawing up the correct dose of albuterol for the inhalation, the practitioner should know the drug to drug interactions. What are they?

Critical Thinking—Correlating Patient Data/Assessment Findings to Plan Care

Suzie should recover and return to home and school and her daily activities. She will need to be scheduled for a PFT before discharge. What information should be provided regarding this test?

Having both the proper care and the right education may help reduce the chance that Suzie may need to be readmitted to the unit. What education will her mom need to properly care for her daughter? What education will Suzie need? What additional needs can you identify?

CASE STUDY 2 • *Ashley*

Ashley is a 9-year-old girl who has sickle cell anemia and is admitted to the medical unit of the local children's hospital with vaso-occlusive crisis pain in her back and right leg; this is her second hospital admission this year.

Ashley lives with her mother and two siblings and is in third grade at the local public elementary school. She is the only child with sickle cell disease. She is active in various school activities and is keeping up with her classes. Now that it is early spring, Ashley has been playing a lot more out of doors, and her mom states that Ashley may be dehydrated with the warm weather.

The practitioner orders the following based on Ashley's weight of 70 pounds:

IV fluids for hydration
Intake and output
Warm compresses to back and right leg, as needed
Morphine sulfate for pain
Folic acid
Activity as tolerated

Cross-Discipline Learning Activities

1. When obtaining blood for a sickle cell test, what may be some interfering factors?
2. When documenting the child's pain and management of the pain, what should be included?
3. What are general measures for well-patient care that need to be addressed with this client?
4. What findings may be found with the physical exam of this child?

Discipline-Specific Learning Activities

Nursing

1. When education should be included in the patient teaching with Ashley, what may the practitioner include in his or her plan of care?
2. What is the most common crisis symptom (and is considered the hallmark of the disease)?
3. When giving morphine sulfate via IV infusion, the child should have a cardiac pulmonary monitor on. What is the rationale for this?
4. When assessing a child's response to pain, what should the practitioner keep in mind?
5. When preparing to place an IV in the child, what equipment should the practitioner have in place?

Medicine/NP/PA

1. What is the purpose of osmotic fragility?
2. The pediatric dosing of morphine sulfate would be how many mg/kg/dose?
3. Diphenhydramine may be administered intravenously. What should the practitioner know about the IV administration?
4. When administering morphine sulfate to the child, what should the practitioner also have on hand at the bedside?
5. What is the life expectancy of a child with sickle cell disease?
6. What are some tests that would aid in a definitive diagnosis of sickle cell disease?
7. How often should a child with sickle cell disease be seen by a pediatric hematologist?
8. List five drugs of choice for a client with sickle cell disease.
9. List the first two possible complications of sickle cell disease.

Physical and Occupational Therapy

Explain the pathophysiology of pain.

Behavioral Health

What may be some barriers to pain assessment and adequate pain management?

Critical Thinking—Correlating Patient Data/Assessment Findings to Plan Care

Ashley is a 9-year-old child who is still learning about how her body responds to her disease process. Clearly, the major goals in the plan of care are to keep her out of the hospital and to help her lead as normal a life as possible. One way to meet these goals is to review with Ashley and her family the signs and symptoms of Ashley's past crisis. Doing so will heighten their awareness of early warning signs, thus enabling them to intervene earlier, possibly avoiding hospitalization or, if necessary, getting Ashley to the hospital *before* she is in severe crisis. Specifically, what are the early warning signs? In addition, what other instructions should the family receive?

CASE STUDY 3 • *Tommy*

Tommy is a 6-year-old boy who was playing with matches and ignited the bed linens. He sustains burns on his chest, right arm, and the front of both legs. He is admitted to the children's burn unit and is now 3 days post admission. Tommy is in bed with the head of the bed elevated, on a cardiac monitor, receiving oxygen via mask, and on a patient-controlled analgesic pump for pain management. He may need skin grafting at a later date.

The orders read:

> Maintain patent airway, oxygen administration
> Bed rest
> Fluid replacement
> Monitor for signs of infection
> Wounds are covered with silver sulfadiazine occlusive dressings
> Provide diet high in calories and protein
> Monitor for signs of Curling's ulcer
> Referral to Social Services
> Referral to Child Life

Cross-Discipline Learning Activities

1. What is Curling's ulcer?
2. What causes the majority of burns?
3. What characteristics are associated with first-, second-, and third-degree burns?
4. Why is the BUN level increased in a client with burns?
5. Why is thorough assessment and documentation of the child's wound appearance so essential?
6. What is the drug classification of sulfadiazine?

Discipline-Specific Learning Activities

Nursing

1. Estimating burn surfaces in adults are done with the rule of nines. The rule of nines is not accurate with infants and children, so what chart may be used for this population?
2. When administering morphine sulfate intravenously, what nursing considerations should the nurse know?
3. What steps should the practitioner take to prevent cross-contamination during wound care?
4. What are key outcomes the nurse should try to attain when caring for the client with burns?

5. What age-related factors are important to remember when dealing with a client with burns?
6. Skin graft failure may result from what?
7. When documenting in the client's chart following skin grafting care, what are important criteria to include?
8. What are "common" side effects of morphine sulfate?

Medicine/NP/PA

Skin is the largest organ of the body protecting us from bacteria and fluid loss. Management of acute burns includes prevention of infection and dehydration. Urinary output is one method by which to monitor adequate hydration in a child suffering with severe burns.

1. What is the acceptable output for a child weighing less than 30 kg?
2. Why should the child be considered for an H_2 blocker medication?
3. The kidneys may be damaged as a result of prolonged tissue destruction. What abnormal findings in the blood and urine may signal kidney failure?
4. What is rhabdomyolysis?
5. What are the therapeutic actions of morphine sulfate?

Critical Thinking—Correlating Patient Data/Assessment Findings to Plan Care

Burns are considered one of the most catastrophic traumas experienced by humans. As with any major trauma, the first considerations are *airway, breathing, and circulation* (ABC). Over the long term, what are the treatment goals for this child? What normal growth and development issues must you consider? What education will this child need? What about the family?

Chapter Summary—Tying It All Together

Pediatric nursing is a complex specialty. A pediatric client can be someone who is less than 5 pounds to a client who may be an adult but is still being cared for in the pediatric facility. Staying attuned to the subtle changes in this client population is critical in the day-to-day care. Therefore, caring for the pediatric client and the extended family makes it vital for the nurse to have the most recent information. As you have learned through the case studies in this chapter, the PDA can be an essential resource for finding this necessary information.

 Visit http://thePoint.LWW.com/cornelius for supplemental information and activities.

ANSWERS TO CASE STUDY QUESTIONS

➤ General Case Studies

CASE STUDY 1 • *James*

1. What is McBurney's sign?

   WUSPeds ➙ Abdominal Pain ➙ Appendicitis

2. Where is McBurney's incision?

   HPND ➙ McBurney's Incision

3. When does perforation commonly occur?

   WUSPeds ➙ Abdominal Pain ➙ Appendicitis

4. When does anorexia usually occur with appendicitis?

   SignsSx ➙ Appendicitis

5. The practitioner is giving a medication via ampule. What are some unexpected situations that he or she may encounter?

   ClinSkills ➙ Ampule:Removing Medications ➙ Unexpected Situations

6. Before starting an IV, the practitioner places EMLA cream over the potential insertion site. What is the total maximum dose that may be given?

   WUSPeds ➙ EMLA ➙ Information

7. James may be started on ampicillin before surgery. What are the IV facts to recall when giving this medication?

   LNDG ➙ Ampicillin ➙ IV Facts

CASE STUDY 2 • *Ms. Behr and Evan*

1. Ms. Behr is concerned with the pearly white papules in Evan's mouth. What is this form of milia called?

   WUSPeds ➙ Neonatal Rashes—Dermatology ➙ Milia

2. Ms. Behr is also questioning the acne on the baby's face. What would you tell her about the acne?

   WUSPeds ➙ Neonatal Rashes—Dermatology ➙ Acne Neonatorum

3. Baby Evan needs some oxygen by mask. What equipment would you need on hand?

   LMNPPr ➔ Administering Oxygen by Simple Face Mask with/without Aerosol ➔ Information

4. Ms. Behr breaks out in her first episode of genital herpes within 24 hours of birthing Evan. If Evan needed to receive acyclovir, what would the route and dosing be for him?

   Nelson ABX ➔ Newborns, Therapy for ➔ Acyclovir

5. You are teaching Evan's mother about administration of acetaminophen. What is the dose for a newborn?

   WUSPeds ➔ Neonatal Drug Recommendations—Formulary ➔ Acetaminophen

6. Evan is noted to have a murmur. What is the definition of a murmur?

   HPND ➔ Murmur

7. While in the hospital recovering from the birth of Evan, Ms. Behr's 18-month-old child is diagnosed with laryngotracheobronchitis. What are the common characteristics of laryngotracheobronchitis or croup?

   NDisCheck ➔ Laryngotracheobronchitis ➔ Overview ➔ Common Characteristics

8. What parent teaching should be given to Ms. Behr regarding caring for her child with laryngotracheobronchitis or croup?

   NDisCheck ➔ Laryngotracheobronchitis ➔ Patient Teaching

CASE STUDY 3 • *Patti*

1. What laboratory diagnosis tools are used to assist with this diagnosis?

   5MCC ➔ Food Poisoning, Bacterial ➔ Diagnosis ➔ Laboratory

2. What are the medications used with this diagnosis?

   5MCC ➔ Food Poisoning, Bacterial ➔ Medications

3. What is the follow-up with Patti's care?

   5MCC ➔ Food Poisoning, Bacterial ➔ Patient Monitoring

4. Patti had a bout of emesis and now needs mouth care. What would you assess during this procedure?

   ClinSkills ➔ Oral Care

5. What are the 10 most common floor calls for fever in a pediatric facility?

   WUSPeds ➔ Fever—Ten Most Common Floor Calls

6. When performing a pediatric abdominal assessment, what focus questions should you ask Patti?

   HlthAssess → Abdominal Assessment → Pediatric Variations Abdominal Assessment → Information

7. What is the definition of *food fever*?

   HPND → Food Fever

➤ Advanced Case Studies

CASE STUDY I • *Suzie*

Cross-Discipline Learning Activities

1. What are the three components that characterize asthma?

   5MCC → Asthma → Database
   NDisCheck → Asthma → Basics

2. What is skin testing?

   HbdxTests → Allergy

3. What are common questions that parents may ask when they have a child who has asthma?

   5MPed → Asthma → Common Questions and Answers
   NDisCheck → Asthma → Patient Teaching
   5MCC → Asthma → Overview and Follow-Up

4. Why is her heart rate elevated when on prednisone (prednisolone)?

   LNDG → Prednisolone → Adverse Effects
   PDH → Prednisolone → Adverse Reactions

Discipline-Specific Learning Activities

Nursing

1. When discussing patient teaching with Suzie and her family, what should you be sure to cover?

   NDisCheck → Asthma → Patient Teaching
   5MCC → Asthma → Follow-Up

2. When hanging a bag of IV fluid ordered, what steps should be implemented for the pediatric client?

   NurProc → Table of Contents → Pediatrics → IV Therapy, Pediatrics → Implementation

3. Suzie is scheduled for PFTs before discharge to home. What patient prep would you give her?

HbdxTests ➝ Pulmonary Capacity Tests ➝ PFT ➝ Patient Preparation

4. What are the special considerations when giving medication to a child?

NurProc ➝ Table of Contents ➝ Pediatrics ➝ Drug Admission, Pediatrics ➝ Special Consideration

5. What is the rationale for cardiac monitoring?

NurProc ➝ Cardiac Monitoring ➝ Introduction

6. What would be a life-threatening reaction to prednisone?

LNDG ➝ Prednisone ➝ Adverse Effects ➝ Shock
PDH ➝ Prednisolone ➝ Adverse Reactions ➝ All Items in Red

Medicine/NP/PA

1. When looking at the interview of a child diagnosed with reactive airway, the practitioner should address the environmental history. What is included in this history?

5MPed ➝ Asthma ➝ Data Gathering
5MCC ➝ Asthma ➝ Follow-Up

2. What is the drug class for methylprednisolone?

LNDG ➝ Methylprednisolone ➝ General ➝ scroll down to Drug Classes
PDH ➝ Methylprednisolone ➝ Classification

3. What is the proper oral dosage for this child?

5MPed ➝ Asthma ➝ Therapy
PDH ➝ Methylprednisolone (Prednisolone) ➝ Indications and Dosages ➝ First Bullet
LNDG ➝ Methylprednisolone ➝ Dosages ➝ scroll down to Pediatric Patients

4. When drawing up the correct dose of albuterol for the inhalation, the practitioner should know the drug to drug interactions. What are they?

LNDG ➝ Albuterol Sulfate ➝ Interventions ➝ Drug-Drug
PDH ➝ Albuterol Sulfate ➝ Adverse Reactions

CASE STUDY 2 • *Ashley*

Cross-Discipline Learning Activities

1. When obtaining blood for a sickle cell test, what may be some interfering factors?

HbDxTests ➝ Table of Contents ➝ Hgb ➝ Sickle Cells ➝ Interfering Factors

2. When documenting the child's pain and management of the pain, what should be included?

   NurProc ➤ Pain Management ➤ Document

3. What are general measures for well-patient care that need to be addressed with this client?

   5MPed ➤ Sickle Cell Disease ➤ Therapy
   5MCC ➤ Sickle Cell Anemia ➤ Treatment
   NDisCheck ➤ Sickle Cell Anemia ➤ Patient Teaching

4. What findings may be found with the physical exam of this child?

   5MPed ➤ Sickle Cell Disease ➤ Physical Examination
   NDisCheck ➤ Sickle Cell Anemia ➤ Assessment
   5MCC ➤ Sickle Cell Anemia ➤ Basics ➤ scroll down to Signs and Symptoms

Discipline-Specific Learning Activities

Nursing

1. When education should be included in the patient teaching with Ashley, what may the practitioner include in his or her plan of care?

   NDisCheck ➤ Sickle Cell Disease ➤ Patient Teaching
   5MCC ➤ Sickle Cell Anemia ➤ Follow-Up
   5MPed ➤ Sickle Cell Anemia ➤ Common Questions and Answers

2. What is the most common crisis symptom (and is considered the hallmark of the disease)?

   5MCC ➤ Sickle Cell Anemia ➤ Basics ➤ scroll down to Signs and Symptoms (fourth bullet)
   NDisCheck ➤ Assessment ➤ scroll down to In Painful Crisis (first bullet)

3. When giving morphine sulfate via IV infusion, the child should have a cardiac pulmonary monitor on. What is the rationale for this?

   LNDG ➤ Morphine Sulfate ➤ Adverse Effects
   PDH ➤ Morphine Sulfate ➤ Adverse Reactions

4. When assessing a child's response to pain, what should the practitioner keep in mind?

   NurProc ➤ Pain Management ➤ Special Considerations

5. When preparing to place an IV in the child, what equipment should the practitioner have in place?

   NurProc ➤ Table of Contents ➤ Pediatrics ➤ Pediatric IV Therapy ➤ Equipment

Medicine/NP/PA

1. What is the purpose of osmotic fragility?

   HbDxTests ➤ Sickle Cell Disease ➤ Osmotic Fragility ➤ Purpose

2. The pediatric dosing of morphine sulfate would be how many mg/kg/dose?

   LNDG ➤ Morphine Sulfate ➤ Dosages
   PDH ➤ Morphine Sulfate ➤ Indications and Dosages

3. Diphenhydramine may be administered intravenously. What should the practitioner know about the IV administration?

   LNDG ➤ Antihistamines ➤ Diphenhydramine ➤ IV
   PDH ➤ Diphenhydramine ➤ Indications and Dosages

4. When administering morphine sulfate to the child, what should the practitioner also have on hand at the bedside?

   LNDG ➤ Morphine Sulfate ➤ Nursing Considerations
   PDH ➤ Morphine Sulfate ➤ Overdose and Treatment

5. What is the life expectancy of a child with sickle cell disease?

   5MPed ➤ Sickle Cell Disease ➤ Database
   5MCC ➤ Sickle Cell Disease ➤ Follow-Up ➤ scroll down to Expected Course and Prognosis

6. What are some tests that would aid in a definitive diagnosis of sickle cell disease?

   5MPed ➤ Sickle Cell Disease ➤ Lab Aids
   5MCC ➤ Sickle Cell Disease ➤ Diagnosis
   NDisCheck ➤ Sickle Cell Disease ➤ Assessment

7. How often should a child with sickle cell disease be seen by a pediatric hematologist?

   5MPed ➤ Sickle Cell Disease ➤ Therapy
   5MCC ➤ Sickle Cell Disease ➤ Follow-Up

8. List five drugs of choice for a client with sickle cell disease.

   5MCC ➤ Anemia, Sickle Cell Disease ➤ Medications
   5MPed ➤ Sickle Cell Disease ➤ Therapy
   NDisCheck ➤ Sickle Cell Disease ➤ Treatment

9. List the first two possible complications of sickle cell disease.

   5MCC ➤ Anemia ➤ Sickle Cell Disease ➤ Follow-Up

NDisCheck ➤ Sickle Cell Disease ➤ Overview
5MPed ➤ Sickle Cell Disease ➤ Database

Physical and Occupational Therapy

Explain the pathophysiology of pain.

PMRRx ➤ Pain, General ➤ General Considerations ➤ Pathophysiology

Behavioral Health

What may be some barriers to pain assessment and adequate pain management?

PsychThrp ➤ Understanding and Assessing Pain and Pain Syndrome ➤ Barriers to Information

CASE STUDY 3 • *Tommy*

Cross-Discipline Learning Activities

1. What is Curling's ulcer?

   5MCC ➤ Burns ➤ Follow-Up ➤ scroll down to Possible Complications
   HPND ➤ Curling Ulcer

2. What causes the majority of burns?

   5MCC ➤ Burns ➤ Basics ➤ scroll down to Causes
   NDisCheck ➤ Burns ➤ Overview ➤ scroll down to Causes

3. What characteristics are associated with first-, second-, and third-degree burns?

   5MCC ➤ Burns ➤ Diagnosis ➤ scroll down to Pathological Findings
   NDisCheck ➤ Burns ➤ Overview ➤ scroll down to Pathophysiology

4. Why is the BUN level increased in a client with burns?

   HbDxTest ➤ Burns
   NDisCheck ➤ Burns ➤ Assessment ➤ scroll down to Laboratory (third bullet)

5. Why is thorough assessment and documentation of the child's wound appearance so essential?

   NurProc ➤ Burn Care ➤ Special Considerations

6. What is the drug classification of sulfadiazine?

   LNDG ➤ Sulfadiazine ➤ General ➤ scroll down to Drug Classes
   PDH ➤ Sulfadiazine ➤ Classification

Discipline-Specific Learning Activities

Nursing

1. Estimating burn surfaces in adults are done with the rule of nines. The rule of nines is not accurate with infants and children, so what chart may be used for this population?

   NurProc → Burn Care → Introduction

2. When administering morphine sulfate intravenously, what nursing considerations should the nurse know?

   LNDG → Morphine Sulfate → Nursing Considerations
   PDH → Morphine Sulfate → Special Considerations

3. What steps should the practitioner take to prevent cross-contamination during wound care?

   NurProc → Burn Care → Preparation of Equipment

4. What are key outcomes the nurse should try to attain when caring for the client with burns?

   NurProc → Burn Care → Introduction

5. What age-related factors are important to remember when dealing with a client with burns?

   5MCC → Burns → Miscellaneous → scroll down to Age-Related Factors

6. Skin graft failure may result from what?

   NurProc → Skin Graft Care → Complications

7. When documenting in the client's chart following skin grafting care, what are important criteria to include?

   NurProc → Skin Graft Care → Documentation

8. What are "common" side effects of morphine sulfate?

   PDH → Morphine Sulfate → Adverse Reactions
   LNDG → Morphine Sulfate → Adverse Effects

Medicine/NP/PA

1. What is the acceptable output for a child weighing less than 30 kg?

   HbDxTest → Burns

2. Why should the child be considered for an H_2 blocker medication?

   5MCC → Burns → Medication

3. The kidneys may be damaged as a result of prolonged tissue destruction. What abnormal findings in the blood and urine may signal kidney failure?

HbDxTest ⤳ Burns

4. What is rhabdomyolysis?

HPND ⤳ Rhabdomyolysis

5. What are the therapeutic actions of morphine sulfate?

PDH ⤳ Morphine ⤳ Pharmacodynamics
LNDG ⤳ Morphine Sulfate ⤳ Therapeutic Actions

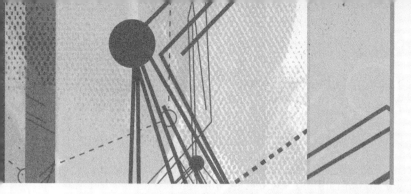

10

Women's Health Case Studies

Patricia Dunphy Suplee

This chapter contains six case studies related to the care of women. Three of them focus on pregnant clients, and the others portray women with signs and symptoms of pelvic inflammatory disease, ovarian cancer, or menopause. These case studies will show you how a multidisciplinary approach can help provide high quality comprehensive care to clients and their families.

➤ General Case Studies

For the following case studies, you will need to download the trial versions of the following references:

- Griffith's 5-Minute Clinical Consult (5MCC)
- Nursing Drug Handbook (NDH)
- Nurse's Quick Check: Diseases (NDisCheck)
- Stedman's Medical Dictionary for the Health Professions and Nursing (HPND)
- Taylor's Clinical Nursing Skills (ClinSkills)
- The Johns Hopkins Manual of Gynecology and Obstetrics (JHUObg)

- The Washington Manual Obstetrics and Gynecology Survival Guide (WUSOBG)

CASE STUDY I • *Sydney*

Sydney is a 26-year-old woman who presents to you with complaints of vaginal bleeding and lower abdominal pain, which is more severe on her left side. Her last menstrual period (LMP) was 3 weeks ago. She states she is dizzy and feels faint when she stands up. A pregnancy test comes back positive, and an ultrasound reveals an ectopic pregnancy. Her hemoglobin is 8.4 and her HCT is 26. She has a blood type of A– .

1. What is an ectopic pregnancy?
2. What is the incidence of an ectopic pregnancy?
3. What are the risk factors associated with ectopic pregnancies?
4. What are the clinical manifestations of an ectopic pregnancy?
5. How would you assess Sydney's blood pressure?
6. What differential diagnosis should be ruled out?
7. What is the medical or surgical management of this patient?
8. What is significant about Rh status and pregnancy?
9. Is Sydney a candidate for Rhogam? If so, how much should be administered?

CASE STUDY 2 • *Madeleine*

Madeleine is a 22-year-old woman who arrives in the emergency room complaining of lower abdominal pain, foul smelling vaginal discharge, fever of 101.3°F, chills, vomiting, and urinary symptoms. She is diagnosed with pelvic inflammatory disease (PID).

1. What is pelvic inflammatory disease?
2. What are the risk factors of pelvic inflammatory disease?
3. What signs and symptoms are associated with pelvic inflammatory disease?
4. What differential diagnosis should the practitioner look for?
5. How is PID treated?
6. What serious consequences could occur if PID is left untreated?
7. Can PID be prevented? If so, how?
8. What information should be shared with a client who is prescribed doxycycline?

CASE STUDY 3 • *Abby*

Abby is a 53-year-old woman who has come to the clinic with complaints of abnormal vaginal bleeding, a bloated pressure-like feeling in her abdomen, and lower back pain. She has been taking Motrin prn for the pain.

1. What is the incidence and mortality rate of ovarian cancer?
2. What are risk factors for ovarian cancer?
3. In addition to the signs and symptoms described by Abby, what other symptoms are associated with ovarian cancer?
4. What screening and diagnostic tests are useful to rule out the diagnosis of ovarian cancer?
5. Is there a genetic association with ovarian cancer? What are the screening tests available to patients?
6. What additional testing should be ordered for Abby once the diagnosis is made?
7. What types of treatments are available to women diagnosed with ovarian cancer?

➤ Advanced Case Studies

For the next three case studies, you will need to download the full versions of the following references:

- Griffith's 5-Minute Clinical Consult (5MCC)
- Handbook of Diagnostic Tests (HbDxTests)
- The Johns Hopkins Manual of Gynecology and Obstetrics (JHUObg)
- Lippincott's Nursing Drug Guide (LNDG) *or* Physician's Drug Handbook (PDH)
- Nurse's Quick Check: Diseases (NDisCheck)
- Stedman's Medical Dictionary for the Health Professions and Nursing (HPND)
- The Washington Manual Obstetrics and Gynecology Survival Guide (WUSOBG)

CASE STUDY I • *Molly*

Molly is a 16-year-old who is 13 weeks pregnant by gestational age. She presents to the clinic for her first obstetric visit with complaints of feeling nauseated for the last 3 weeks and she has vomited two times in the last 48 hours. She had a positive pregnancy test 4 weeks ago in a walk-in clinic that confirmed her pregnancy. As the clinician obtains her history, Molly reveals that her usual diet consists of eating at fast food restaurants, but, for the last couple of weeks, she has "lived on pretzels and soda." She admits to smoking a half pack of cigarettes per day for the last year and denies drug or alcohol use. She denies any medical or surgical history and offers no further complaints at this time. Assessment of Molly reveals the following data:

Height: 5'2"
Weight: 142 lb

Vital signs: Blood Pressure (BP) 116/68, Pulse (P) 76, Respirations (R) 16
Fetal Heart Rate (FHR): 164
Urine: ketones 2+, protein negative, glucose negative
Cervix: long and closed

Cross-Discipline Learning Activities

1. What does *gravida* mean?
2. What does *para* mean?
3. What hormone is elevated in a positive pregnancy test?
4. Identify some health risks to the mother and fetus related to smoking during pregnancy.
5. What percent of pregnant women are affected by nausea and vomiting in early pregnancy?
6. What are ketones?
7. Please calculate Molly's body mass index (BMI). How much weight should this patient be encouraged to gain during her pregnancy?
8. How is a cervix measured?
9. What do the terms "long" and "closed" refer to?

Discipline-Specific Learning Activities

Nursing

1. What are common discomforts of pregnancy that you should discuss with Molly?
2. Identify physiologic changes that occur with pregnancy related to the cardiovascular, respiratory, renal, and endocrine systems.
3. What suggestions might you include in your nutritional counseling for Molly?
4. How often should Molly return for prenatal care?
5. Identify some interventions for smoking cessation counseling.
6. What other types of education should you provide for Molly during this prenatal visit?

Medicine/PA/NP

1. What lab tests would be ordered for Molly during this first prenatal visit?
2. What types of screening tests are offered to women early in their pregnancy?
3. Why might Molly's ketones be elevated in her urine?
4. How would you manage elevated ketones in pregnancy?
5. What nonpharmacologic treatments can be used to manage nausea and vomiting during pregnancy?
6. What medications can be prescribed for Molly for her nausea if she does not get relief from nonpharmacologic measures?

7. What are the side effects of some of these medications?
8. When performing a physical exam, what systems would you evaluate, and what changes would be considered "normal" in pregnancy?
9. Do you feel that Molly requires hospitalization at this time? If so, why?

Behavioral Health

What type of behavior modification can be used to assist Molly with smoking cessation during pregnancy?

Critical Thinking—Correlating Patient Data/Assessment Findings to Plan Care

What additional information would you obtain from the client during this first prenatal visit that would enhance your ability to plan for her future care? What additional educational information could you provide for the client during this visit and subsequent visits?

CASE STUDY 2 • *Caroline*

Caroline is a 54-year-old woman who is being seen for her annual gynecologic (GYN) appointment.

Medical history: hypothyroidism diagnosed 10 years ago, currently taking Synthroid 1 mg/day.

Surgical history: delivered a male infant 30 years ago via cesarean section at term for breech presentation; son is alive and well.

Family history: father deceased at age 64 due to colon cancer; mother has hypertension and is on medications.

Caroline presents with complaints of night sweats and vaginal dryness. She would like more information on hormone replacement therapy (HRT). You suspect that Caroline is experiencing signs/symptoms (s/s) of menopause.

Cross-Discipline Learning Activities

1. What is hypothyroidism?
2. What is breech?
3. Define menopause.
4. What is the average age that women experience menopause?
5. What other condition might Caroline be at risk for due to a decrease in estrogen and bone density?
6. Because of Caroline's family history of colon cancer, is she at risk for developing this type of cancer?

Discipline-Specific Learning Activities

Nursing

1. What are the signs and symptoms of menopause?
2. What would you include in your teaching about menopause to this client?
3. Discuss the risk factors for clients who are prescribed HRT.
4. Are there any specific benefits of HRT for this client?
5. Besides HRT, what nonpharmacologic management options are available for this client?

Medicine/PA/NP

1. What should be included in Caroline's physical exam today?
2. Does this client need a PAP smear performed? If so, why?
3. What are the signs and symptoms of hypothyroidism?
4. What labs should be monitored when a client is taking Synthroid?
5. What is the normal dose of Synthroid? What are the side effects of this drug?
6. What medications can be prescribed for the signs and symptoms of menopause that Caroline is experiencing?
7. What alternative therapies are available for treating signs and symptoms of menopause?
8. Discuss the current recommendations for prescribing HRT.
9. Discuss the screening and diagnostic tests for osteoporosis.

Behavioral Health

Identify three psychosocial needs that should be addressed with this patient.

Critical Thinking—Correlating Patient Data/Assessment Findings to Plan Care

What additional testing should you offer to this client due to her history, age, and menopausal symptoms? What other concerns might this client have related to menopausal symptoms?

CASE STUDY 3 • *Ella*

Ella is a 38-year-old woman (gravida 2, para 1) who is 32 weeks pregnant. She presents to the Labor and Delivery Unit with complaints of abdominal cramping and thigh pressure.

Current OB history (Hx): Amniocentesis performed at 16 weeks gestation—negative for chromosomal abnormalities; at 25 weeks gestation—1-hour glucose tolerance test (GTT), 154; 3-hour GTT, normal.

Past OB Hx: Delivered her first child preterm at 33 weeks gestation after she experienced preterm labor. Infant had Apgars of 6 and 8 and was in the

Neonatal Intensive Care Unit (NICU) for 3 weeks, but is alive and well today.

Medical and Surgical Hx: Denies

Social Hx: Denies drugs, tobacco, alcohol

Assessment:

Vital signs: Blood Pressure (BP) 124/76, Pulse (P) 88, Respiration (R) 18

FHR: 133–138, with accelerations to a rate of 160 seconds, reassuring

Contractions: q3–4 minutes, moderate intensity per palpation, 50–60 second duration

Cervix: 3cms./100% effaced/0 station

Physician orders:

Admit to labor and delivery

IV 1000 cc NS at 75 cc/hr

Magnesium Sulfate ($MgSO_4$) 6 gm IV piggyback over 30 minutes followed by Magnesium Sulfate 2gms./hr IV per protocol

Administer Betamethasone 12 mg IM now and repeat in 24 hours

NPO

Bed rest

Continuous fetal monitoring

Cross-Discipline Learning Activities

1. What is an amniocentesis?
2. Why is this patient at risk for having a fetus with chromosomal abnormalities?
3. What is a glucose tolerance test (GTT)?
4. What does *Apgar* mean?
5. What is preterm labor?
6. What is the primary risk factor that this patient has for developing preterm labor?
7. What is NPO?
8. What is considered a "normal" fetal heart rate at this gestational age?
9. Define effacement and station.
10. If the infant is born at 32 weeks gestation, what are your main physiologic concerns?

Discipline-Specific Learning Activities

Nursing

1. How are contractions assessed?
2. What stage of labor is this patient in?
3. What is the difference between a reassuring and nonreassuring fetal heart rate (FHR) tracing?
4. What are the nursing considerations when administering IV $MgSO_4$?
5. What patient education should you provide at this time?

Medicine/PA/NP

1. When is an amniocentesis usually performed and why?
2. Why was a GTT ordered on this patient?
3. What are the normal parameters for a 1-hour GTT vs. a 3-hour GTT?
4. Describe the normal procedure for performing a 3-hour GTT.
5. List all of the signs and symptoms of preterm labor.
6. What are the causes of preterm labor?
7. What is the mechanism of action for $MgSO_4$?
8. What are the side effects of $MgSO_4$ to the mother and fetus?
9. What is the normal level of magnesium in serum?
10. What is the purpose of administering betamethasone to the patient?

Behavioral Health

If the patient delivers at 32 weeks gestation, what might be some of her psychosocial concerns?

Critical Thinking—Correlating Patient Data/Assessment Findings to Plan Care

What further assessments will be needed while this patient receives IV $MgSO_4$? What would you include in your plan of care if this patient goes on to deliver at 32 weeks gestation?

Chapter Summary—Tying It All Together

As you can see, a multidiscipline team approach to health care, whether it is provided in an office or hospital setting, is always beneficial to the patient. It is vital that health care providers take the time to critically think through cases such as these to provide patients with accurate information, educate them on their current health care needs, and identify preventative measures for them to take in the future. Research continues to identify specific health needs of women. Providing comprehensive education to women will allow them to make more informed health care decisions for themselves and their families.

WebLink. Visit http://thePoint.LWW.com/cornelius for supplemental information and activities.

ANSWERS TO CASE STUDY QUESTIONS

➤ General Case Studies

CASE STUDY 1 • *Sydney*

1. What is an ectopic pregnancy?
   JHUObg ➤ Ectopic Pregnancy ➤ Definition

2. What is the incidence of an ectopic pregnancy?
   JHUObg ➤ Ectopic Pregnancy ➤ Incidence

3. What are the risk factors associated with ectopic pregnancies?
   JHUObg ➤ Ectopic Pregnancy ➤ Etiology

4. What are the clinical manifestations of an ectopic pregnancy?
   JHUObg ➤ Ectopic Pregnancy ➤ Diagnosis ➤ Clinical Manifestations

5. How would you assess Sydney's blood pressure?
   ClinSkills ➤ Blood Pressure ➤ Assessment
   ClinSkills ➤ Blood Pressure ➤ Implementation

6. What differential diagnosis should be ruled out?
   JHUObg ➤ Ectopic Pregnancy ➤ Diagnosis ➤ Differential Diagnosis

7. What is the medical or surgical management of this patient?
   JHUObg ➤ Ectopic Pregnancy ➤ Treatment

8. What is significant about Rh status and pregnancy?
   NDis Check ➤ Rh Incompatibility ➤ Overview

9. Is Sydney a candidate for Rhogam? If so, how much should be administered?
   PDH ➤ RhoGAM ➤ Indications of Dosages

CASE STUDY 2 • *Madeleine*

1. What is pelvic inflammatory disease?
   WUSOBG ➤ Pelvic Inflammatory Disease ➤ Introduction

2. What are the risk factors of pelvic inflammatory disease?
   WUSOBG ➤ Pelvic Inflammatory Disease ➤ Risk Factors

3. What signs and symptoms are associated with pelvic inflammatory disease?

   WUSOBG ➤ Pelvic Inflammatory Disease ➤ History

4. What differential diagnosis should the practitioner look for?

   WUSOBG ➤ Pelvic Inflammatory Disease ➤ Differential Diagnosis

5. How is PID treated?

   JHUObg ➤ Pelvic Inflammatory Disease ➤ Treatment

6. What serious consequences could occur if PID is left untreated?

   WUSObg ➤ Complications

7. Can PID be prevented? If so, how?

   WUOBG ➤ Risk Factors (refer to Table 55-1 Risk Factors and Protective Factors for PID) ➤ Protective Factors

8. What information should be shared with a client who is prescribed doxycycline?

   NDH ➤ Doxycycline ➤ Patient Teaching

CASE STUDY 3 • *Abby*

1. What is the incidence and mortality rate of ovarian cancer?

   JHUObg ➤ Ovarian Cancer ➤ Incidence and Mortality

2. What are risk factors for ovarian cancer?

   JHUObg ➤ Ovarian Cancer ➤ Individual Risk Factors

3. In addition to the signs and symptoms described by Abby, what other symptoms are associated with ovarian cancer?

   JHUObg ➤ Ovarian Cancer ➤ Clinical Evaluation ➤ Presentation

4. What screening and diagnostic tests are useful to rule out the diagnosis of ovarian cancer?

   JHUObg ➤ Ovarian Cancer ➤ Detection and Prevention

5. Is there a genetic association with ovarian cancer? What are the screening tests available to patients?

   JHUObg ➤ Ovarian Cancer ➤ Risk Factors ➤ Family History
   JHUObg ➤ Ovarian Cancer ➤ Detection and Prevention

6. What additional testing should be ordered for Abby once the diagnosis is made?

   JHUObg → Ovarian Cancer → Clinical Evaluation

7. What types of treatment are available to women diagnosed with ovarian cancer?

   JHUObg → Ovarian Cancer → Treatment

➤ Advanced Case Studies

CASE STUDY I • *Molly*

Cross-Discipline Learning Activities

1. What does *gravida* mean?

   HPND → Gravida

2. What does *para* mean?

   HPND → Para

3. What hormone is elevated in a positive pregnancy test?

   HbDxTests → Pregnancy Test

4. Identify some health risks to the mother and fetus related to smoking during pregnancy.

   JHUObg → Smoking → Preeclampsia

5. What percent of pregnant women are affected by nausea and vomiting in early pregnancy?

   WUSOBG → Nausea and Vomiting → Overview

6. What are ketones?

   HPND → Ketones and Ketone body

7. Please calculate Molly's body mass index (BMI). How much weight should this patient be encouraged to gain during her pregnancy?

   NDisCheck → BMI → Measurement
   JHUObg → Preconceptual Counseling → Prenatal Care

8. How is a cervix measured?

   JHUObg → Normal Labor and Delivery → Cervical Examination

9. What do the terms "long" and "closed" refer to?

JHUObg → Normal Labor and Delivery → Cervical Examination

Discipline-Specific Learning Activities

Nursing

1. What are common discomforts of pregnancy that you should discuss with Molly?

JHUObg → Preconceptual Counseling

2. Identify physiologic changes that occur with pregnancy related to the cardiovascular, respiratory, renal, and endocrine systems.

WUSOBG → Pregnancy → Physiologic Changes → Table 2.1

3. What suggestions might you include in your nutritional counseling for Molly?

JHUObg → Preconceptual Counseling → Prenatal Care

4. How often should Molly return for prenatal care?

WUSOBG → Prenatal Care → Visit Interval

5. Identify some interventions for smoking cessation counseling.

JHUObg → Preconceptual Counseling → Prenatal Care

6. What other types of education should you provide for Molly during this prenatal visit?

JHUObg → Preconceptual Counseling → Prenatal Care

Medicine/PA/NP

1. What lab tests would be ordered for Molly during this first prenatal visit?

JHUObg → Pregnancy → Routine Prenatal Testing

2. What types of screening tests are offered to women early in their pregnancy?

WUSOBG → Prenatal Care → Routine Prenatal Care Screening

3. Why might Molly's ketones be elevated in her urine?

JHUObg → Preconception Counseling → Pharmacology → Chapter 16 → Renal Physiologic Changes

4. How would you manage elevated ketones in pregnancy?

5MCC → Hyperemesis Gravidarum → Treatment

5. What nonpharmacologic treatments can be used to manage nausea and vomiting during pregnancy?

WUSOBG ➤ Nausea and Vomiting ➤ Overview
JHUObg ➤ Preconception Counseling ➤ Nonpharmacology

6. What medications can be prescribed for Molly for her nausea if she does not get relief from nonpharmacologic measures?

JHUObg ➤ Preconception Counseling ➤ Nonpharmacology ➤ Chapter 16

7. What are the side effects of some of these medications?

5MCC ➤ Hyperemesis Gravidarum ➤ Medications

8. When performing a physical exam, what systems would you evaluate, and what changes would be considered "normal" in pregnancy?

WUSOBG ➤ Physiologic Changes in Pregnancy

9. Do you feel that Molly requires hospitalization at this time? If so, why?

5MCC ➤ Hyperemesis Gravida ➤ Follow-Up
WUSOBG ➤ Nausea and Vomiting ➤ Overview ➤ Management

Behavioral Health

What type of behavior modification can be used to assist Molly with smoking cessation during pregnancy?

JHUObg ➤ Preconceptual Counseling

CASE STUDY 2 • *Caroline*

Cross-Discipline Learning Activities

1. What is hypothyroidism?

NDisCheck ➤ Hypothyroid ➤ Overview
5MCC ➤ Hypothyroidism ➤ Basics

2. What is breech?

HPND ➤ Breech Presentation

3. Define menopause.

HPND ➤ Menopause

4. What is the average age that women experience menopause?

WUSOBG ➤ Menopause ➤ Introduction
JHUObg ➤ Menopause ➤ Menopause and Hormone Replacement Therapy ➤ Definition

5. What other condition might Caroline be at risk for due to a decrease in estrogen and bone density?

   JHUObg → Menopause → Menopause and Hormone Replacement Therapy → Vasomotor Symptoms
   5MCC → Menopause → Follow-Up

6. Because of Caroline's family history of colon cancer, is she at risk for developing this type of cancer?

   NDisCheck → Colorectal Cancer → Overview
   5MCC → Colorectal Malignancy → Basics

Discipline-Specific Learning Activities

Nursing

1. What are the signs and symptoms of menopause?

   WUSOBG → Menopause → Overview
   5MCC → Menopause → Basics

2. What would you include in your teaching about menopause to this client?

   JHUObg → Menopause and Hormonal Therapy → Overview
   5MCC → Menopause → Follow-Up

3. Discuss the risk factors for clients who are prescribed HRT.

   WUSOBG → Menopause → Hormone Replacement Therapy → Contraindications
   5MCC → Menopause → Medications
   JHUObg → Menopause → Menopause and Hormone Replacement Therapy → Side Effects and Contraindications of Hormone Replacement Therapy

4. Are there any specific benefits of HRT for this client?

   JHUObg → Menopause → Menopause and Hormone Replacement Therapy
   5MCC → Menopause → Treatment

5. Besides HRT, what nonpharmacologic management options are available for this client?

   JHUObg → Menopause → Menopause and Hormone Replacement Therapy → Table 39.3, National Osteoporosis Foundation Guidelines for Prevention and Treatment of Osteoporosis
   5MCC → Menopause → Medication

Medicine/PA/NP

1. What should be included in Caroline's physical exam today?

   5MCC ⇝ Menopause ⇝ Follow-Up

2. Does this client need a PAP smear performed? If so, why?

   5MCC ⇝ Diagnosis and Miscellaneous

3. What are the signs and symptoms of hypothyroidism?

   NDisCheck ⇝ Hypothyroidism ⇝ Assessment
   5MCC ⇝ Hypothyroidism ⇝ Basics

4. What labs should be monitored when a client is taking Synthroid?

   LNDG ⇝ Synthroid ⇝ Nursing Considerations
   PDH ⇝ Synthroid ⇝ Pharmacokinetics

5. What is the normal dose of Synthroid? What are the side effects of this drug?

   LNDG ⇝ Synthroid ⇝ Dosing and Adverse Effects
   PDH ⇝ Synthroid ⇝ Indications and Dosages

6. What medications can be prescribed for the signs and symptoms of menopause that Caroline is experiencing?

   WUSOBG ⇝ Menopause ⇝ Hormone Replacement Therapy
   5MCC ⇝ Menopause ⇝ Medications

7. What alternative therapies are available for treating signs and symptoms of menopause?

   JHUObg ⇝ Menopause ⇝ Menopause and Hormone Replacement
   Therapy ⇝ Topical Outline Alternative Therapies
   5MCC ⇝ Menopause ⇝ Medications

8. Discuss the current recommendations for prescribing HRT.

   JHUObg ⇝ Menopause ⇝ Menopause and Hormone Replacement
   Therapy
   WUSOBG ⇝ Menopause and Hormone Replacement Therapy
   5MCC ⇝ Menopause ⇝ Medications

9. Discuss the screening and diagnostic tests for osteoporosis.

   WUSOBG ⇝ Menopause ⇝ Osteoporosis ⇝ Diagnosis

Behavioral Health

Identify three psychosocial needs that should be addressed with this patient.

JHUObg ⇝ Menopause ⇝ Counseling

CASE STUDY 3 • *Ella*

Cross-Discipline Learning Activities

1. What is an amniocentesis?

   HPND ➤ Amniocentesis

2. Why is this patient at risk for having a fetus with chromosomal abnormalities?

   JHUObg ➤ Preconceptual Counseling ➤ Amniocentesis

3. What is a glucose tolerance test (GTT)?

   HbDxTests ➤ GTT ➤ Introduction

4. What does *Apgar* mean?

   WUSOBG ➤ Labor ➤ Normal ➤ Section Outline ➤ Fetal Assess ➤ Apgar Scores

5. What is preterm labor?

   JHUObg ➤ Preterm Labor
   WUSOBG ➤ Preterm Labor ➤ Section Outline ➤ Definitions

6. What is the primary risk factor that this patient has for developing preterm labor?

   WUSOBG ➤ Preterm Labor ➤ Section Outline ➤ Risk Factors
   JHUObg ➤ Labor

7. What is NPO?

   HPND ➤ NPO

8. What is considered a "normal" fetal heart rate at this gestational age?

   JHUObg ➤ Fetal Heart Rate
   WUSOBG ➤ Intrapartum Fetal Monitoring

9. Define effacement and station.

   WUSOBG ➤ Normal Labor and Delivery ➤ Table 24.1 Evaluation of Mother and Fetus

10. If the infant is born at 32 weeks gestation, what are your main physiologic concerns?

    WUSOBG ➤ Preterm Labor ➤ Management

Discipline-Specific Learning Activities

Nursing

1. How are contractions assessed?

   WUSOBG ⇻ Labor ⇻ Monitoring Intrauterine Contractions

2. What stage of labor is this patient in?

   JHUObg ⇻ Normal Labor and Delivery ⇻ Stages and Phases of Labor

3. What is the difference between a reassuring and nonreassuring fetal heart rate (FHR) tracing?

   JHUObg ⇻ Fetal Monitoring

4. What are the nursing considerations when administering IV MgSO$_4$?

   LNDG ⇻ Magnesium Sulfate ⇻ IV Facts
   PDH ⇻ Magnesium Sulfate ⇻ Special Considerations

5. What patient education should you provide at this time?

   WUSOBG ⇻ Preterm Labor ⇻ Management

Medicine/PA/NP

1. When is an amniocentesis usually performed and why?

   JHUObg ⇻ Amniocentesis
   WUSOBG ⇻ Amniocentesis ⇻ Prenatal Diagnosis

2. Why was a GTT ordered on this patient?

   HbDxTests ⇻ GTT ⇻ Information

3. What are the normal parameters for a 1-hour GTT vs. a 3-hour GTT?

   HbDxTests ⇻ GTT ⇻ Clinical Implications

4. Describe the normal procedure for performing a 3-hour GTT.

   HbDxTests ⇻ GTT ⇻ Procedures

5. List all of the signs and symptoms of preterm labor.

   WUSOBG ⇻ Preterm Labor
   5MCC ⇻ Labor, Premature ⇻ Basics

6. What are the causes of preterm labor?

   JHUObg ⇻ Premature Labor ⇻ Risk Factors
   WUSOBG ⇻ Preterm Labor ⇻ Table 4.1

7. What is the mechanism of action for $MgSO_4$?

   LNDG ➤ Magnesium Sulfate ➤ Therapeutic Action
   PDH ➤ Magnesium Sulfate ➤ Pharmacodynamics

8. What are the side effects of $MgSO_4$ to the mother and fetus?

   WUSOBG ➤ Preterm Labor ➤ Commonly Used Tocolytics ➤ Table 4.2
   PDH ➤ Magnesium Sulfate ➤ Adverse Reactions

9. What is the normal level of magnesium in serum?

   LNDG ➤ Magnesium Sulfate ➤ Nursing Considerations
   HbDxTests ➤ Magnesium ➤ Reference Values

10. What is the purpose of administering betamethasone to the patient?

   WUSOBG ➤ Preterm Labor ➤ Corticosteroids
   5MCC ➤ Labor, Premature ➤ Treatment

Behavioral Health

If the patient delivers at 32 weeks gestation, what might be some of her psychosocial concerns?

JHUObg ➤ Premature Birth ➤ Counseling

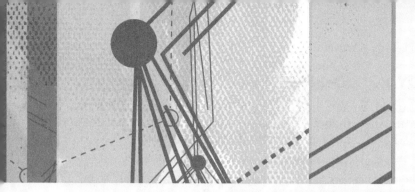

11

Mental Health
Case Studies

Roberta Waite

The case studies in this chapter focus on the care of patients with psychiatric illnesses. Patients with psychiatric ailments often have complex, comorbid issues that require the care of many disciplines. Therefore, a comprehensive, holistic approach to patient care is provided to facilitate optimal functioning and safety.

➤ General Case Studies

For the following three case studies you will need to download trial versions of the following references:

- Griffith's 5-Minute Clinical Consult (5MCC)
- Nurses' Handbook of Health Assessment (HlthAssess)
- Nurse's Quick Check: Diseases (NDisCheck)
- Stedman's Medical Dictionary for the Health Professions and Nursing (HPND)
- The Washington Manual Psychiatry Survival Guide (WUSPsych)

CASE STUDY I • *Debbie*

Debbie, a 32-year-old woman, has been admitted to the unit with a history of sleeping and eating disturbances, with periods of irritability, impulsive actions, delusions, and lethargy; she is diagnosed with bipolar disorder.

1. What is the description of bipolar disorder?
2. If Debbie experiences rapid cycling, when is it most likely to occur?
3. What physical findings are associated with bipolar disorder?
4. What medications are commonly ordered for a patient with bipolar disorder?
5. When Debbie is depressed, what cognitive, behavioral, and physiological signs and symptoms may be present?
6. What recommended reading for depression may be suggested to Debbie?
7. During a manic episode, Debbie twists her ankle. What is the normal range of motion (ROM) for the ankle?
8. Debbie needs a brief psychotic rating scale. What tool would you use to perform this assessment?

CASE STUDY 2 • *Trisha*

Trisha, a 14-year-old girl, has been losing weight for a few months and presents to the clinic with dehydration. Her mother states that she has developed peculiar eating habits, frequently weighing herself, and appears to be losing weight. Trisha is diagnosed with bulimia nervosa.

1. Trisha needs oral rehydration. What is the basic description of oral rehydration?
2. What is the common history of a patient with bulimia nervosa?
3. What are some physical findings associated with bulimia nervosa?
4. Trisha's hemoglobin level is low; she is diagnosed with iron deficiency anemia. What is iron deficiency anemia?
5. What is the treatment for a patient with iron deficiency anemia?
6. During the course of Trisha's therapy, it has been identified that she has been abusing laxatives. What is the description of substance abuse and dependency?
7. Trisha has acne vulgaris. What is this?
8. How will Trisha be treated for acne vulgaris?
9. Trisha complains that her right elbow is hurting her. What is the normal ROM for an elbow?

CASE STUDY 3 • *Roberta*

Roberta, a 22-year-old woman, comes to the local ER with a severe panic attack, is extremely agitated, and appears to be psychotic. She states that she has had some "coke" a few hours ago but is not sure whether she has had any drugs, such as hallucinogens or inhalants.

1. What general information should the practitioner know about anxiety disorders?
2. What are the clinical features of a patient admitted with anxiety disorders?
3. With routine labs, it is found that Roberta has acquired immuno-deficiency syndrome (AIDS). What is the description of AIDS?
4. What physical findings are associated with AIDS?
5. During the course of therapy, it comes out that Roberta was abused as a child. Her stepfather sexually abused her for 6 years, before she ran away from home. What is the description of sexual abuse?
6. Define anxiety reaction.
7. Part of the therapy may be to determine Roberta's perception of her health. What is the purpose of this?
8. While in the unit, Roberta develops a case of the "runs." What is this?
9. What general measures should be offered to Roberta while she is experiencing the symptoms described in question 8?

➤ Advanced Case Studies

For the next three case studies, you will need to download the full versions of the following references:

- Griffith's 5-Minute Clinical Consult (5MCC)
- Manual of Psychiatric Therapeutics (PsychThrp)
- Nurse's Quick Check: Diseases (NDisCheck)
- Nursing Procedures (NurProc)
- Lippincott's Nursing Drug Guide (LNDG) *or* Physician's Drug Handbook (PDH)
- Stedman's Medical Dictionary for the Health Professions and Nursing (HPND)

CASE STUDY I • *Mrs. Gonzalez*

Mrs. Gonzalez is a 30-year-old, married, Hispanic woman who presents to the psychiatric emergency room on an Emergency Involuntary Commitment Petition accompanied by her husband. Mrs. Gonzalez has experienced five distinct episodes of depression and hypomania over the past 9 months and is currently in a depressed state and threatening to kill herself. She has lost 10 pounds over the past 3 weeks, reports insomnia, anxiety, loss of interest in things she once found pleasurable, hopelessness, and reduced energy.

She has been verbally aggressive with her family members and physically aggressive with her neighbors. One week ago, while in a manic state, she sprained her arm fighting with a neighbor. Her husband states that she had experienced similar episodes in the past. However, she has never been physically aggressive and has never presented to be a serious danger to herself or others. The patient has a past history of alcohol abuse but states that she has not used alcohol or drugs in the past 3 years. She reports no symptoms of obsessive-compulsive disorder; denies delusions or hallucinations; verbalizes suicidal ideation, intention, and plan to cut her wrist with a knife; and is not able to contract for safety. She also denies any prior suicide attempts and states that no one in her family has ever attempted suicide and that her religious beliefs as a Roman Catholic usually help her during stressful times. Her level of distress and impairment is marked, and it is unlikely that her symptoms are related to substance abuse.

Her husband reports that her brother has the same disorder and has had a good response to Divalproex. She reports that the medications that she has been treated with in the past were not effective or only partially effective. She recalls that 2 years before she was prescribed Prozac and Klonopin. She discontinued treatment with Prozac on her own because she was feeling agitated. She later discontinued Klonopin because she started using a much higher dosage than was prescribed by her doctor, and, subsequently, her doctor refused to authorize refills on this medication. She also recalls being treated with lithium about 1 year before when she experienced a period of euphoria, spent several thousands dollars on things she did not need, felt like she did not need to sleep, was full of plans and got involved in many projects, and was overly talkative and spoke rapidly and loudly, jumping from idea to idea. She says that she discontinued the medication on her own because of tremors, diarrhea, and increased urination. The patient has been medication-free since then and says that the major reason for this is that her doctor would not listen to her talk about the difficulty tolerating the side effects of therapy and could not do more than suggest that they reduce the dose or other medications to counteract the side effects.

The physician's orders read:

- Axis I: Bipolar I
- Axis II: Deferred
- Axis III: Sprained arm (3 weeks)
- Axis IV: Deferred
- Axis V: 20/50
- One-to-one observation
- Elopement monitoring
- Complete blood count, platelets, liver function tests, electrolytes, blood glucose, lipoprotein profile, lipase, thyroid-stimulating hormone, creatinine, blood urea nitrogen, urinalysis, pregnancy test, and urine drug screen
- Physical/occupational therapy consult for right arm
- Nutrition consult
- Mood stabilizing anticonvulsant agent ordered: divalproex

Cross-Discipline Learning Activities

1. What is the DSM-IV-TR?
2. What is Bipolar I?
3. What is one-to-one observation?
4. What behaviors reflect rapid cycling?

5. What is mania?
6. What is depression?
7. What are mood stabilizing anticonvulsant agents?
8. What is elopement monitoring?

Discipline-Specific Learning Activities

Nursing

1. What nursing considerations are associated with assessment of the patient's mental status and potential for suicide?
2. What mnemonic can be used to assess suicide risk factors?
3. What changes will need to occur within the patient's environment?
4. What are important nursing interventions and documentation measures for a patient on elopement monitoring?
5. What is Divalproex? What is the therapeutic serum level?
6. What adverse gastrointestinal (GI) effects are possible with administration of Divalproex?
7. What inhibitory neurotransmitter does Divalproex (valproate) affect?
8. What must the nurse assess for regarding Mrs. Gonzalez's right arm sprain?
9. What are common characteristics of a sprain?
10. How would nursing aid the patient in promoting interest in food to minimize weight loss?

Medicine/NP/PA

1. What laboratory studies would you expect to order for Mrs. Gonzalez before initiating Divalproex (divalproex sodium)?
2. How much Divalproex should the patient be prescribed initially?
3. What is the therapeutic serum level for Divalproex?
4. When would you expect the onset of action to occur?
5. What imaging tests may be ordered to rule out further complications of the sprain?
6. What medications may be useful to alleviate Mrs. Gonzalez's pain?

Physical and Occupational Therapy

1. What types of hand exercises would be useful for Mrs. Gonzalez?
2. What supportive measures would be useful in promoting comfort to Mrs. Gonzalez?

Behavioral Health

1. Why is a comprehensive psychosocial assessment required for Mrs. Gonzalez?
2. What education is needed for families in recognizing Mrs. Gonzalez's mood liability?

3. Mrs. Gonzalez will receive outpatient treatment after discharge. The couple requests additional information on support groups. What other therapeutic interventions would you suggest as part of the patient discharge planning process?

Critical Thinking—Correlating Patient Data/Assessment Findings to Plan Care

In reflecting on Mrs. Gonzalez's case, consider the following questions. What are other pertinent questions you would want to ask? What staffing considerations are needed for a patient at risk for suicide? Why would they be important to her plan of care? What other diagnostic tests would you consider to further guide your treatment strategies? How would you manage Mrs. Gonzalez's plan of care after initiating divalproex?

CASE STUDY 2   •   *Mrs. Griffin*

Mrs. Griffin, a 55-year-old woman, with NIDDM, increasing discomfort from rheumatoid arthritis and no past psychiatric history, presents with disturbed behavior and profound suspiciousness. The patient lives with her husband, who is similar in age. They have two sons, ages 25 and 20. Her husband runs a small business and her children are in college. The family is quite close, and they have a supportive social network. They have no significant housing concerns and are financially solvent. One month ago, Mrs. Griffin resigned from her job and became reclusive. Despite consultation with the family physician, her symptoms worsened rapidly, and her behavior became progressively more disturbed. She became increasingly fearful of her family and friends, although she was reluctant to discuss the basis of her fears. She began to refuse the food that was prepared for her by her relatives. Her agitation increased to the point that she was urgently referred for inpatient treatment.

The patient accepts admission voluntarily; however, she fails to participate in treatment. She appears guarded, hypervigilant, and suspicious of hospital staff. She repeatedly scrutinizes staff identity cards. Her presentation fluctuates with periods of agitation to profound psychomotor retardation. Her speech is slow, with increased response latency, a lack of spontaneity, and reduced intonation. Mrs. Griffin verbalizes some persecutory delusions and refuses to eat and drink as a result of these delusions. She does not believe she is in the hospital and refuses medication, stating she does not deserve it. She presents with a preoccupied glare and is distracted at times. Her mood is objectively depressed, although upon questioning, she typically states that she is "all right." She denies suicidal ideation; her insight is grossly impaired; and she refuses cognitive assessment, physical examination, and initial serologic investigations.

She is ordered Effexor and olanzapine, and she refuses both. Over the next week, the patient's mental state deteriorates, and she restricts her food and fluid intake significantly. She becomes mildly dehydrated, clinically and biochemically, such that more aggressive treatment is required. Electroconvulsive therapy

(ECT) is proposed, to which she refuses to consent, but her husband agrees with the proposed treatment after the nature of this intervention is explained.

Following ECT, her mental state improves almost immediately, with normalization of mood, eating habits, and motor retardation. She complies with the Effexor and olanzapine treatment. Her suspiciousness resolves, and she becomes adherent to prescribed medication.

The physician's orders read:

- Axis I: Major depression with psychotic features
- Axis II: Deferred
- Axis III: Diabetes
- Axis IV: Deferred
- Axis V: 20/60
- SNRI and atypical antipsychotics: Effexor and olanzapine
- ECT
- Basic metabolic panel
- Daily weights, and intake and output
- Glucosans bid
- Computed tomography (CT) brain scans and EEG

Cross-Discipline Learning Activities

1. What is ECT?
2. What is major depression? What causes it?
3. What are psychotic features?
4. What is computed tomography and EEG?
5. What are atypical antipsychotic medications?
6. What is NIDDM?

Discipline-Specific Learning Activities

Nursing

1. For what changes should the nurse assess in the EEG following ECT?
2. What cognitive changes may be present after ECT?
3. What are Axis I and Axis II disorders according to the DSM-IV-TR?
4. What is an SNRI? What two neurotransmitters are blocked from reuptake?
5. What common side effects occur with patients taking Effexor (venlafaxine)?

Medicine/NP/PA

1. What are some indications that would place a patient at increased risk if he or she received ECT?
2. To minimize the cognitive side effects of ECT, would you use unilateral or bilateral electrode placement? Explain.

3. What medications may increase the seizure threshold, thereby diminishing the efficacy of unilateral ECT?
4. What deviations in laboratory findings are expected of someone who is dehydrated?
5. At what dosage would you initiate both olanzapine and Effexor?

Physical and Occupational Therapy

What mechanisms would serve as a support to facilitate movement and improve balance?

Behavioral Health

1. In addition to psychopharmacologic interventions for depression, what types of psychosocial approaches to treatment are available to Mrs Griffin?
2. What referrals would be helpful in receiving outpatient support?
3. What patient education should occur before discharge?

Critical Thinking—Correlating Patient Data/Assessment Findings to Plan Care

What additional information specific to Mrs. Griffin's case would be helpful before initiating ECT? Identify some therapeutic interventions that would be helpful while working with a suspicious patient. What interventions are appropriate with the patient who is refusing food, fluids, and medications? What is your plan of care for Mrs. Griffin once her suspiciousness resolves and she becomes adherent to prescribed medication?

CASE STUDY 3 • *Mrs. Anderson*

Mrs. Anderson is a physically healthy 32-year-old Caucasian woman with a 15-year history of recurrent depressive disorder. At times she would discontinue her Celexa and take herbal over-the-counter (OTC) medication. She recently experienced acute suicidal thoughts and set herself on fire with a match and kerosene. She acquired second-degree burns on 10% of her body surface area (BSA). After a transfer from the ICU, she is now on a psychiatric medical care unit for treatment of depression and further care for burns. Mrs. Anderson recently broke up with a boyfriend and does not have a good support system. She lives alone in an apartment in a rural area. A standardized rating scale is used as part of the patient's diagnostic assessment.

Mrs. Anderson is taking both 10 mg of Celexa and Hypericum perforatum daily. Initially, after a skin graft operation to her hands and feet, Mrs. Anderson was taking IV morphine for pain relief; however, she is currently comfortably maintained on 50 mg/day of tramadol for pain relief. Subsequently, she developed serotonin syndrome.

The physician's orders read:

- Axis I: Major depression
- Axis II: Deferred
- Axis III: S/P 2nd-degree skin burns
- Axis IV: Poor social supports
- Axis V: 20/55
- Monitor vital signs every 4 hours while awake
- Dressing changes daily
- Antibiotic ointments daily with dressing change
- Initiate an SSRI
- Laboratory tests

Cross-Discipline Learning Activities

1. What is serotonin syndrome? What are the symptoms?
2. What does SSRI indicate?
3. What is a standardized rating scale?
4. What is a second-degree burn?
5. What is BSA?

Discipline-Specific Learning Activities
Nursing

1. What are some common side effects of SSRIs?
2. What education must be provided regarding discontinuation of SSRIs?
3. Why is there a contraindication with patients taking Hypericum perforatum and SSRIs?
4. What rating scale could be used in identifying depressed patients?
5. What educational interventions are necessary for the patient's continued compliance even when she feels better?
6. What assessments are needed when caring for a patient with a second-degree burn?
7. What self-care teaching should occur with the patient?

Medicine/NP/PA

1. What dosage of medication would be prescribed for the patient?
2. If treatment is adequate, what is the approximate time period before depression improves?
3. What topical cream may be ordered to apply to the burn site?
4. What laboratory test might you order?
5. How would you ensure proper nutritional interventions?

Physical and Occupational Therapy

1. Why is movement important for Mrs. Anderson?

2. What documentation by physical/occupational therapist should occur for a patient with second-degree burns?
3. What is the activity goal for such a patient?

Behavioral Health

1. Besides psychopharmacologic interventions, what other measures (psychosocial) would be prescribed to assist the patient in restoring her normal level of well-being?
2. In arranging the patient's outpatient follow-up, what relevance does the therapeutic alliance have in the success of treatment for depression?

Critical Thinking—Correlating Patient Data/Assessment Findings to Plan Care

What additional information specific to Mrs. Anderson's case (physical, emotional, and medications) would be helpful to know to facilitate effective intervention? How could Mrs. Anderson's environmental surroundings be altered (modified) to facilitate self-care?

Chapter Summary—Tying It All Together

You have explored several psychiatric patient scenarios that are typical for acute care settings. Each case presented a patient requiring interventions for a comorbid illness with psychiatric concerns being most acute. The DSM-IV-TR serves as a guide to understanding psychiatric care concerns and identifying behavioral dynamics that are reflected in a patient's presentation. Axis I diagnoses involving mood disorders—bipolar disorder, major depression, psychotic disorders—were discussed as well as contemporary treatments for managing their symptoms, such as ECT, SSRIs, SNRIs, and atypical antipsychotics.

Additionally, many patients present with medical issues. We addressed a patient with a sprained arm, NIDDM, and a burn. Because of the interplay between the physiologic and psychological treatments, a multidisciplinary approach is useful in providing the patient with optimal care. Also, this approach promotes collaboration between individuals during the course of the patient's treatment. These factors are essential when providing the best possible outcomes for our patients.

WebLink. | Visit http://thePoint.LWW.com/cornelius for supplemental information and activities.

ANSWERS TO CASE STUDY QUESTIONS

➤ General Case Studies

CASE STUDY 1 • *Debbie*

1. What is the description of bipolar disorder?

   5MCC ➣ Bipolar Disorder ➣ Basics

2. If Debbie experiences rapid cycling, when is it most likely to occur?

   5MCC ➣ Bipolar Disorder ➣ Basics

3. What physical findings are associated with bipolar disorder?

   NDisCheck ➣ Bipolar Disorder ➣ Assessment

4. What medications are commonly ordered for a patient with bipolar disorder?

   5MCC ➣ Bipolar Disorder ➣ Medications

5. When Debbie is depressed, what cognitive, behavioral, and physiological signs and symptoms may be present?

   NDisCheck ➣ Bipolar Disorder ➣ Overview

6. What recommended reading for depression may be suggested to Debbie?

   5MCC ➣ Depression ➣ Treatment

7. During a manic episode, Debbie twists her ankle. What is the normal range of motion (ROM) for the ankle?

   HlthAssess ➣ Ankles, Normal Range of Motion

8. Debbie needs a brief psychotic rating scale. What tool would you use to perform this assessment?

   WUSPsych ➣ Brief Psychotic Rating Scale ➣ Section Outline ➣ Hamilton Rating Scale for Depression

CASE STUDY 2 • *Trisha*

1. Trisha needs oral rehydration. What is the basic description of oral rehydration?

   5MCC ➣ Oral Rehydration ➣ Basics

2. What is the common history of a client with bulimia nervosa?

   5MCC ➣ Bulimia Nervosa ➣ Basics

3. What are some physical findings associated with bulimia nervosa?

   NDisCheck ➤ Bulimia Nervosa ➤ Assessment ➤ Physical Findings

4. Trisha's hemoglobin level is low; she is diagnosed with iron deficiency anemia. What is iron deficiency anemia?

   5MCC ➤ Iron Deficiency Anemia ➤ Basics

5. What is the treatment for a patient with iron deficiency anemia?

   5MCC ➤ Iron Deficiency Anemia ➤ Treatment

6. During the course of Trisha's therapy, it has been identified that she has been abusing laxatives. What is the description of substance abuse and dependency?

   NDisCheck ➤ Substance Abuse and Dependency ➤ Overview

7. Trisha has acne vulgaris. What is this?

   5MCC ➤ Acne Vulgaris ➤ Basics

8. How will Trisha be treated for acne vulgaris?

   5MCC ➤ Acne Vulgaris ➤ Treatment

9. Trisha complains that her right elbow is hurting her. What is the normal ROM for an elbow?

   HlthAssess ➤ Elbow, Normal Range of Motion

CASE STUDY 3 • *Roberta*

1. What general information should the practitioner know about anxiety disorders?

   5MCC ➤ Anxiety ➤ Basics

2. What are the clinical features of a patient admitted with anxiety disorders?

   WUSPsych ➤ Anxiety Disorders ➤ Clinical Features

3. With routine labs, it is found that Roberta has acquired immunodeficiency syndrome (AIDS). What is the description of AIDS?

   NDisCheck ➤ Acquired Immunodeficiency Syndrome ➤ Overview

4. What physical findings are associated with AIDS?

   5MCC ➤ HIV Infection and AIDS ➤ Basics

5. During the course of therapy, it comes out that Roberta was abused as a child. Her stepfather sexually abused her for 6 years, before she ran away from home. What is the description of sexual abuse?

   5MCC ➤ Child Abuse ➤ Basics

6. Define anxiety reaction.

   HPND ➤ Anxiety Reaction

7. Part of the therapy may be to determine Roberta's perception of her health. What is the purpose of this?

   HlthAssess ➤ Health Perception, Health Management Pattern, Components of the Nursing Health History ➤ Information

8. While in the unit, Roberta develops a case of the "runs." What is this?

   5MCC ➤ Runs, the ➤ Basics

9. What general measures should be offered to Roberta while she is experiencing the symptoms described in question 8?

   5MCC ➤ Runs, the ➤ Treatment

➤ Advanced Case Studies

CASE STUDY I • *Mrs. Gonzalez*

Cross-Discipline Learning Activities

1. What is the DSM-IV-TR?

   HPND ➤ DSM ➤ Definition

2. What is Bipolar I?

   PsychThrp ➤ Main Index ➤ scroll down to Manic Depressive States ➤ Diagnosis of, Criteria for ➤ General Diagnostic Considerations

3. What is one-to-one observation?

   5MCC ➤ Main Index ➤ Suicide ➤ Treatment ➤ scroll down to Activity

4. What behaviors reflect rapid cycling?

   PsychThrp ➤ Main Index ➤ Manic Depressive States ➤ General Diagnostic Considerations ➤ scroll down to Rapid Cycling Mania

5. What is mania?

   PsychThrp ➤ Main Index ➤ scroll down to Manic Depressive States ➤ Diagnosis of, Criteria for ➤ General Diagnostic Considerations ➤ scroll down to Manic Episodes ➤ Table 19.1
   NDisCheck ➤ Mania ➤ Overview

6. What is depression?

PsychThrp → Main Index → scroll down to Manic Depressive States → Diagnosis of, Criteria for → General Diagnostic Considerations → scroll down to Depressive Episodes → Table 18.1
NDisCheck → Depression → Bipolar Disorder → Overview
5MCC → Depression → Basics

7. What are mood stabilizing anticonvulsant agents?

PsychThrp → Main Index → scroll down to Manic Depressive States → Mood Stabilizing Anticonvulsant Agents

8. What is elopement monitoring?

NurProc → Index → Elopement Monitoring → Introduction

Discipline-Specific Learning Activities

Nursing

1. What nursing considerations are associated with assessment of the patient's mental status and potential for suicide?

PsychThrp → Main Index → scroll down to Suicide and Risk of . . . → Mental Status Examination
NDisCheck → Suicide Prevention Guidelines → Information

2. What mnemonic can be used to assess suicide risk factors?

5MCC → Main Index → Suicide → scroll down to SAD PERSONS

3. What changes will need to occur within the patient's environment?

5MCC → Main Index → Suicide → Treatment
NDisCheck → Suicide Prevention Guidelines → scroll to Provide a Safe Environment

4. What are important nursing interventions and documentation measures for a patient on elopement monitoring?

NurProc → Index → Elopement Monitoring → Implementation → Documentation

5. What is Divalproex? What is the therapeutic serum level?

PsychThrp → Main Index → scroll down to Manic Depressive States → Mood Stabilizing Anticonvulsant Agents → Divalproex (Valproate)
PDH → Divalproex Sodium → Trade Name → Pharmacodynamics
LNDG → Divalproex Sodium → Nursing Considerations → scroll down to Interventions (last bullet)

6. What adverse gastrointestinal (GI) effects are possible with administration of Divalproex?

   PsychThrp → Main Index → scroll down to Manic Depressive States → Mood Stabilizing Anticonvulsant Agents → Divalproex (Valproate)
   PDH → Divalproex Sodium → Adverse Reactions
   LNDG → Divalproex Sodium → Adverse Effects

7. What inhibitory neurotransmitter does Divalproex (valproate) affect?

   PsychThrp → Main Index → Valproate → Pharmacologic Treatments → Valproate (second bullet) GABA
   PDH → Divalproex Sodium → Pharmacodynamics
   LNDG → Divalproex Sodium → Therapeutic Actions

8. What must the nurse assess for regarding Mrs. Gonzalez's right arm sprain?

   NDisCheck → Sprains and Strains → Monitoring → Edema, Pain Control, ROM, Response to Treatment
   5MCC → Sprains and Strains → Follow-Up

9. What are common characteristics of a sprain?

   NDisCheck → Sprains and Strains → Outline → scroll down to Common Characteristics → Localized Pain, Swelling and Warmth, Progressive Loss of Motion, and Ecchymosis
   5MCC → Sprains and Strains → Basics

10. How would nursing aid the patient in promoting interest in food to minimize weight loss?

    NurProc → Index → Feeding → Introduction → Identifying Food Preferences

Medicine/NP/PA

1. What laboratory studies would you expect to order for Mrs. Gonzalez before initiating Divalproex (divalproex sodium)?

   PsychThrp → Main Index → Bipolar Disorders → Treatment of, Pharmacotherapy, Divalproate
   PDH → Divalproex Sodium → Effects on Lab Test Results
   LNDG → Divalproex Sodium → Nursing Considerations → scroll down to Assessment (second bullet)

2. How much Divalproex should the patient be prescribed initially?

   PsychThrp → Main Index → Manic Depressive States → Valproate
   PDH → Divalproex Sodium → Indications and Dosages
   LNDG → Divalproex Sodium → Dosages

3. What is the therapeutic serum level for Divalproex?

PsychThrp → Main Index → Manic Depressive States → Valproate
PDH → Divalproex Sodium → Pharmacokinetics
LNDG → Divalproex Sodium → Nursing Considerations → scroll down to
Interventions (last bullet)

4. When would you expect the onset of action to occur?

PsychThrp → Main Index → Bipolar Disorder → Treatment of, Pharma-
cotherapy, Divalproate
PDH → Divalproex Sodium → Pharmacokinetics
LNDG → Divalproex Sodium → Pharmacodynamics

5. What imaging tests may be ordered to rule out further complications of the sprain?

NDisCheck → Sprains → Assessment → scroll down to Imaging → X-ray
to r/o (rule out) Fracture and Confirm Damage to Ligaments
5MCC → Sprains and Strains → Diagnosis

6. What medications may be useful to alleviate Mrs. Gonzalez's pain?

NDisCheck → Sprains → Medication → Analgesics → Nonsteroidal Anti-
inflammatory Drugs
5MCC → Sprains and Strains → Medications

Physical and Occupational Therapy

1. What types of hand exercises would be useful for Mrs. Gonzalez?

NDisCheck → Sprains → Treatment → ROM Exercises

2. What supportive measures would be useful in promoting comfort to Mrs. Gonzalez?

NDisCheck → Sprains → Treatment → Wrapping in Elastic Bandage
5MCC → Sprains and Strains → Treatment

Behavioral Health

1. Why is a comprehensive psychosocial assessment required for Mrs. Gonzalez?

PsychThrp → Manic Depressive → Epidemiology of → Increase
Understanding of Shortened Periods Between Episodes of Bipolar Disorder

2. What education is needed for families in recognizing Mrs. Gonzalez's mood liability?

PsychThrp → Bipolar Disorder → Treatment of, Psycho Education → Life Chart
PsychThrp → Main Index → Manic Depressive States → Introduction to →
General Treatment Considerations

3. Mrs. Gonzalez will receive outpatient treatment after discharge. The couple requests additional information on support groups. What other therapeutic interventions would you suggest as part of the patient discharge planning process?

   Psych Thrp → Main Index → scroll down to Manic Depressive States → Introduction to → General Treatment Considerations

CASE STUDY 2 • *Mrs. Griffin*

Cross-Discipline Learning Activities

1. What is ECT?

   PsychThrp → ECT → scroll down to Overview → Introduction
   HPND → ECT

2. What is major depression? What causes it?

   PsychThrp → Depression → Clinical Features of → Diagnostic Features of Major Depressive Disorder → Depressed Mood, Change in Appetite
   5MCC → Depression → Description
   PsychThrp → Depression → Etiology of → Biologic/Psychosocial Theories
   5MCC → Depression → Description
   NDisCheck → Depression → Major Depression → Overview → scroll down to Causes

3. What are psychotic features?

   PsychThrp → Psychosis → Delusions, Hallucinations, Disorganized Speech, Catatonic Behavior

4. What is computed tomography and EEG?

   HPND → Computed Tomography → CAT, Computed Tomography
   HPND → EEG → Electroencephalogram

5. What are atypical antipsychotic medications?

   5MCC → Schizophrenia → Treatment → Medications → Atypical

6. What is NIDDM?

   HPND → Diabetes → NIDDM → Non-Insulin Dependent Diabetes Mellitus
   5MCC → NIDDM → Basics

Discipline-Specific Learning Activities

Nursing

1. For what changes should the nurse assess in the EEG following ECT?

   PsychThrp → ECT → Complications of → Cardiovascular Effects → ST Segment Depression, T-Wave Inversion

2. What cognitive changes may be present after ECT?

PsychThrp → ECT → Complications of → Adverse Cognitive Effects → Anterograde/Retrograde Amnesia

3. What are Axis I and Axis II disorders according to the DSM-IV-TR?

HPND → DSM → Definition → Axis I Clinical Disorders, Axis II Personality Disorders and Mental Retardation

4. What is an SNRI? What two neurotransmitters are blocked from reuptake?

5MCC → Depression → Rx → Others → Venlafaxine → Serotonin Norepinephrine Reuptake Inhibitor

5. What common side effects occur with patients taking Effexor (venlafaxine)?

5MCC → Depression → Rx → Others → Venlafaxine → Serotonin Norepinephrine Reuptake Inhibitor → Insomnia, Anorexia, Anxiety
PsychThrp → Olanzapine → Psychotic Depression → Venlafaxine → Nausea, Drowsiness

Medicine/NP/PA

1. What are some indications that would place a patient at increased risk if he or she received ECT?

PsychThrp → ECT → Indications → Medical Conditions Associated with Increased Risk → Recent MI, Unstable Angina

2. To minimize the cognitive side effects of ECT, would you use unilateral or bilateral electrode placement? Explain.

PsychThrp → ECT → Indications → scroll down to Modifications in Electrode Placement and Treatment Frequency

3. What medications may increase the seizure threshold, thereby diminishing the efficacy of unilateral ECT?

PsychThrp → ECT → Indications → Modifications in Electrode Placement and Treatment Frequency → Benzodiazepines, Barbiturates, Anticonvulsants

4. What deviations in laboratory findings are expected of someone who is dehydrated?

5MCC → Dehydration, Hypertonic → Diagnosis → Laboratory → Elevated Sodium (Na)

5. At what dosage would you initiate both olanzapine and Effexor?

PsychThrp → Olanzapine → Psychotic Depression → Venlafaxine → 75–375 mg/day or a modal dose of 250 mg/day
5MCC → Schizophrenia → Olanzapine → 7.5–25 mg/day

Physical and Occupational Therapy

What mechanisms would serve as a support to facilitate movement and improve balance?

NurProc ➤ Canes ➤ Introduction ➤ Supports Walking, Decreases Strain on Weight Bearing Joints
NDisCheck ➤ Arthritis ➤ Rheumatoid ➤ Treatment ➤ Splinting, ROM, Moist Heat

Behavioral Health

1. In addition to psychopharmacologic interventions for depression, what types of psychosocial approaches to treatment are available to Mrs. Griffin?

   PsychThrp ➤ Depression ➤ Psychosocial Treatment for ➤ Psychodynamic Therapies, Experiential-Expressive Therapies, Cognitive Behavior Therapies, Interpersonal Therapy

2. What referrals would be helpful in receiving outpatient support?

   NDisCheck ➤ Arthritis, Rheumatoid ➤ Patient Teaching ➤ Discharge Planning ➤ Refer for PT, OT, Arthritis Foundation

3. What patient education should occur before discharge?

   5MCC ➤ Depression ➤ Treatment ➤ Patient Education ➤ Teach about Each Medication, Referrals to Support Groups, Stress Need for Long-Term Treatment and Follow-Up
   5MCC ➤ Arthritis, Rheumatoid ➤ Follow-Up ➤ Patient Monitoring
   NDisCheck ➤ Arthritis, Rheumatoid ➤ Patient Teaching

CASE STUDY 3 • *Mrs. Anderson*

Cross-Discipline Learning Activities

1. What is serotonin syndrome? What are the symptoms?

   5MCC ➤ Main Index ➤ Suicide ➤ Rx ➤ Significant Possible Interactions
   PsychThrp ➤ Olanzapine ➤ Overdose, Discussion and Treatment of ➤ Toxic Serotonin Syndrome

2. What does SSRI indicate?

   5MCC ➤ Main Index ➤ Suicide ➤ Rx ➤ Drug(s) of Choice

3. What is a standardized rating scale?

   5MCC ➤ Main Index ➤ Depression ➤ Diagnostic Procedures ➤ Validated Standard Rating Scales ➤ Zung's Self-Rating Depression Scale

4. What is a second-degree burn?

HPND → Burn → Second Degree → Burn Involving the Epidermis and Dermis
5MCC → Burns → Basics → Involves Varying Degrees of the Epidermis
NDisCheck → Burns → Overview

5. What is BSA?

5MCC → Burns → Treatment → BSA
HPND → BSA

Discipline-Specific Learning Activities

Nursing

1. What are some common side effects of SSRIs?

5MCC → Depression → Medications (Rx) → Insomnia, Anxiety

2. What education must be provided regarding discontinuation of SSRIs?

5MCC → Depression → Medications (Rx) → Precautions → SSRIs: Abrupt
Discontinuation May Result in Withdrawal Symptoms

3. Why is there a contraindication with patients taking Hypericum perforatum
and SSRIs?

PsychThrp → Olanzapine → Overdose, Discussion, and Treatment of →
scroll down to Toxic Serotonin Syndrome

4. What rating scale could be used in identifying depressed patients?

5MCC → Depression → Diagnosis → scroll down to Diagnostic Procedures →
Validated Rating Scales → BDI, CES-D

5. What educational interventions are necessary for the patient's continued
compliance even when she feels better?

5MCC → Depression → Follow-Up → Explain that the Treatment Must Continue Even after Improvement
NDisCheck → Depression → Major Depression → Patient Teaching

6. What assessments are needed when caring for a patient with a second-
degree burn?

5MCC → Burns → Diagnosis → Pathological Findings → Second Degree:
The Degree of Coagulation Necrosis, Skin Appendages Intact
NDisCheck → Burns → Nursing Considerations → scroll down to Monitoring

7. What self-care teaching should occur with the patient?

NurProc → Burn Care → Patient Teaching → Successful Burn Care after
Discharge → Self Care → Eat Well-Balanced Meals; Avoid Tobacco, Alcohol,

Caffeine Because They Constrict Peripheral Flow

NDisCheck → Burns → Patient Teaching

5MCC → Burns → Treatment → scroll down to Patient Education

Medicine/NP/PA

1. What dosage of medication would be prescribed for the patient?

    PsychThrp → Depression → Pharmacotherapy for → Selective Serotonin Reuptake Inhibitor → Some SSRI Pharmacokinetic and Dosage Data → Daily Dose Range 20–40 mg/day

2. If treatment is adequate, what is the approximate time period before depression improves?

    5MCC → Depression → Follow-Up → 4 Weeks after Initiating Treatment

3. What topical cream may be ordered to apply to the burn site?

    5MCC → Burns → Medication (Rx) → Drug(s) of Choice → Silvadene

4. What laboratory test might you order?

    5MCC → Burns → Diagnosis → scroll down to Diagnostic Procedures → Bronchoscopy

5. How would you ensure proper nutritional interventions?

    5MCC → Burns → Treatment → Diet → High Protein, High Calorie

    NurProc → Burn Care → Special Considerations → Extra Protein and Carbohydrates

Physical and Occupational Therapy

1. Why is movement important for Mrs. Anderson?

    5MCC → Burns → Follow-Up → Possible Complications → Decreased Mobility May Promote Future Flexion Contractures

2. What documentation by the physical/occupational therapist should occur for a patient with second-degree burns?

    NurProc → Burn Care → Documentation → Wound Condition, Special Dressing Change Techniques, Topical Medications

3. What is the activity goal for such a patient?

    5MCC → Burns → Treatment → scroll down to Activity

Behavioral Health

1. Besides psychopharmacologic interventions, what other measures (psychosocial) would be prescribed to assist the patient in restoring her normal level of well-being?

   NurProc → Burn Care → Patient Teaching → Encouragement and Emotional Support, Burn Survivor Support Group
   NDisCheck → Burns → Patient Teaching → scroll down to Discharge Planning
   PsychThrp → National Alliance for the Mentally III → Information → Support Group

2. In arranging the patient's outpatient follow-up, what relevance does the therapeutic alliance have in the success of treatment for depression?

   5MCC → Depression → Follow-Up → Patient Monitoring → Therapeutic Alliance is Very Important

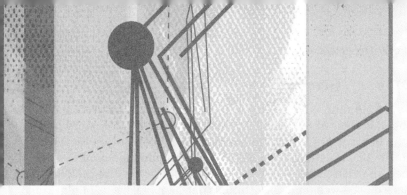

12

Community Health and Home Care Case Studies

Francine Gelo

C ommunity health nurses act as advocates and educators for individuals, families, and communities. They are in a unique position to assess the factors that contribute to the health of the community and to develop health promotion and health education programs to address those needs; they provide health care to diverse populations anywhere in the community—in schools, churches, health clinics, social service agencies, and the home.

➤ General Case Studies

For the following three case studies you will need to download and install the trial versions of these references:

- Griffith's 5-Minute Clinical Consult (5MCC)
- Nurse's Quick Check: Diseases (NDisCheck)
- Nursing Drug Handbook (NDH)
- Nurses' Handbook of Health Assessment (HlthAssess)

CASE STUDY 1 • *George*

George is a 34-year-old man who has come to the clinic with gastrointestinal problems that have increased over the last few weeks. He has a history of hypertension for the last 3 years, which he has medication for, but, in his words, he doesn't need. He has a plethoric facies and poor oral and personal hygiene. When questioned, he does state that he drinks at least a six-pack every evening, and more on the weekend, and thinks that he has periods of blacking out. He has not had a drink in 2 days and believes he is having withdrawal symptoms.

1. Is there a genetic correlation with alcohol abuse?
2. What is the predominant age of alcohol abuse?
3. What are some risk factors with a patient who has a substance abuse and dependency problem?
4. What are associated conditions with a patient with a diagnosis of alcohol abuse?
5. George is given Campral. What is the drug class of this medication?
6. What contraindications and cautions should be evaluated before administering Campral to George?
7. If George were given an abdominal assessment, what should be included in the objective data?

CASE STUDY 2 • *Chip*

Chip is a 24-year-old man who presents to the clinic with severe fatigue, frequent infections and fevers lasting more than 1 month, unexplained weight loss, and persistent diarrhea. He is sexually active, having sex with both men and women, without protection on occasion. He is diagnosed with human immunodeficiency virus (HIV).

1. What is the description of HIV?
2. What is the classification of AZT?
3. How is a diagnosis of HIV made?
4. When treating a patient with HIV, what diet education should be given?
5. What opportunistic infections may a patient with HIV acquire?
6. Chip is also diagnosed with pneumocystis pneumonia (PCP). What is PCP?
7. What patient monitoring should be included in someone diagnosed with PCP?
8. What are the drugs of choice for a patient diagnosed with HIV?

CASE STUDY 3 • *Eileen*

Eileen, a 31-year-old police officer in a local suburban community, presents to you with a chief complaint of chronic diarrhea, muscle cramps, unintended weight loss, fatigue, and general malaise. She is diagnosed with celiac disease.

1. What is the description of celiac disease?
2. What are the signs and symptoms of celiac disease?
3. Eileen will need patient teaching regarding a gluten-free diet. What are alternatives?
4. What are possible complications in a patient who is diagnosed with celiac disease?
5. What medication may be used in cases of refractory sprue?
6. Education of a patient with celiac disease is very important. Where should a patient be directed for additional support?
7. Eileen states that she has allergic rhinitis. When you look at her, what common physical findings do you note?
8. What is the course of treatment for a patient with allergic rhinitis?

➤ Advanced Case Studies

For the next three case studies, you will need to download full versions of the following references:

- Griffith's 5-Minute Clinical Consult (5MCC)
- Handbook of Diagnostic Tests (HbDxTests)
- Lippincott's Nursing Drug Guide (LNDG) *or* Physician's Drug Handbook (PDH)
- Manual of Psychiatric Therapeutics (PsychThrp)
- Nurses' Handbook of Health Assessment (HlthAssess)
- Nurse's Quick Check: Diseases (NDisCheck) *or* 5MCC
- Nursing Procedures (NurProc)
- Physical Medicine and Rehabilitation Pocketpedia (PMRRx)
- Stedman's Medical Dictionary for the Health Professions and Nursing (HPND)
- Taylor's Clinical Nursing Skills (ClinSkills)

CASE STUDY 1 • *Kim*

Kim is a 38-year-old African American single mother of two children, living in public housing with her boyfriend in a two-story apartment. This is her first visit to her community health clinic in 14 months; she presents complaining of depression, fatigue, intermittent and transient weakness of her extremities, and a sudden blurring of vision in one eye for 2 to 3 months. Her weakened physical condition and money problems have left her frustrated and anxious about her symptoms. She does not want any member of her family to know her diagnosis for fear that they may interfere with her children. Review of her medical records reveals a diagnosis of multiple sclerosis (MS) after an MRI and lab studies. She was given a referral to a neurologist, but she has never followed up. On exam today she had decreased distal strength in legs, blurred vision with pain in left eye, and a positive Babinski's sign on the right.

Cross-Discipline Learning Activities

1. What is MS?
2. In an adult neurologic assessment, what are two focus questions asked to elicit subjective data?
3. What is a Babinski's sign?
4. What are possible causes of MS?

Discipline-Specific Learning Activities

Nursing

1. Kim is at risk for falls in her home; what teaching should she receive?
2. Kim is sexually active and has not had a PAP test in over 3 years. Give three examples of objective data obtained from a routine GYN exam.
3. What does PAP stand for?
4. Kim will need to give herself weekly injections of Avonex; explain the technique for intramuscular injections.

Medicine/NP/PA

1. What is present in an MRI that suggests a diagnosis of MS?
2. Beta interferon is used to treat MS; what is the action of this class of drug?
3. What are two differential diagnoses for MS?

Physical and Occupational Therapy

1. What are some goals of rehabilitation management for patients with MS?
2. Define range of motion (ROM) exercises.

Behavioral Health

Kim's MS may mask signs of depression. A mental status exam should be done. What are four elements of a mental status exam?

Critical Thinking—Correlating Patient Data/Assessment Findings to Plan Care

Kim is a high risk patient who refuses to return to the clinic for her care. She continues to bring her children to see the primary care provider and remains friendly with the staff, but denies any problems. She does not want any help from her family and refuses to share her diagnosis with them. What is the core of the principle of patient-provider confidentiality? What community resources may be available to Kim?

CASE STUDY 2 • *Florence*

Florence is a 45-year-old African American woman who is distressed about fatigue, vision problems, and frequent vaginal yeast infections over the last year. Teary and anxious, she reports feeling depressed and not sleeping well. Her history reveals irregular menstrual periods, frequent urination, thirst, and tingling in her feet. She has asthma that has been controlled with inhalers as needed. However, at least once a year Florence has needed steroids to control an acute episode. On exam, she is obese with dry skin, and lungs reveal wheezing. She suspects that she has symptoms of "sugar," which runs in her family. Assessment finds the following data: weight 245 lb, height 5'3", random glucose 234, BP 152/88, HR 86.

Florence is diagnosed with type II diabetes, asthma, hypertension, and obesity. During the discussion of planning for her care, she states, "Everyone in my family dies young; there is nothing that can be done."

Cross-Discipline Learning Activities

1. What is type II diabetes mellitus (DM)?
2. What conditions are associated with type II DM?
3. What is the plan for follow-up for patients with DM?

Discipline-Specific Learning Activities

Nursing

1. What are the three "Ps" of symptoms of type II diabetes?
2. What equipment is needed to perform blood glucose testing?
3. What are the educational needs of a patient with diabetes?
4. Florence needs a nutritional assessment; what are two components of this type of assessment?
5. What are two nursing diagnoses that illustrate Florence's self-management ability?

Medicine/PA/NP

1. What lab tests need to be done to evaluate Florence's DM?
2. Diabetics can suffer many complications; list three.
3. Glucophage (metformin hydrochloride) is commonly used in the treatment of type II DM; how does it work?
4. Florence needs methylprednisolone (Medrol) at times for acute asthma; what effect does this drug have on blood sugar?

Physical and Occupational Therapy

1. How do diabetics benefit from aerobic exercise?
2. What is aerobic exercise?
3. What are the therapeutic benefits of exercise for patients with diabetes?

Behavioral Health

Depression can limit a patient's ability to be actively involved in his or her medical treatment.

1. What are the symptoms of depression?
2. What kind of subjective data should be obtained from Florence about how she manages health concerns?

Critical Thinking—Correlating Patient Data/Assessment Findings to Plan Care

Florence suffers from diabetes, asthma, hypertension, and obesity. It is important to help her understand that she can influence the course of her medical conditions. What strategies could you use to help Florence? What should you consider next in a comprehensive plan of care? Discuss components of a multidisciplinary approach to assist Florence.

CASE STUDY 3   •   *Tom*

During a community screening for hypertension (HTN), Tom, a 59-year-old man, is found to have a blood pressure (BP) of 164/88 on his left arm and 178/96 on his right. He denies any symptoms and reveals that high BP runs in his family and that it has never really been a problem. He has not been to a medical provider in many years and has no insurance. Tom is overweight, a smoker, and appears slightly short of breath (SOB) with activity. He is strongly encouraged to visit a primary care provider as soon as possible and is directed to a community health center; he refuses because he cannot afford the costs without insurance.

Two weeks later he walks in to the health center asking for care and seems anxious and worried about his health. His vital signs are as follows: BP 176/94 on the left, 192/100 on the right, heart rate 108; respirations 16; weight 240 lb, height 5'9".

Cross-Discipline Learning Activities

1. What is hypertension?
2. What is the difference between primary and secondary hypertension?
3. Hypertension can cause serious medical problems; list three.

Discipline-Specific Learning Activities

Nursing

1. What elements of care must be monitored in a patient with high blood pressure?
2. What dietary information does Tom need?
3. How does the size of the blood pressure cuff affect the reading?

Medicine/NP/PA

The treatment of hypertension is aimed at decreasing vascular resistance (making the artery larger and more pliant). Two classes of drugs that are used to decrease vascular resistance are angiotensin receptor blockers (ARBs) and angiotensin-converting enzymes (ACE). The following questions relate to this treatment modality.

1. What lab tests should be ordered for this patient in a clinic visit?
2. What is the therapeutic action of Cozaar?
3. What is an example of an ACE inhibitor-type drug?

Physical and Occupational Therapy

Tom expressed a desire to change his lifestyle, lose weight, stop smoking, and change his diet. He was given a referral to a physical/occupational therapist for an exercise program and decided to try hypnosis for smoking and anxiety.

1. What are isometric exercises?
2. Why should isometric exercises be avoided in patients with hypertension?

Behavioral Health

1. What is the purpose of assessing a patient's coping and stress tolerance pattern?
2. Give an example of a hypnosis technique used to reduce anxiety.

Critical Thinking—Correlating Patient Data/Assessment Findings to Plan Care

Tom has made lifestyle choices that contributed to his development of hypertension, and he is scared and anxious. He has expressed readiness to change bad habits and is asking for help; he is at risk for heart disease, stroke, diabetes, and lung disease. Tom's strongest asset is his willingness to change his habits. Discuss additional considerations that would help Tom succeed in his efforts to change his behavior.

Chapter Summary—Tying It All Together

You have explored several patient scenarios typical for a community setting. In each case, the patient presented with complex health problems that are not uncommon in this setting. Providing care to patients in community settings requires a multidisciplinary approach to ensure that all aspects—physiologic and psychosocial—are addressed. This setting poses additional challenges because services from the different disciplines are often dispersed, geographically and across agencies, making communication between providers more difficult. As in other health care settings, it is imperative that providers strive to maintain interdisciplinary collaboration to provide optimal care with the goal of improving the patient's quality of life and supporting their self management goals.

 Visit http://thePoint.LWW.com/cornelius for supplemental information and activities.

ANSWERS TO CASE STUDY QUESTIONS

➤ General Case Studies

CASE STUDY 1 • *George*

1. Is there a genetic correlation with alcohol abuse?

   5MCC ➤ Alcohol Use Disorder ➤ Basics ➤ Genetics

2. What is the predominant age of alcohol abuse?

   5MCC ➤ Alcohol Use Disorders ➤ Basics ➤ Predominant Age

3. What are some risk factors with a patient who has a substance abuse and dependency problem?

   NDisCheck ➤ Substance Abuse and Dependency ➤ Overview ➤ Risk Factors

4. What are associated conditions with a patient with a diagnosis of alcohol abuse?

   5MCC ➤ Alcohol Use Disorders ➤ Miscellaneous

5. George is given Campral. What is the drug class of this medication?

   NDH ➤ Campral ➤ General

6. What contraindications and cautions should be evaluated before administering Campral to George?

   NDH ➤ Campral ➤ Contraindications and Cautions

7. If George were given an abdominal assessment, what should be included in the objective data?

   HlthAssess ➤ Adult Assessment, Abdominal Assessment ➤ Information ➤ Objective Data: Assessment Techniques

CASE STUDY 2 • *Chip*

1. What is the description of HIV?

   5MCC ➤ HIV Infection and AIDS ➤ Basics

2. What is the classification of AZT?

   NDH ➤ AZT ➤ Classification

3. How is a diagnosis of HIV made?

   5MCC ➤ HIV Infection and AIDS ➤ Diagnosis

4. When treating a patient with HIV, what diet education should be given?

   5MCC ➤ HIV Infection and AIDS ➤ Treatment

5. What opportunistic infections may a patient with HIV acquire?

   5MCC ➤ HIV Infection and AIDS ➤ Miscellaneous

6. Chip is also diagnosed with pneumocystis pneumonia (PCP). What is PCP?

   5MCC ➤ Pneumonia, Pneumocystis ➤ Basics

7. What patient monitoring should be included in someone diagnosed with PCP?

   5MCC ➤ Pneumonia, Pneumocystis ➤ Follow-Up

8. What are the drugs of choice for a patient diagnosed with HIV?

   5MCC ➤ HIV Infection and AIDS ➤ Medications

CASE STUDY 3 • *Eileen*

1. What is the description of celiac disease?

   5MCC ➤ Celiac Disease ➤ Basics

2. What are the signs and symptoms of celiac disease?

   5MCC ➤ Celiac Disease ➤ Basics

3. Eileen will need patient teaching regarding a gluten-free diet. What are alternatives?

   5MCC ➤ Celiac Disease ➤ Treatment

4. What are possible complications in a patient who is diagnosed with celiac disease?

   5MCC ➤ Celiac Disease ➤ Follow-Up

5. What medication may be used in cases of refractory sprue?

5MCC ➤ Celiac Disease ➤ Medication

6. Education of a patient with celiac disease is very important. Where should a patient be directed for additional support?

5MCC ➤ Celiac Disease ➤ Treatment

7. Eileen states that she has allergic rhinitis. When you look at her, what common physical findings do you note?

NDisCheck ➤ Allergic Rhinitis ➤ Assessment ➤ Physical Findings

8. What is the course of treatment for a patient with allergic rhinitis?

NDisCheck ➤ Allergic Rhinitis ➤ Treatment

➤ Advanced Case Studies

CASE STUDY I • *Kim*

Cross-Discipline Learning Activities

1. What is MS?

5MCC ➤ Multiple Sclerosis ➤ Basics
NDisCheck ➤ Overview

2. In an adult neurologic assessment, what are two focus questions asked to elicit subjective data?

HlthAssess ➤ Main Index ➤ Neurologic Assessment ➤ Adult

3. What is a Babinski's sign?

HPND ➤ Babinski's Sign

4. What are possible causes of MS?

NDisCheck ➤ Main Index ➤ Multiple Sclerosis ➤ Causes
5MCC ➤ Multiple Sclerosis ➤ Basics

Discipline-Specific Learning Activities

Nursing

1. Kim is at risk for falls in her home; what teaching should she receive?

NurProc ➤ Procedure Index ➤ Fall Prevention ➤ Patient Teaching ➤ scroll down to Promoting Safety in the Home

2. Kim is sexually active and has not had a PAP smear in over 3 years. Give three examples of objective data obtained from a routine GYN exam.

   HlthAssess ⇀ Table of Contents ⇀ Genitourinary-Reproductive Assessment ⇀ Adult Assessment

3. What does PAP stand for?

   HPND ⇀ PAP

4. Kim will need to give herself weekly injections of Avonex; explain the technique for intramuscular injections.

   ClinSkills ⇀ Intramuscular Injection

Medicine/NP/PA

1. What is present in an MRI that suggests a diagnosis of MS?

   HbDxTests ⇀ Main Index ⇀ Multiple Sclerosis

2. Beta interferon is used to treat MS; what is the action of this class of drug?

   LNDG ⇀ Drug Index ⇀ Beta Interferon
   PDH ⇀ Beta Interferon ⇀ Classification

3. What are two differential diagnoses for MS?

   5MCC ⇀ Multiple Sclerosis ⇀ Basics ⇀ Diagnosis

Physical and Occupational Therapy

1. What are some goals of rehabilitation management for patients with MS?

   PMRRx ⇀ Multiple Sclerosis ⇀ Clinical Categories and Treatment

2. Define range of motion (ROM) exercises.

   HPND ⇀ Range of Motion

Behavioral Health

Kim's MS may mask signs of depression. A mental status exam should be done. What are four elements of a mental status exam?

PsychThrp ⇀ Main Index ⇀ Mental Status Exam

CASE STUDY 2 • *Florence*

Cross-Discipline Learning Activities

1. What is type II diabetes mellitus (DM)?

   5MCC ⇀ Adult Onset Diabetes ⇀ Basics
   NDisCheck ⇀ Diabetes Mellitus ⇀ Overview

2. What conditions are associated with type II DM?

   5MCC → Diabetes → Miscellaneous
   NDisCheck → Diabetes Mellitus → Overview → Risk Factors

3. What is the plan for follow-up for patients with DM?

   5MCC → Diabetes, Adult Onset → Follow-Up
   NDisCheck → Diabetes Mellitus → Patient Teaching → scroll down
   to Discharge Planning

Discipline-Specific Learning Activities

Nursing

1. What are the three "Ps" of symptoms of type II diabetes?

   5MCC → Diabetes Adult → Basics → scroll down to Signs and Symptoms
   NDisCheck → Overview → scroll down to Common Characteristics

2. What equipment is needed to perform blood glucose testing?

   NurProc → Blood Glucose Test → Equipment

3. What are the educational needs of a patient with diabetes?

   5MCC → Diabetes Adult → Treatment
   NDisCheck → Diabetes → Patient Teaching

4. Florence needs a nutritional assessment; what are two components of this type of assessment?

   HlthAssess → Table of Contents → Nutritional Assessment

5. What are two nursing diagnoses that illustrate Florence's self-management ability?

   HlthAssess → Table of Contents → Health Perception—Health
   Management → Diagnosis

Medicine/PA/NP

1. What lab tests need to be done to evaluate Florence's DM?

   HbDxTest → Diabetes
   5MCC → Diabetes → Follow-Up → scroll down to Patient Monitoring (second
   through fourth bullets)
   NDisCheck → Diabetes → Treatment → scroll down to General (fourth bullet)

2. Diabetics can suffer many complications; list three.

   NDisCheck → Diabetes → Overview → scroll down to Complications
   5MCC → Diabetes → Follow-Up → scroll down to Complications

3. Glucophage (metformin hydrochloride) is commonly used in the treatment of type II DM; how does it work?

    LNDG ➔ Glucophage ➔ Therapeutic Actions
    PDH ➔ Glucophage ➔ Pharmacodynamics

4. Florence needs methylprednisolone (Medrol) at times for acute asthma; what effect does this drug have on blood sugar?

    LNDG ➔ Methylprednisolone ➔ Adverse Effects
    PDH ➔ Methylprednisolone ➔ Adverse Reactions

Physical and Occupational Therapy

1. How do diabetics benefit from aerobic exercise?

    PMRRx ➔ Table of Contents ➔ Therapeutic Exercise

2. What is aerobic exercise?

    HPND ➔ Aerobics

3. What are the therapeutic benefits of exercise for patients with diabetes?

    PMRRx ➔ Table of Contents ➔ Therapeutic Exercise Aerobic

Behavioral Health

1. What are the symptoms of depression?

    PsychThrp ➔ Depression

2. What kind of subjective data should be obtained from Florence about how she manages health concerns?

    HlthAssess ➔ Table of Contents ➔ Health Perception—Health Management

CASE STUDY 3 • *Tom*

Cross-Discipline Learning Activities

1. What is hypertension?

    NDisCheck ➔ Hypertension ➔ Overview
    5MCC ➔ Hypertension ➔ Basics
    HPND ➔ Hypertension

2. What is the difference between primary and secondary hypertension?

    5MCC ➔ Hypertension ➔ Basics ➔ scroll down to Causes (first and second bullets)
    NDisCheck ➔ Hypertension ➔ Assessment

3. Hypertension can cause serious medical problems; list three.

   5MCC → Hypertension → Follow-Up → scroll down to Complications
   NDisCheck → Hypertension → Overview → scroll down to Complications

Discipline-Specific Learning Activities

Nursing

1. What elements of care must be monitored in a patient with high blood pressure?

   5MCC → Hypertension → Follow-Up → scroll down to Patient Monitoring
   NDisCheck → Hypertension → Nursing Considerations

2. What dietary information does Tom need?

   NDisCheck → Hypertension → Treatment → scroll down to General (third bullet)
   5MCC → Hypertension → Treatment

3. How does the size of the blood pressure cuff affect the reading?

   NurProc → Blood Pressure

Medicine/PA/NP

1. What lab tests should be ordered for this patient in a clinic visit?

   5MCC → Hypertension → Diagnosis
   NDisCheck → Hypertension → Assessment → scroll down to Laboratory

2. What is the therapeutic action of Cozaar?

   LNDG → Cozaar → Therapeutic Action
   PDH → Cozaar → Pharmacodynamics

3. What is an example of an ACE inhibitor-type drug?

   LNDG → Drug Class Index → Angiotensin-Converting Enzyme Inhibitor → General
   PDH → Angiotensin-Converting Enzyme Inhibitor → Drugs

Physical and Occupational Therapy

1. What are isometric exercises?

   PMRRx → Therapeutic Exercise → Strength Training

2. Why should isometric exercises be avoided in patients with hypertension?

   PMRRx → Table of Contents → Therapeutic Exercise

Behavioral Health

1. What is the purpose of assessing a patient's coping and stress tolerance pattern?

   HlthAssess ⇀ Table of Contents ⇀ Components of Nursing Health History

2. Give an example of a hypnosis technique used to reduce anxiety.

   PsychThrp ⇀ Table of Contents ⇀ Medical Uses of Hypnosis

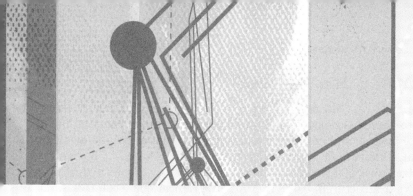

13

Gerontologic Case Studies

Judith L. Draper

The case studies in this chapter focus on the care of older patients with specialized needs. As with the previous case studies, these patients are complex and have additional concerns and needs beyond the primary gerontologic issues. The goal of health care providers working with patients with gerontologic health issues is to provide comprehensive care to enhance the quality of life for those affected by changes in functional levels and chronic illness. This type of care requires a multidisciplinary approach to achieve success.

➤ General Case Studies

For the following three case studies, you will need to download the trial versions of these references:

- Lippincott's Nursing Drug Guide (LNDG)
- Manual of Psychiatric Therapeutics (PsychThrp)
- Nurse's Quick Check: Diseases (NDisCheck)
- Physician's Drug Handbook (PDH)
- Stedman's Medical Dictionary for the Health Professions and Nursing (HPND)

CASE STUDY 1 • *Mrs. Paulson*

Mrs. Paulson is a 77-year-old married woman of Northern European descent who is bought to the emergency room by her husband. She is complaining of weakness, a sore tongue, and numbness and tingling in her arms and legs. She also reports that she has had nausea, vomiting, and diarrhea that has gotten worse over the last several days. Mrs. Paulson has a history of osteoarthritis for which she follows a structured water therapy program at the local YMCA, although she reports that she has been too tired to participate in the program for the past week. She is otherwise healthy, with no significant medical history other than insomnia, for which her family physician has prescribed chloral hydrate 500 mg p.o. (by mouth) h.s. (at bedtime). The physician on call gives a diagnosis of pernicious anemia and orders a nutritionist consult for diet counseling. Mr. and Mrs. Paulson have many questions about this new diagnosis.

1. What is pernicious anemia?
2. What is the cause of pernicious anemia?
3. What is the incidence of pernicious anemia? As an elderly woman of Northern European descent, is Mrs. Paulson at risk for this disorder?
4. What is the standard treatment for Mrs. Paulson?
5. What is the therapeutic action of chloral hydrate?
6. Are there any contraindications or precautions associated with it?
7. What are special considerations for the elderly when prescribing it?
8. What should you include in your instructions to Mrs. Paulson regarding chloral hydrate?
9. What should you consider in your discharge planning?

CASE STUDY 2 • *Mrs. DeKyper*

Mrs. DeKyper is a 72-year-old woman who presents in the emergency room very distraught and complaining of severe back pain. She reports that she has not been able to sleep or eat and she "just wants it all to end." Her daughter, with whom Mrs. DeKyper lives, reports that Mrs. DeKyper is depressed and is concerned for her safety. The pain has been a long-standing problem for Mrs. DeKyper, and she has had extensive diagnostic tests to determine the cause of her pain; no underlying cause of her pain has been identified, so she has been diagnosed with chronic pain syndrome.

1. What is chronic pain?
2. What are the barriers to effective pain assessment and management?
3. Is depression a common occurrence among patients with chronic pain?
4. What are the principles to consider when treating a person with severe chronic pain?

The attending physician orders pain medication. In addition to an opiate, acetaminophen, a nonsteroidal anti-inflammatory drug (NSAID) is also prescribed; you know that NSAIDs are frequently used to treat pain.

5. What are NSAIDs?

6. Mrs. DeKyper has difficulty swallowing and would prefer a liquid medication. Is acetaminophen available in liquid form?
7. What instruction related to acetaminophen should you provide Mrs. DeKyper?
8. What are some nonpharmacologic treatments for chronic pain?

The physician makes a referral to the on-call psychiatrist who, after evaluating Mrs. DeKyper, prescribes Desyrel.

9. What is Desyrel (what kind of medication is it)?
10. What is Desyrel prescribed for? What are some of the other uses for it?
11. What are the side effects of Desyrel?
12. What are special considerations for the elderly patient?

CASE STUDY 3 • *Mr. Jones*

Mr. Jones is an 84-year-old man who lives with his son and daughter-in-law. Mr. Jones has a history of chronic constipation and uses lactulose to manage this problem. His family reports that he has recently become more forgetful and has exhibited loss of coordination; he is also complaining of gastric discomfort. His son brings him in for evaluation, and it is determined that he is in the early stages of Alzheimer's disease.

1. What is Alzheimer's disease?
2. What are the common characteristics of Alzheimer's disease?
3. What are the environmental factors linked to Alzheimer's disease?

The attending physician orders memantine hydrochloride (Magaldrate).

4. For what is memantine hydrochloride prescribed?
5. What are the side effects associated with memantine hydrochloride?
6. Why was memantine hydrochloride prescribed for Mr. Jones?
7. What should the son and daughter-in-law be taught about it?

As stated earlier, Mr. Jones has been taking lactulose to manage his chronic constipation.

8. What are the potential side effects associated with lactulose?

➤ Advanced Case Studies

For the next three case studies, you will need to download the full versions of the following references:

- Griffith's 5-Minute Clinical Consult (5MCC)
- Handbook of Diagnostic Tests (HbDxTests)
- Lippincott's Nursing Drug Guide (LNDG)
- Nurse's Quick Check: Diseases (NDisCheck)
- Nursing Procedures (NurProc)
- Physical Medicine and Rehabilitation Pocketpedia (PMRRx)
- Stedman's Medical Dictionary for the Health Professions and Nursing (HPND)

CASE STUDY I • *Ms. Ling*

Ms. Jenny Ling is a 65-year-old woman who lives in a senior high-rise apartment building in the city. She is retired from her job as an administrative assistant and leads a very active life in her neighborhood. She volunteers at a local hospital, sings in her church choir, and works part-time at an adult day care center. She calls for an appointment at her physician's office today, stating that she has had fever and chills for 2 days, with nausea and a poor appetite, and is always sleeping. After completing an assessment on Ms. Ling, her physician wants her to go straight to the hospital for admission. Ms. Ling's temperature and white cell count are elevated, and she appears dehydrated and very weak.

At the hospital, Ms. Ling has a chest x-ray that shows right lower lobe pneumonia. She is started on intravenous fluids for her dehydration and is given intravenous Levaquin for her community-acquired pneumonia; she also has a history of diabetes mellitus and takes Humulin 70/30 insulin subcutaneously twice a day. At home she monitors her blood sugar in the morning and evening. Upon admission, her blood sugar is over 500 mg/dL. She tells you that her blood sugar is always within the normal range when she is at home.

You are assigned to care for Ms. Ling. She is very distressed about her blood sugar and does not understand why it is elevated.

The physician's orders read:

Monitor blood sugars q.i.d. with Humulin R insulin coverage subcutaneously
0.45 NSS 1000 mL intravenously every 12 hours
Encourage p.o. fluids
Levaquin 500 mg IV daily × 10 days
Humulin 70/30 insulin b.i.d.

Cross-Discipline Learning Activities

You want to be sure that you understand the history and recent course of events for this patient, so you consult your PDA to answer the following questions:

1. What is a white blood cell count?
2. What is pneumonia?
3. What age cohort of patients has the highest incidence and mortality from pneumonia?
4. What is diabetes mellitus?
5. What class of medication is Levaquin?
6. What is the normal range for an adult's fasting blood sugar?
7. What is an Accu-Check (blood glucose test)?
8. Why is an intravenous solution given to a patient with pneumonia?

Discipline-Specific Learning Activities

Nursing

1. What would you hear upon auscultation of lung sounds in a patient with pneumonia?

2. Why would the patient with diabetes be more prone to developing pneumonia?
3. What is the usual dosage of Levaquin for an older adult with normal renal function?
4. When the nurse is administering IV Levaquin, what is important to note about how the infusion is administered?
5. How often does the IV tubing for an IV line need to be changed?

Medicine/PA/NP

1. What would you hear upon auscultation of lung sounds on a patient with pneumonia?
2. What are the symptoms of the three types of pneumonia?
3. What is the usual dosage of Levaquin for an older adult with normal renal function?
4. What laboratory values should be monitored for potential adverse effects of Levaquin?
5. What are the onset, peak, and duration of action for Humulin R insulin?
6. How do the onset, peak, and duration of action of Humulin R compare to those of Humulin 70/30?
7. Why would the patient with diabetes be more prone to developing pneumonia?

Physical and Occupational Therapy

1. In the general treatment of a patient with pneumonia, what treatment recommendation might concern the therapist in regard to mobility?
2. What might the therapist want to assess for in a patient's history of diabetes mellitus related to mobility issues?
3. What type of exercise is recommended to be included in the treatment of diabetes mellitus?

Behavioral Health

1. When a patient has pneumonia, what is an important referral to make before discharge, if the patient is a smoker?
2. In the patient with pneumonia, what is an important psychosocial intervention?
3. When a patient has a chronic disease like diabetes mellitus, what are some important psychosocial interventions?

Critical Thinking—Correlating Patient Data/Assessment Findings to Plan Care

What additional information specific to this case (physical assessment, diagnostic testing, and medications) would you need to know to further your assessment of the patient's needs and to guide your interventions?

What is your plan of care for this patient (what should you do next)?

CASE STUDY 2 • *Mr. Green*

Mr. Morris Green is an 87-year-old African American man who lives in a nursing home. He has a history of prostatic cancer without metastasis and Alzheimer's dementia, which was diagnosed 5 years ago. At his baseline, he is experiencing mild to moderate symptoms of Alzheimer's disease. He wears an alarm that will go off if he attempts to leave the facility, and he is on a secure, closed unit with an outside garden area where he can safely wander. He ambulates around the facility all day long and is usually safe unassisted; however, lately his gait and balance have been challenged and he fell 2 days ago; there appears to be no injury. He always wears an adult brief for urinary and fecal incontinence and has a bed monitor at night for safety. He has been taking Aricept for several years.

Since his fall, Mr. Green has been moaning and is unable to ambulate without assistance. As his condition worsens, it is determined that he should be evaluated further at the local hospital. In the emergency department, Mr. Green becomes very combative and screams intermittently. X-rays of the hips and pelvic area reveal a fractured pelvis; treatment will require bed rest and pain management while the fracture heals.

You are assigned to care for Mr. Green. He is moaning and calling out and combative as anyone approaches his bedside.

The physician's orders read:

> Vest restraints and full side rails up as needed to prevent injury
> Ativan 0.25 mg Q 6 hours p.r.n. agitation
> Percocet 5–325 mg 1–2 tablets Q 4–6 hours p.r.n. pain
> Complete bed rest
> Sequential compression stockings
> Heparin 5000 units subcutaneous t.i.d.

Cross-Discipline Learning Activities

You want to be sure that you understand the history and recent course of events for this patient, so you consult your PDA to answer the following questions:

1. What are the risk factors for developing prostatic cancer?
2. What is metastasis?
3. What are the common characteristics of Alzheimer's disease?
4. What two tests may be performed on the patient to aid in diagnosing Alzheimer's disease?
5. What are some complications that may result from urinary and fecal incontinence?
6. What are the indications for the use of tacrine?
7. What class of medication is Ativan?
8. What are the two active ingredients in Percocet?
9. What are sequential compression stockings?

Discipline-Specific Learning Activities

Nursing

1. What interventions can the nurse implement to aid in preventing patients from falling?
2. To assess the functional level of an older adult, which two widely used scales should the nurse complete?
3. What equipment will the nurse need to assist with incontinence management?
4. What is the procedure for applying a vest restraint?
5. How does the nurse determine the proper size of the sequential compression sleeve?
6. Should the nurse administer tacrine with meals or on an empty stomach?

Medicine/PA/NP

1. What medications might affect bowel activity, causing or worsening fecal incontinence?
2. How soon must the physician evaluate a patient after restraint use is initiated?
3. What is the initial geriatric dosing range for Ativan?
4. If the patient experiences severe side effects from tacrine, what special considerations must be given to discontinuing the medication?
5. Name several unlabeled uses for heparin sodium.
6. Which laboratory tests may show abnormally increased results when the patient is receiving heparin?

Physical and Occupational Therapy

1. What physical finding with Alzheimer's disease relates directly to a mobility issue?
2. What assessment scale might the therapist use to determine a patient's physical functional abilities?

Behavioral Health

1. Name several negative personality changes that may occur with Alzheimer's disease.
2. What are some important interventions related to communication with a patient who has Alzheimer's disease?
3. To whom should the patient and family or caregivers be referred before discharge for continued support?

Critical Thinking—Correlating Patient Data/Assessment Findings to Plan Care

What additional information specific to this case (physical assessment, diagnostic testing, and medications) would you need to know to further your assessment of the patient's needs and to guide your interventions?

What is your plan of care for this patient (what should you do next)?

CASE STUDY 3   •   *Mr. Ward*

Mr. Ronald Ward is a 94-year-old, non-Hispanic man who lives in the assisted living section of a retirement community. He has a history of high cholesterol and osteoarthritis and has problems sleeping at night. He is scheduled for diagnostic testing and evaluation for obstructive sleep apnea and is sometimes incontinent of urine and ambulates using a rolling walker. He has full upper and lower dentures and always wears glasses. He has macular degeneration and glaucoma and takes eye drops twice a day. He is independent with most of his personal hygiene and makes his own breakfast; he attends lunch and dinner in the dining room of the assisted living facility.

Two days ago, he experienced an episode of epistaxis. Yesterday, he complained of a headache in the occipital area, and the nurse dispensing medications took his blood pressure. His blood pressure was 220/100, and he was immediately taken to the area medical center for evaluation. He was admitted to an inpatient unit with the diagnosis of new onset of severe hypertension and started on several intravenous medications to slowly lower his elevated blood pressure.

Today, you are caring for Mr. Ward. He is very concerned about his new diagnosis and questions how he got this disease at his age; he is also very anxious to go home and does not see what all of the fuss is about because he is feeling just fine right now.

The physician's orders read:

> Cozaar 50 mg p.o. daily
> Zestril 5 mg p.o. daily
> Lipitor 40 mg p.o. daily
> Zetia 10 mg p.o. daily
> Monitor oxygen saturation Q shift
> Monitor blood pressure Q 4 hours while awake
> Take blood pressure lying, sitting, and standing once daily and record
> Physical therapy evaluation and treatment for ambulation dysfunction

Cross-Discipline Learning Activities

You want to be sure that you understand the history and recent course of events for this patient, so you consult your PDA to answer the following questions:

1. What is obstructive sleep apnea?
2. What is the predominant age and sex of a person with obstructive sleep apnea?
3. What is macular degeneration?

4. What is glaucoma?
5. What is epistaxis?
6. What is a normal blood pressure range for an older adult?
7. What is the difference in the terms *severe hypertension, hypertensive crisis,* and *hypertensive emergencies?*
8. What laboratory work is needed to assess a patient's cholesterol for hypercholesterolemia?
9. What is oxygen saturation?

Discipline-Specific Learning Activities

Nursing

1. What should the nurse stress when conducting an education session with a patient experiencing obstructive sleep apnea?
2. When the nurse is assessing the patient for obstructive sleep apnea, what signs and symptoms would be expected findings?
3. What symptoms displayed by Mr. Ward would be most indicative of hypertension?
4. When teaching a patient about hypertension, what over-the-counter medications should he or she avoid?
5. What is the reason for ordering the blood pressure to be taken with the patient in different positions?

Medicine/PA/NP

1. What special tests may be ordered to assist in the diagnosis of obstructive sleep apnea?
2. If obstructive sleep apnea results in death, what are the usual causes?
3. What interventions aid in the prevention or avoidance of macular degeneration?
4. What is the usual dosage of methazolamide (GlauTabs), which is given to treat glaucoma?
5. What is an important consideration when determining the initial dose of Zestril for an older patient?

Physical and Occupational Therapy

1. In preparing a patient with new onset of hypertension for discharge, what mobility instructions are important?
2. What would be a typical exercise prescription for duration/frequency for a patient who is deconditioned and experiencing ambulation dysfunction?

Behavioral Health

1. In preparing a patient with new onset of hypertension for discharge, what behavioral health referral is important to offer?
2. When a patient is complaining of sleep deprivation, how should the behavioral health therapist approach evaluation and diagnosis of this problem?

Critical Thinking—Correlating Patient Data/Assessment Findings to Plan Care

What additional information specific to this case (physical assessment, diagnostic testing, and medications) would you need to know to further your assessment of the patient's needs and to guide your interventions?

What is your plan of care for this patient (what should you do next)?

Chapter Summary—Tying It All Together

You have explored several patient scenarios that are typical of the complex care involving the older adult. In each case, the patient presented with at least one chronic health care problem and a new acute illness/condition requiring medical evaluation and treatment. Infections of the urinary or respiratory systems as well as fractures are very common in this age group. Often a mental health problem like dementia or depression will add to the challenges of care while the patient is hospitalized. The gerontologic population, like the rehabilitation group, also requires a multidisciplinary approach to its complex care to aid in ensuring successful outcomes.

 Visit http://thePoint.LWW.com/cornelius for supplemental information and activities.

ANSWERS TO CASE STUDY QUESTIONS

➤ General Case Studies

CASE STUDY I • *Mrs. Paulson*

1. What is pernicious anemia?

   NDisCheck ➙ Pernicious Anemia ➙ Overview

2. What is the cause of pernicious anemia?

   NDisCheck ➙ Pernicious Anemia ➙ Overview ➙ scroll down to Causes

3. What is the incidence of pernicious anemia? As an elderly woman of Northern European descent, is Mrs. Paulson at risk for this disorder?

   NDisCheck ➙ Pernicious Anemia ➙ Overview ➙ scroll down to Incidence

4. What is the standard treatment for Mrs. Paulson?

   NDisCheck → Pernicious Anemia → Treatment

5. What is the therapeutic action of chloral hydrate?

   PDH → Chloral Hydrate → Therapeutic Actions

6. Are there any contraindications or precautions associated with it?

   PDH → Chloral Hydrate → Contraindications and Cautions

7. What are special considerations for the elderly when prescribing it?

   PDH → Chloral Hydrate → Special Considerations (scroll down to Geriatric Patients)

8. What should you include in your instructions to Mrs. Paulson regarding chloral hydrate?

   PDH → Chloral Hydrate → Nursing Considerations → Patient Education

9. What should you consider in your discharge planning?

   NDisCheck → Pernicious Anemia → Patient Teaching → Discharge Planning

CASE STUDY 2 • *Mrs. DeKyper*

1. What is chronic pain?

   PsychThrp → Pain Syndromes → scroll down to Definitions → select Chronic Pain

2. What are the barriers to effective pain assessment and management?

   PsychThrp → Pain Syndromes → scroll down to Barriers to Effective Pain Assessment and Management

3. Is depression a common occurrence among patients with chronic pain?

   PsychThrp → Pain Syndromes → scroll down to Barriers to Effective Pain Assessment and Management

4. What are the principles to consider when treating a person with severe chronic pain?

   PsychThrp → Pain Syndromes → scroll down to Principles Behind

5. What are NSAIDs?

   PsychThrp → Pain Syndromes → scroll down to Pharmacologic Treatment of . . .

6. Mrs. DeKyper has difficulty swallowing and would prefer a liquid medication. Is acetaminophen available in liquid form?

   PDH → Acetaminophen → Available Forms

7. What instruction related to acetaminophen should you provide Mrs. DeKyper?

    PDH → Acetaminophen → Patient Education

8. What are some nonpharmacologic treatments for chronic pain?

    PsychThrp → Pain Syndromes → scroll down to Nonpharmacologic Treatment of...

9. What is Desyrel (what kind of medication is it)?

    LNDG → Desyrel → General (scroll down to Drug Class)

10. What is Desyrel prescribed for? What are some of the other uses for it?

    LNDG → Desyrel → Indications

11. What are the side effects of Desyrel?

    LNDG → Desyrel → Adverse Effects

12. What are special considerations for the elderly patient?

    LNDG → Desyrel → Dosages (scroll down to Geriatric Patients)

CASE STUDY 3 • *Mr. Jones*

1. What is Alzheimer's disease?

    HPND → Alzheimer's Disease

2. What are the common characteristics of Alzheimer's disease?

    NDisCheck → Alzheimer's Disease → Overview (scroll down to Common Characteristics)

3. What are the environmental factors linked to Alzheimer's disease?

    NDisCheck → Alzheimer's Disease → Overview (scroll down to Environmental)

4. For what is memantine hydrochloride prescribed?

    PDH → Memantine Hydrochloride → Indications and Dosage

5. What are the side effects associated with memantine hydrochloride?

    PDH → Memantine Hydrochloride → Adverse Reactions

6. Why was memantine hydrochloride prescribed for 0Mr. Jones?

    LNDG → Memantine Hydrochloride → Indications and Dosages

7. What should the son and daughter-in-law be taught about it?

    LNDG → Memantine Hydrochloride → Patient Teaching

8. What are the potential side effects associated with lactulose?

    LNDG → Lactulose → Adverse Effects

➤ Advanced Case Studies

CASE STUDY 1 • *Ms. Ling*

Cross-Discipline Learning Activities

1. What is a white blood cell count?

   HbDxTests ➤ White Blood Cell Count ➤ Introduction

2. What is pneumonia?

   NDisCheck ➤ Pneumonia... ➤ <u>Pneumonia</u> ➤ Overview

3. What age cohort of patients has the highest incidence and mortality from pneumonia?

   NDisCheck ➤ Pneumonia... ➤ <u>Pneumonia</u> ➤ Overview ➤ Incidence ➤ Age Issue

4. What is diabetes mellitus?

   NDisCheck ➤ Diabetes Mellitus ➤ Overview

5. What class of medication is Levaquin?

   LNDG ➤ Levaquin ➤ General

6. What is the normal range for an adult's fasting blood sugar?

   HbDxTests ➤ Fasting Blood Sugar ➤ Normal Findings

7. What is an Accu-Check (blood glucose test)?

   NurProc ➤ Blood Glucose Tests ➤ Introduction

8. Why is an intravenous solution given to a patient with pneumonia?

   NDisCheck ➤ Pneumonia... ➤ <u>Pneumonia</u> ➤ Nursing Considerations

Discipline-Specific Learning Activities

Nursing

1. What would you hear upon auscultation of lung sounds in a patient with pneumonia?

   NDisCheck ➤ Pneumonia... ➤ <u>Pneumonia</u> ➤ Assessment ➤ Physical Findings

2. Why would the patient with diabetes be more prone to developing pneumonia?

   NDisCheck ➤ Diabetes Mellitus ➤ Overview ➤ Complications

3. What is the usual dosage of Levaquin for an older adult with normal renal function?

   LNDG → Levaquin → Dosages

4. When the nurse is administering IV Levaquin, what is important to note about how the infusion is administered?

   LNDG → Levaquin → IV Facts → Infusion

5. How often does the IV tubing for an IV line need to be changed?

   NurProc → I.V. Therapy Preparation → Special Considerations

Medicine/PA/NP

1. What would you hear upon auscultation of lung sounds on a patient with pneumonia?

   NDisCheck → Pneumonia ... → <u>Pneumonia</u> → Assessment → Physical Findings

2. What are the symptoms of the three types of pneumonia?

   NDisCheck → Overview → Assessment

3. What is the usual dosage of Levaquin for an older adult with normal renal function?

   LNDG → Levaquin → Dosages

4. What laboratory values should be monitored for potential adverse effects of Levaquin?

   LNDG → Levaquin → Adverse Effects

5. What are the onset, peak, and duration of action for Humulin R insulin?

   LNDG → Humulin R → Pharmacokinetics

6. How do the onset, peak, and duration of action of Humulin R compare to those of Humulin 70/30?

   LNDG → Humulin 70/30 → Pharmacokinetics

7. Why would the patient with diabetes be more prone to developing pneumonia?

   NDisCheck → Diabetes Mellitus → Overview → Complications

Physical and Occupational Therapy

1. In the general treatment of a patient with pneumonia, what treatment recommendation might concern the therapist in regard to mobility?

   NDisCheck → Pneumonia . . . → <u>Pneumonia</u> → Treatment → General

2. What might the therapist want to assess for in a patient's history of diabetes mellitus related to mobility issues?

   NDisCheck → Diabetes Mellitus → Assessment → History → Weakness; Fatigue

3. What type of exercise is recommended to be included in the treatment of diabetes mellitus?

   NDisCheck → Diabetes Mellitus → Treatment → General

Behavioral Health

1. When a patient has pneumonia, what is an important referral to make before discharge, if the patient is a smoker?

   NDisCheck → Pneumonia . . . → <u>Pneumonia</u> → Patient Teaching → Discharge Planning

2. In the patient with pneumonia, what is an important psychosocial intervention?

   NDisCheck → Pneumonia . . . → <u>Pneumonia</u> → Nursing Considerations → Nursing Interventions → scroll down to second bullet from bottom

3. When a patient has a chronic disease like diabetes mellitus, what are some important psychosocial interventions?

   NDisCheck → Diabetes Mellitus → Nursing Considerations → Nursing Interventions → scroll down to last three bullets

CASE STUDY 2 • *Mr. Green*

Cross-Discipline Learning Activities

1. What are the risk factors for developing prostatic cancer?

   NDisCheck → Prostatic Cancer → Overview → scroll down to Risk Factors

2. What is metastasis?

   HPND → Metastasis

3. What are the common characteristics of Alzheimer's disease?

NDisCheck → Alzheimer's Disease → Overview → scroll down to Common Characteristics

4. What two tests may be performed on the patient to aid in diagnosing Alzheimer's disease?

HbDxTests → Alzheimer's Disease → Tests for Alzheimer's Disease

5. What are some complications that may result from urinary and fecal incontinence?

NurProc → Incontinence Management → Complications

6. What are the indications for the use of tacrine?

LNDG → Indications

7. What class of medication is Ativan?

LNDG → Ativan → General → Drug Classes

8. What are the two active ingredients in Percocet?

LNDG → Percocet → Percocet [Appendix G] → Active Ingredients

9. What are sequential compression stockings?

NurProc → Sequential Compression Therapy → Introduction

Discipline-Specific Learning Activities

Nursing

1. What interventions can the nurse implement to aid in preventing patients from falling?

NurProc → Fall Prevention and Management → Implementation → Preventing Falls

2. To assess the functional level of an older adult, which two widely used scales should the nurse complete?

NurProc → Functional Assessment → Introduction

3. What equipment will the nurse need to assist with incontinence management?

NurProc → Incontinence Management → Equipment

4. What is the procedure for applying a vest restraint?

NurProc ➤ Restraint Application ➤ Implementation ➤ Applying a Vest Restraint

5. How does the nurse determine the proper size of the sequential compression sleeve?

NurProc ➤ Sequential Compression Therapy ➤ Implementation ➤ To Determine the Proper Size of Sleeve

6. Should the nurse administer tacrine with meals or on an empty stomach?

LNDG ➤ Tacrine ➤ Nursing Considerations ➤ Interventions ➤ scroll down to fourth bullet

Medicine/PA/NP

1. What medications might affect bowel activity, causing or worsening fecal incontinence?

NurProc ➤ Incontinence Management ➤ Implementation ➤ Interventions ➤ For Fecal Incontinence ➤ scroll down to fourth bullet

2. How soon must the physician evaluate a patient after restraint use is initiated?

NurProc ➤ Restraint Application ➤ Implementation

3. What is the initial geriatric dosing range for Ativan?

LNDG ➤ Ativan ➤ Dosages ➤ scroll down to bottom

4. If the patient experiences severe side effects from tacrine, what special considerations must be given to discontinuing the medication?

LNDG ➤ Tacrine ➤ Nursing Considerations ➤ Interventions ➤ scroll down to sixth bullet

5. Name several unlabeled uses for heparin sodium.

LNDG ➤ Heparin ➤ Indications ➤ scroll down to last bullet

6. Which laboratory tests may show abnormally increased results when the patient is receiving heparin?

LNDG ➤ Heparin ➤ Interactions ➤ Drug-Lab Test

Physical and Occupational Therapy

1. What physical findings with Alzheimer's disease relates directly to a mobility issue?

NDisCheck ➤ Alzheimer's Disease ➤ Assessment ➤ Physical Findings

2. What assessment scale might the therapist use to determine a patient's physical functional abilities?

NurProc → Functional Assessment → Introduction → Katz Index

Behavioral Health

1. Name several negative personality changes that may occur with Alzheimer's disease.

NDisCheck → Alzheimer's Disease → Assessment → History → scroll down to tenth bullet

2. What are some important interventions related to communication with a patient who has Alzheimer's disease?

NDisCheck → Alzheimer's Disease → Nursing Considerations → Nursing Interventions → scroll down to first three bullets

3. To whom should the patient and family or caregivers be referred before discharge for continued support?

NDisCheck → Alzheimer's Disease → Patient Teaching → Discharge Planning

CASE STUDY 3 • *Mr. Ward*

Cross-Discipline Learning Activities

1. What is obstructive sleep apnea?

5MCC → Obstructive, Sleep Apnea → Basics

2. What is the predominant age and sex of a person with obstructive sleep apnea?

5MCC → Obstructive, Sleep Apnea → Basics → Incidence/Prevalence in USA

3. What is macular degeneration?

5MCC → Macular Degeneration, Senile → Basics

4. What is glaucoma?

HPND → Glaucoma

5. What is epistaxis?

HPND → Epistaxis

6. What is a normal blood pressure range for an older adult?

NurProc → Blood Pressure Assessment → Effects of Age on Blood Pressure

7. What is the difference in the terms *severe hypertension, hypertensive crisis,* and *hypertensive emergencies?*

   5MCC ➤ Hypertension, Severe and Hypertensive Crisis/Emergencies ➤ Hypertensive Emergencies ➤ Basics

8. What laboratory work is needed to assess a patient's cholesterol for hypercholesterolemia?

   5MCC ➤ Hypercholesterolemia ➤ Diagnosis

9. What is oxygen saturation?

   HPND ➤ Oxygen Saturation

Discipline-Specific Learning Activities

Nursing

1. What should the nurse stress when conducting an education session with a patient experiencing obstructive sleep apnea?

   5MCC ➤ Obstructive, Sleep Apnea ➤ Treatment ➤ Patient Education

2. When the nurse is assessing the patient for obstructive sleep apnea, what signs and symptoms would be expected findings?

   5MCC ➤ Obstructive, Sleep Apnea ➤ Basics ➤ Signs and Symptoms

3. What symptoms displayed by Mr. Ward would be most indicative of hypertension?

   NDisCheck ➤ Hypertension ... ➤ Hypertension ➤ Assessment ➤ History

4. When teaching a patient about hypertension, what over-the-counter medications should he or she avoid?

   NDisCheck ➤ Hypertension ... ➤ Hypertension ➤ Patient Teaching ➤ scroll down to fifth bullet

5. What is the reason for ordering the blood pressure to be taken with the patient in different positions?

   NurProc ➤ Blood Pressure Assessment ➤ Special Considerations ➤ scroll down to sixth bullet

Medicine/PA/NP

1. What special tests may be ordered to assist in the diagnosis of obstructive sleep apnea?

   5MCC ➤ Obstructive, Sleep Apnea ➤ Diagnosis ➤ Special Tests

2. If obstructive sleep apnea results in death, what are the usual causes?

   5MCC ➤ Obstructive, Sleep Apnea ➤ Follow-Up ➤ scroll down to last bullet

3. What interventions aid in the prevention or avoidance of macular degeneration?

   5MCC ➤ Macular Degeneration, Senile ➤ Follow-Up ➤ Prevention/Avoidance

4. What is the usual dosage of methazolamide (GlauTabs), which is given to treat glaucoma?

   LNDG ➤ Methazolamide ➤ Dosages

5. What is an important consideration when determining the initial dose of Zestril for an older patient?

   LNDG ➤ Zestril ➤ Dosages ➤ Geriatric Patients and Patients with Renal Impairment

Physical and Occupational Therapy

1. In preparing a patient with new onset of hypertension for discharge, what mobility instructions are important?

   NDisCheck ➤ Hypertension ➤ Patient Teaching ➤ scroll down to seventh bullet

2. What would be a typical exercise prescription for duration/frequency for a patient who is deconditioned and experiencing ambulation dysfunction?

   PMRRx ➤ Exercise Prescription ➤ Info ➤ scroll down to last bullet

Behavioral Health

1. In preparing a patient with new onset of hypertension for discharge, what behavioral health referral is important to offer?

   NDisCheck ➤ Hypertension ➤ Patient Teaching ➤ Discharge Planning

2. When a patient is complaining of sleep deprivation, how should the behavioral health therapist approach evaluation and diagnosis of this problem?

   5MCC ➤ Insomnia ➤ Treatment ➤ General Measures

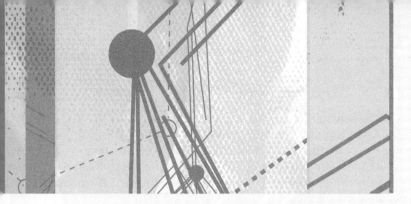

Critical Care
Case Studies

Faye A. Pearlman • Magdeleine Vasso

The case studies in this chapter focus on the care of patients in critical care situations. As with the previous case studies, these patients are complex and have additional concerns and needs beyond the initial emergency care interventions. The goal of health care providers working with patients in emergency and critical care situations is to provide comprehensive care that will reduce or prevent mortality and morbidity resulting from sustained injuries. As always, this type of care requires a multidisciplinary approach to achieve success.

➤ General Case Studies

For the following three case studies, you will need to download the trial versions of these references:

- Griffith's 5-Minute Clinical Consult (5MCC)
- Lippincott's Nursing Drug Guide (LNDG)
- Nurse's Quick Check: Diseases (NDisCheck)
- Rosen and Barkin's 5-Minute Emergency Medicine Consult (5MEmerg)
- Physician's Drug Handbook (PDH)
- Stedman's Medical Dictionary for the Health Professions and Nursing (HPND)

CASE STUDY I • *Mrs. Andrews*

Mrs. Andrews is a 48-year-old, married woman with a history of insulin-dependent diabetes who presents in the emergency room with significant paresthesia of feet and hands starting 3 days before. She is now complaining of acute, symmetric weakness of all four extremities. Past medical history indicates that she recently received the rabies vaccination due to her employment as an animal control officer. The lab results indicate that she has an elevated protein with normal white blood count (albuminocytological dissociation); the attending physician makes the preliminary diagnosis of Guillain-Barré syndrome.

1. What is a syndrome?
2. What is Guillain-Barré syndrome?
3. What causes Guillain-Barré syndrome?
4. Is Mrs. Andrews' job as an animal control officer linked in any way to her current illness?
5. Does Mrs. Andrews have any risk factors associated with this illness?

The attending physician wants to admit Mrs. Andrews to monitor her respiratory function. You explain to Mrs. Andrews that she is at risk for acute respiratory failure and that she may need to be intubated and mechanically ventilated. You tell her that the device is called an *endotracheal tube*.

6. What is acute respiratory failure?
7. What is an endotracheal tube?
8. If Mrs. Andrews is intubated, she will need to be mechanically ventilated; what factors must be closely monitored?
9. What are the psychosocial complications associated with Guillain-Barré syndrome?
10. Mrs. Andrews asks about her prognosis. What is her prognosis?

CASE STUDY 2 • *Mr. Samuelson*

Mr. Samuelson is admitted to the emergency room with a fever and severe left leg pain. On exam, there is a 2-inch gash on the inner aspect of the calf, which he obtained 2 days earlier; the surrounding tissue is necrotic, and his entire calf is swollen and reddened. Mr. Samuelson has been taking acetaminophen for the pain and reports that his pain has been so severe that he has taken four tablets every 2 hours for the past 10 hours without relief. Now he is also experiencing nausea. The attending physician is concerned about acetaminophen poisoning and orders gastric decontamination.

1. What is gastric decontamination?
2. What is activated charcoal?

The attending physician also makes the diagnosis of necrotizing fasciitis.

3. What is necrotizing fasciitis?
4. How does someone get necrotizing fasciitis?
5. How is necrotizing fasciitis treated?

Mr. Samuelson is hospitalized for treatment of the necrotizing fasciitis. The disease progresses rapidly, and amputation of the lower leg is necessary to stop the progression and to prevent death. Postoperatively, Mr. Samuelson develops a deep vein thrombosis (blood clot) for which the physician orders heparin and orders penicillin for respiratory infection.

6. What are the contraindications for giving penicillin?

CASE STUDY 3 • *Mr. Jefferies*

Mr. Jefferies is a 38-year-old landscaper who is brought to the emergency room by his coworkers after being stung by several bees. He and his coworkers had been clearing land for a building project and apparently disturbed a nearby bees nest. Mr. Jefferies was stung repeatedly on his arms and face. The affected areas are very swollen and inflamed. Mr. Jefferies is complaining of pain, itchiness, and difficulty breathing, and he is very anxious. The physician's diagnosis is anaphylaxis, related to bee stings.

1. What is anaphylaxis?
2. What are the signs and symptoms associated with an allergic reaction to an insect bite?
3. What is the immediate treatment for anaphylaxis?
4. The physician orders epinephrine 1.5 mg subcutaneous (SQ). What are side effects of epinephrine?
5. What drug interactions are associated with epinephrine?
6. Insect bites are a common emergency. What is the incidence of this type of emergency, and what age group does it affect?
7. What possible complications are associated with insect bites and stings?

Mr. Jefferies is discharged with a prescription and instructions for an Epi-Pen. He is instructed to keep the Epi-Pen with him when working outdoors. He is also given a prescription for Benadryl.

8. What should Mr. Jefferies be instructed regarding Benadryl?

➤ Advanced Case Studies

For the next three case studies, you will need to download full versions of the following references:

- Griffith's 5-Minute Clinical Consult (5MCC)
- Handbook of Diagnostic Tests (HbDxTests)
- Lippincott's Nursing Drug Guide (LNDG)
- Manual of Laboratory and Diagnostic Tests (LabTests)
- Manual of Psychiatric Therapeutics (PsychThrp)
- Nurse's Quick Check: Diseases (NDisCheck)
- Nursing Procedures (NurProc)

- Rosen and Barkin's 5-Minute Emergency Medicine Consult (5MEmerg)
- Physical Medicine and Rehabilitation Pocketpedia (PMRRx)
- Physician's Drug Handbook (PDH)
- Stedman's Medical Dictionary for the Health Professions and Nursing (HPND)

CASE STUDY I • *Mrs. Tighe*

Mrs. Tighe is a 58-year-old Caucasian woman who weighs 195 pounds and is 5 feet, 1½ inches tall. She has smoked approximately two packs of cigarettes per day since age 20. She has a history of hypertension, has not seen a physician for several years, and denies any other significant medical history. Her mother died suddenly at age 60 from unknown causes. Her father, who also had hypertension, died from a massive stroke at age 68. Mrs. Tighe works as a housekeeper for an industrial cleaning company and has lately been under an increased amount of stress due to rumored layoffs by her employer. Her husband is on partial disability, but he has a part-time job in a local convenience store and does qualify for health benefits.

Mrs. Tighe has not been feeling well for the past several days, experiencing weakness, fatigue, and gastrointestinal (GI) upset. She assumed that she had a case of the flu and treats herself with over-the-counter medications, Tylenol Flu and Maalox, with minimal relief. After dinner this evening, she experiences worsening epigastric pain that radiated to her jaw; she also experienced diaphoresis and nausea, which worsened despite the use of Tums. Her husband insisted that she go to the emergency room.

Upon arrival to the emergency room, Mrs. Tighe rates her pain as 8 on a 1–10 scale. She is immediately placed on a cardiac monitor. Her initial vital signs are blood pressure 160/90, heart rate 72, and unlabored respirations at a rate of 26 breaths per minute. Her pulse oximetry on room air is 96%. She appears pale and anxious and is immediately placed on oxygen via nasal cannula at a rate of 2 L per minute. An 18-gauge angiocath is placed in her right antecubital vein infusing 0.9% normal saline. A second IV access is obtained and blood is sent to the laboratory for analysis. Mrs. Tighe is medicated with sublingual nitroglycerin and 325 mg aspirin p.o. Her EKG reveals normal sinus rhythm with ST segment elevations in Leads V2, V3, and V4, indicating an acute anterior myocardial infarction. The cardiac catheterization lab will not be available until the next morning.

After receiving the sublingual nitroglycerin, Mrs. Tighe reports that her pain is still present but decreased to a rating of 2. The emergency department physician orders 2 mg morphine to be administered by IV push and asks that a nitroglycerin infusion and heparin infusion be started as soon as possible. Because the cardiac catheterization lab is not available until morning, the physicians decide to treat Mrs. Tighe with the coronary reperfusion medication alteplase intravenously as soon as possible. The pharmacy is notified to send the medication immediately to the emergency department.

Cross-Discipline Learning Activities

1. What is a myocardial infarction?
2. What physical signs and symptoms does Mrs. Tighe display that are consistent with a diagnosis of acute myocardial infarction (AMI)?
3. What is the difference between a Q-wave and non–Q-wave infarction?
4. What is a thrombus?
5. What is the definition of *transmural*?
6. After receiving the sublingual nitroglycerin, Mrs. Tighe complains of a headache. She asks if it means something else is wrong with her. What patient education information is important to share with Mrs. Tighe to relieve her anxiety?

Discipline-Specific Learning Activities

Nursing

You have been asked to perform serial EKGs on Mrs. Tighe.

1. To ensure accurate test results it is extremely important to position the chest electrodes in the correct anatomic position. Electrode V_1 is positioned in the fourth intercostal space at the right border of the sternum. Electrode V_2 is positioned in the fourth intercostal space at the left border of the sternum. Electrode V_4 is placed in the fifth intercostal space at the midclavicular line. What is the correct position for electrode V_3?
2. As the nurse caring for Mrs. Tighe, your responsibility is to monitor her response to treatment. What are the important considerations for patients receiving thrombolytic therapy? What adverse cardiovascular effects are possible with the administration of the medication alteplase?
3. Several potential life-threatening adverse effects are associated with the administration of an opioid agonist analgesic such as IV morphine. Major cardiovascular problems include circulatory depression, shock, and cardiac arrest. What are the three major adverse effects involving the respiratory system?
4. During report, the nurse who cared for Mrs. Tighe during the previous shift informs you that the patient appeared to be slightly confused at times. You decide to do a mini-mental state examination using the Short Portable Mental Status Questionnaire as part of your general assessment of Mrs. Tighe. What are the first three questions you would ask her?
5. Another nursing intervention is the assessment and documentation of Mrs. Tighe's pain on an ongoing basis. What is important for you to document about pain related to AMI?
6. Ms. Tighe is still receiving a nitroglycerin infusion. Is it possible to infuse nitroglycerin and alteplase through the same line using a Y-site IV connection?

7. It is also important to monitor coagulation studies in patients receiving alteplase. The prothrombin time (PT) and Activated Partial Thromboplastin time (APTT) should be less than two times the control value. The normal reference value for APTT is 21–35 seconds. What is the normal reference value for PT?

Medicine/PA/NP

1. What laboratory studies would you expect to order to diagnose AMI?
2. What is the significance of an elevated Troponin I level?
3. Because the cardiac catheterization lab is not available, the patient will be receiving the coronary reperfusion medication alteplase via an accelerated infusion. How will this medication be administered to Mrs. Tighe?
4. Another treatment option for diagnosis of occluded coronary arteries and treatment of AMI is an invasive procedure called percutaneous transluminal coronary angioplasty (PTCA). What is PTCA?
5. Why are nitroglycerin and heparin used during the procedure?
6. What is the emphasis of the clinician's role in the pretest phase of any diagnostic testing?

Physical and Occupational Therapy

Mrs. Tighe is scheduled to begin a cardiac rehabilitation program before she is discharged from the hospital.

1. What elements may be included in a comprehensive cardiac rehabilitation program?
2. How is submaximal stress testing used during phase I of cardiac rehabilitation?
3. What types of exercises should be emphasized in the rehabilitation plan?
4. During your initial evaluation of Mrs. Tighe, you notice that she is not wearing antiembolism stockings despite her limited mobility at this time. Why is it important to suggest this treatment modality to the nurses and physicians caring for Mrs. Tighe?
5. Mrs. Tighe has been prescribed a beta-blocker medication, Toprol XL 100 mg by mouth twice a day. What common central nervous system (CNS) adverse effects should you monitor during her cardiac rehabilitation sessions?

Behavioral Health

1. Mrs. Tighe and her husband have asked how they can receive additional printed information about myocardial infarction and lifestyle changes to prevent future heart attacks. You are aware that the American Heart Association has various information available to the public that would be useful for them to receive. What contact information could you give them to request such information?

2. You have been asked to assist in developing the discharge plan for Mrs. Tighe. Any type of supportive care that Mrs. Tighe will receive in the home will require information related to her inpatient diagnosis and recent hospitalization. What is the ICD-9 code associated with an anterior wall myocardial infarction?
3. You are aware that the physician is planning to refer Mrs. Tighe for ongoing cardiac rehabilitation after discharge from the hospital. What other referrals would you suggest as part of the patient teaching and discharge planning process?
4. The doctors inform Mrs. Tighe that she will need a cardiac catheterization as an outpatient after she returns home and regains her strength. She confides in you that, although the doctors and nurses do their best to explain things thoroughly, she still does not understand the purpose of this test and asks if you can explain the procedure in layman's terms. What can you tell her?

Critical Thinking—Correlating Patient Data/Assessment Findings to Plan Care

What additional information specific to this case (physical assessment, diagnostic testing, and medications) would you need to know to further your assessment of the patient's needs and to guide your interventions? What is your plan of care for this patient (what should you do next)?

CASE STUDY 2 • *Mr. Steinman*

Mr. Steinman, A 31-year-old glazier, who is not wearing a safety harness while working on a man lift, is dropped 10 feet to the concrete below due to equipment malfunction. EMS is activated, and he is airlifted to a Level One Trauma Center.

During transport, the patient is intubated with an endotracheal tube and is placed on a transport ventilator. Two large bore IVs were started in his antecubital veins infusing lactated Ringer's.

Upon arrival to the hospital he is unconscious, pale, and has poor capillary refill. ECG monitoring reveals sinus tachycardia with a rate of 130 beats per minute. His blood pressure is 80/40. Multiple radiological studies were performed in addition to a diagnostic peritoneal lavage. The following injuries are identified: closed head injury, including subdural and epidural hematoma, multiple rib fractures with a flail chest, right hemothorax and a left tension pneumothorax, pelvic fractures, and bilateral femur fractures.

You have just started your clinical rotation in the emergency department. You recognize that this patient is in critical condition and will require the coordinated effort of the specialized interdisciplinary trauma team. Although you will not have primary responsibility for caring for this patient, you want to maximize your learning opportunities and understanding of the complex care required for this patient. In addition, you want to be prepared to assist in the care of this patient or his family if you are called upon to do so. Your PDA will be a valuable resource to help you achieve your goals.

Cross-Discipline Learning Activities

1. You understand that the Glasgow Coma Score is used to evaluate level of consciousness in a patient. However, you hear the residents discussing this patient's Trauma Score. What is "Trauma Score," and why is it applicable in the care of this patient?
2. In addition to having a subdural hematoma, which is tearing of the subdural veins and bleeding into the subdural space, this patient is diagnosed as having an epidural hematoma. What is an epidural hematoma?
3. In addition to the injuries that resulted to the head, this patient has multiple other traumatic injuries. When assessing a multisystem trauma patient, a primary survey using the ABCDE order is conducted on arrival in the emergency department. This primary survey is done in a systematic and focused way to determine immediate patient care priorities. After consulting your PDA, you realize that

   "A" stands for assessment of the patient's airway and stabilization of the cervical spine
   "B" stands for assessment of the patient's breathing status
   "C" stands for assessment of the patient's circulation

   What critical element does the "D" step of the primary assessment involve?

4. The patient has experienced a significant amount of internal bleeding, and his vital signs indicate that he is experiencing decompensated hemorrhagic shock. When does decompensated hemorrhagic shock occur?
5. The patient has multiple fractures, including a flail chest. What is the description of a flail chest, and what is the most common cause?
6. A diagnostic peritoneal lavage (DPL) is often performed in the emergency department on all patients with blunt chest trauma. Why is this procedure performed?
7. What is the pathophysiology associated with hemothorax?

Discipline-Specific Learning Activities

Nursing

1. When caring for a patient with head trauma that results in an epidural hematoma, positioning of the patient is an important component of care. What is the appropriate position of the bed?
2. What happens when a patient experiences increased intracranial pressure (ICP)?
3. The patient is transferred to ICU after surgery. Although his hemodynamic status is somewhat improved, there is still significant risk of increased ICPs. An ICP bolt is placed in the OR so that ICPs could be monitored frequently. What is the most common complication of ICP monitoring?

4. The nurse is the person most likely to identify complications occurring in a patient with ICP monitoring. What are the signs of impending or overt decompensation that should be reported to the physician immediately?
5. The patient also returned from the OR with chest tubes in place. You have been asked to accompany the patient to x-ray for follow-up CT studies. What special considerations are important when transporting a patient with chest tubes?

Medicine/PA/NP

1. You are impressed by how quickly and efficiently each member of the trauma team carries out his or her individual responsibilities. Yet you wonder why a chest tube is placed before the technician completes processing the multiple trauma x-rays. What is the rationale for this treatment action with blunt chest trauma?
2. What are the mandatory x-rays that are an essential part of the diagnostic workup for all patients with multisystem trauma?
3. What are the emergency department treatment priorities with multisystem trauma patients?
4. What is a classic symptom that distinguishes an epidural hematoma from other types of intracranial bleeds when you are obtaining a history on a patient with blunt head trauma?
5. What laboratory tests are typically ordered as part of the diagnostic workup for patients who present with blunt head trauma?

Physical and Occupational Therapy

1. As a therapist, you care for many patients with a history of traumatic brain injury. What are the dynamic processes associated with traumatic brain injury?
2. You notice that a significant number of your patients in therapy for posttraumatic brain injury have seizure disorders. Is this patient at risk for developing seizures?
3. What gross assessment techniques are used to assess for disability related to spinal cord injuries in a patient with multisystem trauma during the primary survey conducted immediately upon arrival in the emergency department?
4. This patient has multiple femur fractures. When assessing the degree of comminution, the Winquist and Hansen classification system may be used. What is a grade III fracture according to this classification?
5. Passive range-of-motion exercises are often indicated for patients with temporary or permanent loss of mobility sensation or consciousness. Are there ever situations where passive range-of-motion exercises are contraindicated?

Behavioral Health

It is not uncommon for patients and families who experience traumatic events to experience posttraumatic stress disorder (PTSD). In this disorder, symptoms do not exist before the trauma and persist for at least 1 month following the trauma. There are three classifications of PTSD based on the onset of symptoms: acute PTSD, chronic PTSD, and delayed onset PTSD. Because the onset of PTSD can be variable, there are important implications for ongoing follow-up with both patients and families who are at risk.

1. What are the criteria for onset of symptoms in delayed onset PTSD?
2. What is the role of crisis intervention shortly after the traumatic event?
3. You are aware that the Minnesota Multiphasic Personality Inventory (MMPI) is sometimes used to diagnose PTSD by evaluating an individual's personality dysfunction and level of stress. What are the elements that compose the MMPI?
4. In some circumstances, a patient with PTSD will present with amnesia about the traumatic event. What special treatment modalities may be used to assist in the examination and interview of these patients during the diagnostic phase of treatment?
5. You are aware that a patient who has experienced an epidural hematoma has had a significant cerebral insult that will require attention of an interdisciplinary care team after discharge from the hospital. What are two key elements that you will suggest that the nurses include in the planning of care for this patient?

Critical Thinking—Correlating Patient Data/Assessment Findings to Plan Care

What additional information specific to this case (physical assessment, diagnostic testing, and medications) would you need to know to further your assessment of the patient's needs and to guide your interventions?

What is your plan of care for this patient (what should you do next)?

CASE STUDY 3 • *Mr. Kiomato*

Mr. Kiomato is a 52-year-old construction worker brought to the emergency department after being rescued from a house fire at the work site. He was trapped for approximately 15 minutes in a room engulfed by flames and dense smoke before firefighters were able to reach him. He is confused and lethargic; he has singed nose hair, an overall cherry-red appearance, and is coughing up sooty sputum. Mr. Kiomato has second- and third-degree burns over an estimated 30% of his body; his estimated weight is 90 kg.

You have never taken care of a burn patient and consult your PDA for general information to help you identify priorities in caring for Mr. Kiomato.

Cross-Discipline Learning Activities

1. What are two important factors to consider in anticipating the extent of injury in a burn patient?
2. What criteria did the paramedics use to determine that Mr. Kiomato should be transported to your hospital, which is a regional burn center?
3. Are there age-related factors that impact Mr. Kiomato's overall prognosis?
4. Patients with severe burns present complex challenges that require the dedication and expertise of a specialized interdisciplinary group of professionals. What are the five major goals of care for a patient with severe burns?
5. When should an interdisciplinary approach to discharge planning be started for Mr. Kiomato?

Discipline-Specific Learning Activities

Nursing

1. Maintaining fluid and electrolyte balance is a critical priority for burn patients. Monitoring intake and output is an important part of this nursing activity. What criteria should be used to monitor urine output in an adult burn patient?
2. You recognize that carboxyhemoglobin is formed when hemoglobin is exposed to carbon monoxide during excessive smoke inhalation and that the affinity of hemoglobin for carbon monoxide is 240 times greater than that for oxygen causing hypoxia. What physical characteristic does Mr. Kiomato exhibit that suggests his carboxyhemoglobin level is elevated and that his confusion and lethargy are related to hypoxia?
3. Twice daily dressing changes are common in the care of severely burned patients. What are the two ways burn dressings encourage healing?
4. Dressing changes for burn patients can be an extremely painful experience. How should you schedule the administration of pain medication in relation to the timing of the scheduled dressing changes?
5. The physician has decided to place an endotracheal tube in Mr. Kiomato to protect his airway and has ordered that 2 mg Versed be given as IV push for sedation and amnesia. How will you implement the administration of this initial infusion?

Medicine/PA/NP

1. Mr. Kiomato's singed nose hairs and his lethargy and confusion cause you to think about smoke inhalation as a differential diagnosis when considering airway management. What laboratory tests would you order to evaluate the severity of smoke inhalation in a patient?

2. To estimate the body surface area (BSA) involved in burn injuries, a technique called "rule of nines" is often used. If Mr. Kiomato presented with burns over both lower extremities, what percent of BSA would you estimate his injuries represent?
3. Fluid resuscitation is an important aspect of care for a burn patient. What formula would you use to calculate Mr. Kiomato's fluid requirements for the first 24 hours? How much of that total amount should be administered during the first 8 hours, after the burn injury occurred?
4. Pain management is an important consideration in the care of burn patients. What is the drug of choice in adults, and what dosage is recommended?
5. When reviewing lab results you notice that Mr. Kiomato has an elevated blood urea nitrogen (BUN). Other than dehydration, what is another common cause of an elevated BUN in burn patients?

Physical and Occupational Therapy

1. What is the typical approach to burn therapy for severe burns that is largely within the practice domain of physical therapy?
2. What is the activity goal of therapy once a burn patient is stabilized?
3. Mr. Kiomato remains on a ventilator and is heavily sedated. He has an extensive third-degree circumferential burn on his left leg. The doctors are concerned about necrotic tissue affecting the peripheral circulation to his lower extremity and have asked Mr. Kiomato's wife for permission to perform an escharotomy. She states that she has a basic understanding and has given her consent for the needed treatment, but that she is uncomfortable explaining the purpose of the procedure to her daughter and asks for your assistance. How would you respond?
4. What are possible complications of extensive burns that can be prevented or minimized by early and ongoing physical and occupational therapy intervention and treatment?
5. First-degree burns tend to resolve completely. Less severe second-degree burns will begin the process of epithelialization within 10–14 days. What is the expected course/prognosis for deep second- and third-degree burns?
6. What patient teaching is required for prevention and avoidance of complications of involved burn sites after discharge?

Behavioral Health

1. Mr. Kiomato's condition is stabilized in the emergency department, and he has been transferred into the ICU. While you are providing emotional support to the family, Mr. Kiomato's daughter asks how long her father will remain in the ICU and when can they expect that he will be discharged from the hospital. How would you respond?

2. Discharge planning will be an important part of the treatment plan for Mr. Kiomato. What three referral sources should be included in his discharge plan?

3. Both nursing and behavioral disciplines will identify a common key outcome that Mr. Kiomato and his family will demonstrate effective coping techniques. The nursing staff has consulted you for advice on how best to achieve this goal. What nursing intervention would you suggest?

4. Mr. Kiomato's family is concerned about Mr. Kiomato's ability to return to work after he recovers. They tell you that he is a proud man who takes great pride in his work. What statistical information can you provide?

5. Mr. Kiomato's family does not understand why they are asked to wear a gown and mask when entering his room. You understand that these precautions are used to help prevent infection. Why is it especially important to prevent infection in burn patients?

Critical Thinking—Correlating Patient Data/Assessment Findings to Plan Care

What additional information specific to this case (physical assessment, diagnostic testing, and medications) would you need to know to further your assessment of the patient's needs and to guide your interventions?

What is your plan of care for this patient (what should you do next)?

Mr. Kiomato is facing a long and difficult recovery from his injuries. What measures can be put into place to help prepare Mr. Kiomato and his family for what lies ahead?

Chapter Summary—Tying It All Together

You have explored several patient scenarios typical for the critical care setting. In each case, the patient presented with an acute diagnosis requiring multiple diagnostic studies and interventions requiring the attention and care of various health care providers to achieve a successful course of treatment. As in the earlier case studies, it is essential that the care delivered is a collaborative and a multidisciplinary approach (physicians, nurses, physical and occupational therapists, and behavioral health). Remember, the primary goal is to provide comprehensive care that will reduce or prevent mortality and morbidity resulting from sustained injuries.

 Visit http://thePoint.LWW.com/cornelius for supplemental information and activities.

ANSWERS TO CASE STUDY QUESTIONS

➤ General Case Studies

CASE STUDY I • *Mrs. Andrews*

1. What is a syndrome?

   HPND → Syndrome

2. What is Guillain-Barré syndrome?

   5MCC → Basics

3. What causes Guillain-Barré syndrome?

   5MCC → Basics → scroll down to Causes

4. Is Mrs. Andrews' job as an animal control officer linked in any way to her current illness?

   5MCC → Basics → scroll down to Causes (third bullet)

5. Does Mrs. Andrews have any risk factors associated with this illness?

   5MCC → Basics → scroll down to Risk Factors (second bullet)

6. What is acute respiratory failure?

   NDisCheck → Acute Respiratory Failure → Overview

7. What is an endotracheal tube?

   HPND → Endotracheal Tube

8. If Mrs. Andrews is intubated, she will need to be mechanically ventilated; what factors must be closely monitored?

   NDisCheck → Acute Respiratory Failure → Nursing Considerations → scroll down to Monitoring: If patient requires mechanical ventilation

9. What are the psychosocial complications associated with Guillain-Barré syndrome?

   5MCC → Guillain-Barré Syndrome → Follow-Up → scroll down to Possible Complications

10. Mrs. Andrews asks about her prognosis. What is her prognosis?

    5MCC → Guillain-Barré Syndrome → Follow-Up → scroll down to Expected Course/Prognosis

CASE STUDY 2 • *Mr. Samuelson*

1. What is gastric decontamination?

   5MEmerg ➤ Acetaminophen Poisoning ➤ Treatment

2. What is activated charcoal?

   PDH ➤ Activated Charcoal

3. What is necrotizing fasciitis?

   NDisCheck ➤ Necrotizing Fasciitis ➤ Overview

4. How does someone get necrotizing fasciitis?

   NDisCheck ➤ Necrotizing Fasciitis ➤ Overview ➤ scroll down to Pathophysiology

5. How is necrotizing fasciitis treated?

   NDisCheck ➤ Necrotizing Fasciitis

6. What are the contraindications for giving penicillin?

   LNDG ➤ Penicillin ➤ Contraindications and Cautions

CASE STUDY 3 • *Mr. Jefferies*

1. What is anaphylaxis?

   NDisCheck ➤ Anaphylaxis ➤ Overview

2. What are the signs and symptoms associated with an allergic reaction to an insect bite?

   NDisCheck ➤ Anaphylaxis ➤ Assessment ➤ scroll down to Physical Findings

3. What is the immediate treatment for anaphylaxis?

   NDisCheck ➤ Anaphylaxis ➤ Treatment ➤ scroll down to Medication

4. The physician orders epinephrine 1.5 mg subcutaneous (SQ). What are side effects of epinephrine?

   LNDG ➤ Epinephrine ➤ Adverse Effects

5. What drug interactions are associated with epinephrine?

   LNDG ➤ Epinephrine ➤ Interactions

6. Insect bites are a common emergency. What is the incidence of this type of emergency and what age group does it affect?

   5MCC → Insect Bites and Stings → Basics → scroll down to Incidence/Prevalence in USA and Predominant Age

7. What possible complications are associated with insect bites and stings?

   5MCC → Insect Bites and Stings → Follow-Up → scroll down to Possible Complications

8. What should Mr. Jefferies be instructed regarding Benadryl?

   LNDG → Benadryl → Nursing Considerations → scroll down to Teaching Points

---

➤ Advanced Case Studies

CASE STUDY I • *Mrs. Tighe*

Cross-Discipline Learning Activities

1. What is a myocardial infarction?

   5MCC → Myocardial Infarction → Basics → Description

2. What physical signs and symptoms does Mrs. Tighe display that are consistent with a diagnosis of acute myocardial infarction (AMI)?

   5MCC → Myocardial Infarction → Basics → scroll down to Signs and Symptoms

3. What is the difference between a Q-wave and non–Q-wave infarction?

   5MCC → Myocardial Infarction → Basics → Description → scroll down to third bullet

4. What is a thrombus?

   HPND → Thrombus

5. What is the definition of *transmural*?

   HPND → Transmural

6. After receiving the sublingual nitroglycerin, Mrs. Tighe complains of a headache. She asks if it means something else is wrong with her. What patient education information is important to share with Mrs. Tighe to relieve her anxiety?

   PDH → Nitroglycerin → Patient Education → scroll down to ninth bullet

Discipline-Specific Learning Activities

Nursing

1. To ensure accurate test results it is extremely important to position the chest electrodes in the correct anatomic position. Electrode V_1 is positioned in the fourth intercostal space at the right border of the sternum. Electrode V_2 is positioned in the fourth intercostal space at the left border of the sternum. Electrode V_4 is placed in the fifth intercostal space at the midclavicular line. What is the correct position for electrode V_3?

   NurProc ➤ Cardiac Monitoring ➤ Positioning Chest Electrodes

2. As the nurse caring for Mrs. Tighe, it is your responsibility to monitor her response to treatment. What adverse cardiovascular effects are possible with the administration of the medication alteplase?

   LNDG ➤ Alteplase, Recombinant ➤ Adverse Effects ➤ CV

3. Several potential life-threatening adverse effects are associated with the administration of an opioid agonist analgesic such as IV morphine. Major cardiovascular problems include circulatory depression, shock, and cardiac arrest. What are the three major adverse effects involving the respiratory system?

   LNDG ➤ Opioid Agonist Analgesic ➤ Morphine Sulfate ➤ Adverse Effects ➤ Major Hazards

4. During report, the nurse who cared for Mrs. Tighe during the previous shift informs you that the patient appeared to be slightly confused at times. You decide to do a mini-mental state examination using the Short Portable Mental Status Questionnaire as part of your general assessment of Mrs. Tighe. What are the first three questions you would ask her?

   PsychThrp ➤ Mental Status Exam ➤ Index ➤ Use of Short Portable Mental Status Questionnaire ➤ scroll down to Questions or Tasks

5. Another nursing intervention is the assessment and documentation of Mrs. Tighe's pain on an ongoing basis. What is important for you to document about pain related to AMI?

   NDisCheck ➤ Myocardial Infarction ➤ Nursing Considerations ➤ Nursing Interventions ➤ scroll down to first bullet

6. Ms. Tighe is still receiving a nitroglycerin infusion. Is it possible to infuse nitroglycerin and alteplase through the same line using a Y-site IV connection?

   LNDG ➤ Alteplase, Recombinant ➤ IV Facts ➤ Y Site Incompatibilities

7. It is also important to monitor coagulation studies in patients receiving alteplase. The prothrombin time (PT) and Activated Partial Thromboplastin

time (APTT) should be less than two times the control value. The normal reference value for APTT is 21–35 seconds. What is the normal reference value for PT?

LabTests → Prothrombin Time → Reference Values → Normal → PT

Medicine/PA/NP

1. What laboratory studies would you expect to order to diagnose AMI?

   5MCC → Myocardial Infarction → Diagnosis → Laboratory

2. What is the significance of an elevated Troponin I level?

   HbDxTests → Myocardial Infarction → Information → scroll down to fourth bullet

3. Because the cardiac catheterization lab is not available, the patient will be receiving the coronary reperfusion medication alteplase via an accelerated infusion. How will this medication be administered to Mrs. Tighe?

   PDH → Alteplase → Indications and Dosages → Accelerated Infusion

4. Another treatment option for diagnosis of occluded coronary arteries and treatment of AMI is an invasive procedure called percutaneous transluminal coronary angioplasty (PTCA). What is PTCA?

   LabTests → Cardiac ... → Tests → Invasive Procedures → Percutaneous Transluminal Coronary Angioplasty → scroll down to first bullet

5. Why are nitroglycerin and heparin used during the procedure?

   LabTests → Cardiac ... → Tests → Invasive Procedures → Percutaneous Transluminal Coronary Angioplasty → scroll down to second bullet

6. What is the emphasis of the clinician's role in the pretest phase of any diagnostic testing?

   LabTests → Diagnostic Testing → Pretest Phase

Physical and Occupational Therapy

1. What elements may be included in a comprehensive cardiac rehabilitation program?

   PMRRx → Cardiac Rehabilitation → Introduction → scroll down to first bullet

2. How is submaximal stress testing used during phase I of cardiac rehabilitation?

   PMRRx → Cardiac Rehabilitation → Phases of CR → Phase I → scroll down to third bullet

3. What types of exercises should be emphasized in the rehabilitation plan?

   PMRRx → Cardiac Rehabilitation → Exercise Rx → scroll down to second bullet

4. During your initial evaluation of Mrs. Tighe, you notice that she is not wearing antiembolism stockings despite her limited mobility at this time. Why is it important to suggest this treatment modality to the nurses and physicians caring for Mrs. Tighe?

   NurProc → Table of Contents → Antiembolism Stockings → Introduction

5. Mrs. Tighe has been prescribed a beta-blocker medication, Toprol XL 100 mg by mouth twice a day. What common central nervous system (CNS) adverse effects should you monitor during her cardiac rehabilitation sessions?

   PDH → Toprol XL → Adverse Reactions → CNS

Behavioral Health

1. Mrs. Tighe and her husband have asked how they can receive additional printed information about myocardial infarction and lifestyle changes to prevent future heart attacks. You are aware that the American Heart Association has various information available to the public that would be useful for them to receive. What contact information could you give them to request such information?

   5MCC → Myocardial Infarction → Patient Information

2. You have been asked to assist in developing the discharge plan for Mrs. Tighe. Any type of supportive care that Mrs. Tighe will receive in the home will require information related to her inpatient diagnosis and recent hospitalization. What is the ICD-9 code associated with and anterior wall myocardial infarction?

   5MCC → Myocardial Infarction → Miscellaneous → ICD-9

3. You are aware that the physician is planning to refer Mrs. Tighe for ongoing cardiac rehabilitation after discharge from the hospital. What other referrals would you suggest as part of the patient teaching and discharge planning process?

   NDisCheck → Myocardial Infarction → Patient Teaching → Discharge Planning

4. The doctors inform Mrs. Tighe that she will need a cardiac catheterization as an outpatient after she returns home and regains her strength. She confides in you that, although the doctors and nurses do their best to

explain things thoroughly, she still does not understand the purpose of this test and asks if you can explain the procedure in layman's terms. What can you tell her?

HbDxTests → Cardiac Catheterization → Patient Preparation

CASE STUDY 2 • *Mr. Steinman*

Cross-Discipline Learning Activities

1. You understand that the Glasgow Coma Score is used to evaluate level of consciousness in a patient. However, you hear the residents discussing this patient's Trauma Score. What is "Trauma Score," and why is it applicable in the care of this patient?

   HPND → Trauma Score → scroll down to first two sentences

2. In addition to having a subdural hematoma, which is tearing of the subdural veins and bleeding into the subdural space, this patient is diagnosed as having an epidural hematoma. What is an epidural hematoma?

   5MEmerg → Head Trauma, Blunt → Epidural Hematoma

3. In addition to the injuries that resulted to the head, this patient has multiple other traumatic injuries. When assessing a multisystem trauma patient a primary survey using the ABCDE order is conducted on arrival in the emergency department. This primary survey is done in a systematic and focused way to determine immediate patient care priorities. After consulting your PDA, you realize that

   "A" stands for assessment of the patient's airway and stabilization of the cervical spine

   "B" stands for assessment of the patient's breathing status

   "C" stands for assessment of the patient's circulation

   What critical element does the "D" step of the primary assessment involve?

   5MEmerg → Trauma, Multiple → Clinical Presentation → Primary Survey

4. The patient has experienced a significant amount of internal bleeding, and his vital signs indicate that he is experiencing decompensated hemorrhagic shock. When does decompensated hemorrhagic shock occur?

   5MEmerg → Clinical Presentation → Mechanism /Description → scroll down to fourth bullet

5. The patient has multiple fractures, including a flail chest. What is the description of a flail chest, and what is the most common cause?

   5MEmerg → Flail Chest → Clinical Presentation → scroll down to first and second bullets

6. A diagnostic peritoneal lavage (DPL) is performed in the emergency department on all patients with blunt chest trauma. Why is this procedure performed?

   5MEmerg → Chest Trauma, Blunt → Treatment → ED Treatment → scroll down to fourth bullet

7. What is the pathophysiology associated with hemothorax?

   NDisCheck → Hemothorax → Pathophysiology → scroll down to first and second bullets

Discipline-Specific Learning Activities

Nursing

1. When caring for a patient with head trauma that results in an epidural hematoma, positioning of the patient is an important component of care. What is the appropriate position of the bed?

   NDisCheck → Head Trauma → Epidural Hematoma → Treatment → scroll down to third bullet

2. What happens when a patient experiences increased intracranial pressure (ICP)?

   NDisCheck → Intracranial Pressure Elevation → What happens with . . .

3. The patient is transferred to ICU after surgery. Although his hemodynamic status is somewhat improved, there is still significant risk of increased ICPs. An ICP bolt is placed in the OR so that ICPs could be monitored frequently. What is the most common complication of ICP monitoring?

   NurProc → Intracranial Pressure Monitoring → Complications

4. The nurse is the person most likely to identify complications occurring in a patient with ICP monitoring. What are the signs of impending or overt decompensation that should be reported to the physician immediately?

   NurProc → Intracranial Pressure Monitoring → Complications

5. The patient also returned from the OR with chest tubes in place. You have been asked to accompany the patient to x-ray for follow-up CT studies. What special considerations are important when transporting a patient with chest tubes?

   NurProc → Chest Tube Insertion → Special Considerations

Medicine/PA/NP

1. You are impressed by how quickly and efficiently each member of the trauma team carries out his or her individual responsibilities. Yet you wonder why a

chest tube is placed before the technician completes processing the multiple trauma x-rays. What is the rationale for this treatment action with blunt chest trauma?

5MEmerg ➤ Chest Trauma, Blunt ➤ Treatment ➤ scroll down to fourth bullet

2. What are the mandatory x-rays that are an essential part of the diagnostic workup for all patients with multisystem trauma?

5MEmerg ➤ Trauma, Multiple ➤ Diagnosis ➤ Essential Workup ➤ scroll down to second bullet

3. What are the emergency department treatment priorities with multisystem trauma patients?

5MEmerg ➤ Trauma Multiple ➤ Treatment ➤ ED Treatment

4. What is a classic symptom that distinguishes an epidural hematoma from other types of intracranial bleeds when you are obtaining a history on a patient with blunt head trauma?

5MEmerg ➤ Head Trauma, Blunt ➤ Epidural Hematoma

5. What laboratory tests are typically ordered as part of the diagnostic workup for patients who present with blunt head trauma?

5MEmerg ➤ Head Trauma, Blunt ➤ Diagnosis ➤ Laboratory

Physical and Occupational Therapy

1. As a therapist, you care for many patients with a history of traumatic brain injury. What are the dynamic processes associated with traumatic brain injury?

5MCC ➤ Brain Injury, Traumatic ➤ Description

2. You notice that a significant number of your patients in therapy for post-traumatic brain injury have seizure disorders. Is this patient at risk for developing seizures?

5MCC ➤ Brain Injury, Traumatic ➤ Follow-Up

3. What gross assessment techniques are used to assess for disability related to spinal cord injuries in a patient with multisystem trauma during the primary survey conducted immediately upon arrival in the emergency department?

5MEmerg ➤ Trauma, Multiple ➤ Clinical Presentation ➤ Disability ➤ scroll down to third bullet

4. This patient has multiple femur fractures. When assessing the degree of comminution, the Winquist and Hansen classification system may be used. What is a grade III fracture according to this classification?

   5MEmerg → Femur Fracture → Clinical Presentation → Degree of Comminution → Winquist and Hansen Classification

5. Passive range-of-motion exercises are often indicated for patients with temporary or permanent loss of mobility sensation or consciousness. Are there ever situations where passive range-of-motion exercises are contraindicated?

   NurProc → Passive Range of Motion Exercises → Introduction → scroll down to second paragraph

Behavioral Health

1. What are the criteria for onset of symptoms in delayed onset PTSD?

   5MCC → Post Traumatic Stress Disorder → Basics → Description → scroll down to 5th bullet

2. What is the role of crisis intervention shortly after the traumatic event?

   5MCC → Post Traumatic Stress Disorder → Treatment → General Measures

3. You are aware that the Minnesota Multiphasic Personality Inventory (MMPI) is sometimes used to diagnose PTSD by evaluating an individual's personality dysfunction and level of stress. What are the elements that compose the MMPI?

   HPND → Minnesota Multiphasic Personality Inventory → Definition

4. In some circumstances a patient with PTSD will present with amnesia about the traumatic event. What special treatment modalities may be used to assist in the examination and interview of these patients during the diagnostic phase of treatment?

   5MCC → Post Traumatic Stress Disorder → Diagnosis → Special Tests → scroll down to 5th bullet

5. You are aware that a patient who has experienced an epidural hematoma has had a significant cerebral insult that will require attention of an inter-disciplinary care team after discharge from the hospital. What are two key elements that you will suggest that the nurses include in the planning of care for this patient?

   NDisCheck → Epidural Hematoma → Discharge Planning

CASE STUDY 3 • *Mr. Kiomato*

Cross-Discipline Learning Activities

1. What are two important factors to consider in anticipating the extent of injury in a burn patient?

   5MCC → Burns → Basics → Description

2. What criteria did the paramedics use to determine that Mr. Kiomato should be transported to your hospital, which is a regional burn center?

   5MCC → Burns → Treatment → Appropriate Health Care → scroll down to second bullet and second item

3. Are there age-related factors that impact Mr. Kiomato's overall prognosis?

   5MCC → Burns → Miscellaneous → Age-Related Factors → Expected Course/ Prognosis

4. Patients with severe burns present complex challenges that require the dedication and expertise of a specialized interdisciplinary group of professionals. What are the five major goals of care for a patient with severe burns?

   NurProc → Burn Care → Introduction → scroll down to first sentence

5. When should an interdisciplinary approach to discharge planning be started for Mr. Kiomato?

   NurProc → Burn Care → Patient Teaching → scroll down to first bullet

Discipline-Specific Learning Activities

Nursing

1. Maintaining fluid and electrolyte balance is a critical priority for burn patients. Monitoring intake and output is an important part of this nursing activity. What criteria should be used to monitor urine output in an adult burn patient?

   NDisCheck → Burns → Treatment → General → scroll down to fourth bullet

2. You recognize that carboxyhemoglobin is formed when hemoglobin is exposed to carbon monoxide during excessive smoke inhalation and that the affinity of hemoglobin for carbon monoxide is 240 times greater than that for oxygen causing hypoxia. What physical characteristic does Mr. Kiomato exhibit that suggests his carboxyhemoglobin level is elevated and that his confusion and lethargy are related to hypoxia?

   LabTests → Carboxyhemoglobin → Information → scroll down to fourth bullet

3. Twice daily dressing changes are common in the care of severely burned patients. What are the two ways burn dressings encourage healing?

NurProc ➤ Burn Care ➤ Introduction ➤ Toward bottom of paragraph

4. Dressing changes for burn patients can be an extremely painful experience. How should you schedule the administration of pain medication in relation to the timing of the scheduled dressing changes?

NurProc ➤ Burn Care ➤ Implementation ➤ scroll down to first bullet

5. The physician has decided to place an endotracheal tube in Mr. Kiomato to protect his airway and has ordered that 2 mg Versed be given as IV push for sedation and amnesia. How will you implement the administration of this initial infusion?

LNDG ➤ Versed (will automatically direct you to the generic name heading of midazolam hydrochloride) ➤ IV Facts ➤ Infusion

Medicine/PA/NP

1. Mr. Kiomato's singed nose hairs and his lethargy and confusion cause you to think about smoke inhalation as a differential diagnosis when considering airway management. What laboratory tests would you order to evaluate the severity of smoke inhalation in a patient?

5MCC ➤ Burns ➤ Diagnosis ➤ Special Tests ➤ scroll down to second bullet

2. To estimate the body surface area (BSA) involved in burn injuries, a technique called "rule of nines" is often used. If Mr. Kiomato presented with burns over both lower extremities, what percent of BSA would you estimate his injuries represent?

5MCC ➤ Burns ➤ Treatment ➤ General Measures ➤ scroll down to first bullet

3. Fluid resuscitation is an important aspect of care for a burn patient. What formula would you use to calculate Mr. Kiomato's fluid requirements for the first 24 hours?

5MCC ➤ Burns ➤ Treatment ➤ General Measures ➤ Burn Fluid Resuscitation ➤ scroll down to first bullet

How much of that total amount should be administered during the first 8 hours, after the burn injury occurred?

5MCC ➤ Burns ➤ Treatment ➤ General Measures ➤ Burn Fluid Resuscitation ➤ scroll down to first bullet

4. Pain management is an important consideration in the care of burn patients. What is the drug of choice in adults, and what dosage is recommended?

5MCC ➤ Burns ➤ Medications ➤ Drugs of Choice ➤ scroll down to first bullet

5. When reviewing lab results you notice that Mr. Kiomato has an elevated blood urea nitrogen (BUN). Other than dehydration, what is another common cause of an elevated BUN in burn patients?

HbDxTests ➙ Burns ➙ Information ➙ scroll down to seventh bullet

Physical and Occupational Therapy

1. What is the typical approach to burn therapy for severe burns that is largely within the practice domain of physical therapy?

5MCC ➙ Burns ➙ Treatment ➙ General Measures (half way through paragraph)

2. What is the activity goal of therapy once a burn patient is stabilized?

5MCC ➙ Burns ➙ Treatment ➙ Activity

3. Mr. Kiomato remains on a ventilator and is heavily sedated. He has an extensive third-degree circumferential burn on his left leg. The doctors are concerned about necrotic tissue affecting the peripheral circulation to his lower extremity and have asked Mr. Kiomato's wife for permission to perform an escharotomy. She states that she has a basic understanding and has given her consent for the needed treatment, but that she is uncomfortable explaining the purpose of the procedure to her daughter and asks for your assistance. How would you respond?

HPND ➙ Escharotomy

4. What are possible complications of extensive burns that can be prevented or minimized by early and ongoing physical and occupational therapy intervention and treatment?

5MCC ➙ Burns ➙ Possible Complications ➙ scroll down to fourth bullet

5. First-degree burns tend to resolve completely. Less severe second-degree burns will begin the process of epithelialization within 10–14 days. What is the expected course/prognosis for deep second- and third-degree burns?

5MCC ➙ Burns ➙ Expected Course/Prognosis

6. What patient teaching is required for prevention and avoidance of complications of involved burn sites after discharge?

5MCC ➙ Burns ➙ Prevention/Avoidance

Behavioral Health

1. Mr. Kiomato's condition is stabilized in the emergency department, and he has been transferred into the ICU. While you are providing emotional support to the family, Mr. Kiomato's daughter asks how long her father will

remain in the ICU and when they can expect that he will be discharged from the hospital. How would you respond?

5MCC ➤ Burns ➤ Expected Course/Prognosis ➤ scroll down to fourth bullet

2. Discharge planning will be an important part of the treatment plan for Mr. Kiomato. What three referral sources should be included in his discharge plan?

NDisCheck ➤ Burns ➤ Discharge Planning

3. Both nursing and behavioral disciplines will identify a common key outcome that Mr. Kiomato and his family will demonstrate effective coping techniques. The nursing staff has consulted you for advice on how best to achieve this goal. What nursing intervention would you suggest?

NDisCheck ➤ Burns ➤ Nursing Intervention ➤ scroll down to last bullet

4. Mr. Kiomato's family is concerned about Mr. Kiomato's ability to return to work after he recovers. They tell you that he is a proud man who takes great pride in his work. What statistical information can you provide?

5MCC ➤ Burns ➤ Follow-Up ➤ scroll down to last bullet

5. Mr. Kiomato's family does not understand why they are asked to wear a gown and mask when entering his room. You understand that these precautions are used to help prevent infection. Why is it especially important to prevent infection in burn patients?

NurProc ➤ Burn Care ➤ Introduction ➤ scroll down half way through paragraph

Unit 3

ADVANCED FUNCTIONALITIES— LETTING THE TECHNOLOGY DO THE HEAVY LIFTING

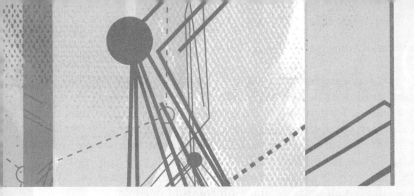

15

What Next? Putting Your PDA to Work

Frances H. Cornelius

Key Terms

Folders • In Pocket PC/Windows CE devices, places where you can organize and store items (documents, images, and applications) for easy access

Shared folder • The folder on the computer desktop that permits Pocket PC/Windows CE users to access and edit, on the computer, documents housed on the PDA (Notes, Word, Excel)

Template • A set of predesigned formats for text and graphics used to eliminate the need to recreate the same forms repeatedly; using a template saves time by speeding up the data entry process

Now that you have learned the basics about your PDA and have become more proficient in navigating some of the resources within your PDA to access information, you are ready to move on to new challenges. In this chapter, we discuss and demonstrate techniques that you can easily use to put this powerful tool to work—letting the technology "do the heavy lifting" by streamlining the work you do. Mastering the content in this chapter will help you organize your PDA according to your individual preferences. It will help you manage your information needs more efficiently and effectively.

Organizing and Managing Files/Applications

As with any information management system, establishing an organized file system can save you time and frustration and make it easier for you to locate important information. Both the Palm and the Pocket PC PDAs offer you a way to do this. Each device allows you to create files for your applications/tools and then move these applications/tools into the files. Palm users organize the filing system by categories, whereas Pocket PC users use **folders**, which is the standard Windows terminology. Although each device offers slightly different functionalities, the end result is the same—a better organized PDA that streamlines your workflow!

Pocket PC Folders

As stated earlier, the Pocket PC is a Windows OS, so it provides similar functionalities for creating and organizing folders. You can create folders from your desktop view or from the PDA view.

Creating a Folder Through ActiveSync

To create a folder from the desktop view, you must have your device connected to your computer. Using the ActiveSync window, click on Explore → My Pocket PC → Windows → Start Menu. This will get you to the area where you can place folders on your Start drop-down menu for quick access to your favorite tools and applications. Think a moment about how you want to set this up and decide what would best meet your needs. In the following exercises, you will set up several folders and move various applications into these folders. First, to keep things simple, remove all of the current items on your Start Menu.

On the Today screen of your PDA, tap on Start → Settings → Menus and remove the check mark from all of the boxes. Be sure to scroll through the entire list. When you have finished, tap on OK in the upper right corner of the screen. Now you are ready to create a folder on the Start Menu of your PDA.

Test Drive . . . .

To create a folder, follow the steps outlined below and illustrated in Figure 15.1.

1. Open ActiveSync on your desktop. (Be sure your PDA is connected.)
2. Using the ActiveSync window as shown in Figure 15.1A, click on Explore, located on the toolbar.
3. Select My Pocket PC as shown in Figure 15.1B.
4. Scroll down to select and open the Windows folder (see Figure 15.1C).
5. Scroll down to select and open the Start Menu folder (see Figure 15.1D).
6. Your screen should look like Figure 15.1E. Using standard Windows tools, create a new folder and give it the name Calculators. The following are two ways to create a new folder in this window:

   * Using the toolbar, select File ➤ New Folder
   * Right-click in the white area of the window and select New Folder

7. The Start Menu screen should look like Figure 15.1F.

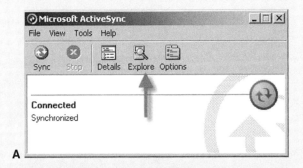

A

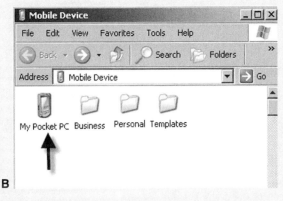

B

Figure 15.1 A–F Creating a new folder on the Start menu using ActiveSync—Pocket PC.

(Continued)

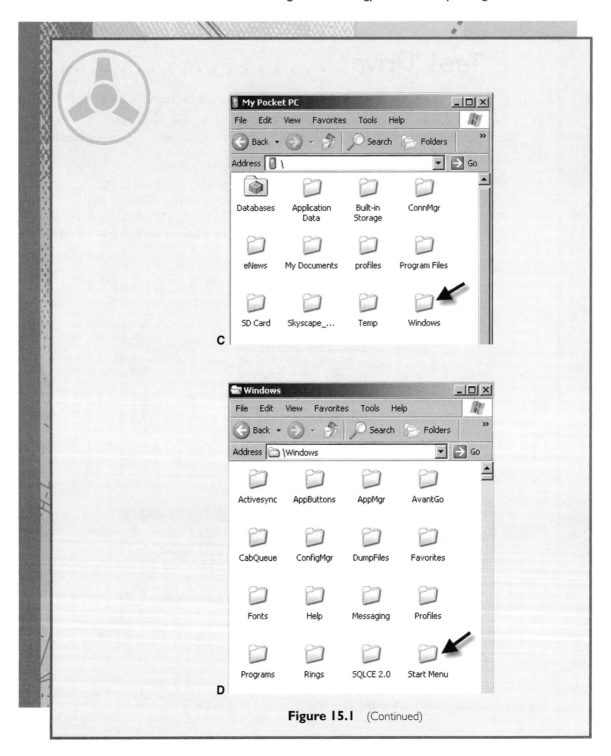

Figure 15.1   (Continued)

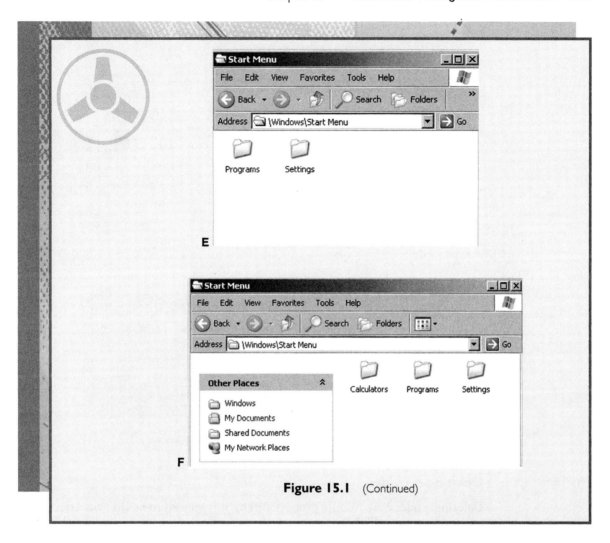

Figure 15.1 (Continued)

Now take a look at the Start Menu from your PDA. To do this, tap on Start on your Today screen. You should now see the Calculators folder on the dropdown menu as depicted in Figure 15.2. You can create additional folders using the same method.

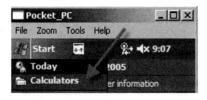

Figure 15.2 PDA view of the new folder on the Start menu—Pocket PC.

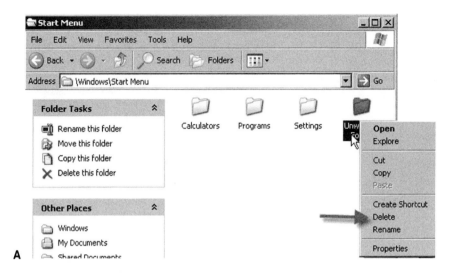

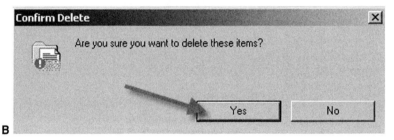

Figure 15.3 A–B Deleting a folder—Pocket PC.

Deleting a Folder

Deleting a folder is a simple process. Again, it is easiest to do this via ActiveSync on your computer. To begin, repeat steps 1 through 5 above and follow the steps below.

1. In the Start Menu folder, locate the folder you wish to delete.
2. *Before* you delete the folder, look inside the folder to make sure that you are not deleting anything that you wish to keep.
3. To proceed with the deletion, highlight and right-click on the folder.
4. From the drop-down menu, select Delete as shown in Figure 15.3A.
5. You will then see a delete-file confirmation message as depicted in Figure 15.3B. Click Yes to confirm the deletion.

Grouping Applications/Tools/References

Now that you have created a folder, it is time to move an item into the folder. Again, this process is very similar to moving items on your computer in a Windows environment. The first five steps are the same as for creating a new folder; subsequent steps are illustrated in Figure 15.4.

Test Drive . . . .

1. Open ActiveSync on your desktop (again, be sure your PDA is connected).
2. Using the ActiveSync window, click on Explore located on the toolbar.
3. Select My Pocket PC.
4. Scroll down to select and open the Windows folder.
5. Scroll down to select and open the Start Menu folder.
6. Select Programs as shown in Figure 15.4A.
7. Locate and highlight Calculator as shown in Figure 15.4B.
8. Right-click on Calculator and select Cut from the drop-down menu (see Figure 15.4C). *Note that cutting will remove the shortcut from the Programs folder. If you se-lect Copy, the shortcut will be available in both the Programs and the Calculator folders. Opting to use Copy instead of Cut thus defeats the purpose of moving items to decrease clutter in any particular area.*
9. Using the Back button on the upper left corner, go back to the Start Menu screen and open the Calculators folder (see Figure 15.4D).
10. Right-click in the white area of the folder and select Paste from the drop-down menu shown in Figure 15.4E.
11. Your screen should look like Figure 15.4F.

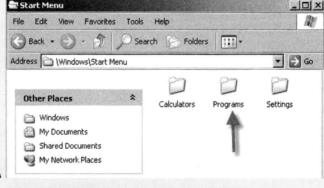

A

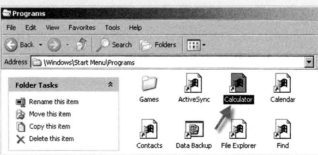

B

Figure 15.4 A–F Moving applications—Pocket PC.

(Continued)

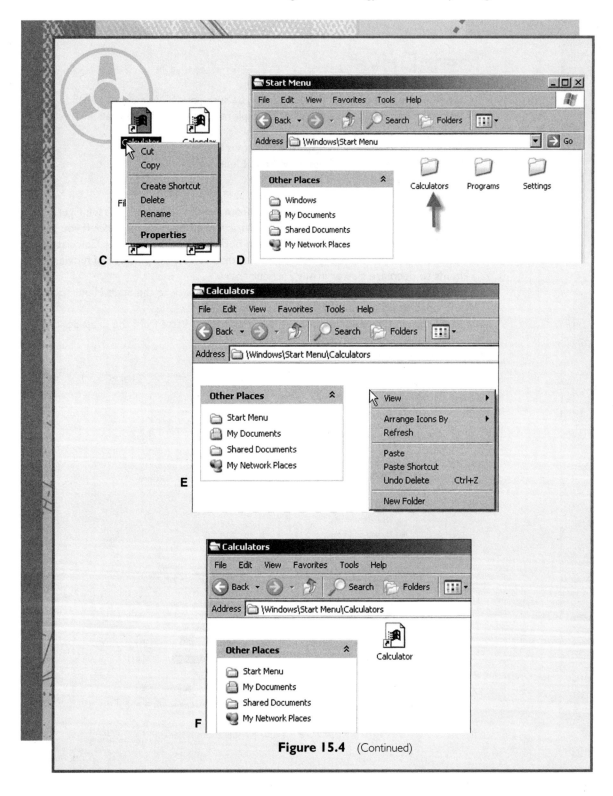

Figure 15.4 (Continued)

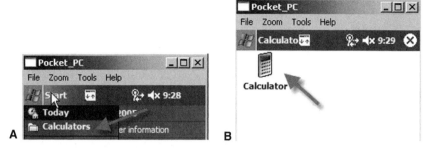

Figure 15.5 A–B PDA view of moved applications—Pocket PC.

Now return to your PDA. Tap on Start → Calculators (see Figure 15.5A), and you will be taken directly to the calculator application (see Figure 15.5B). As you can see, this speeds up access to programs that you frequently use, allowing you to access the program with only a few taps. Now you know how to easily organize your PDA according to your individual preferences. Using this process will help you efficiently and quickly access frequently used applications at the point-of-care, which, after all, is the purpose of bringing these handy and powerful tools to the health care arena!

Palm Categories

In Palm devices, creating folders that organize your tools and applications is a very simple process. This simple measure provides you with a means to quickly and easily access programs and tools you want to use. The Palm system refers to these folders as categories and offers the following default categories: Games, Main, System, Utilities, and Unfiled (see Figure 15.6). As you can see, Palm offers a broad category—All—which includes all of the tools and applications on the device as well as the capability to add or remove categories via the Edit Categories feature. For example, you may wish to add a new category, such as Calculators, to allow you to quickly access your PDA references. You can easily do this using the Edit Categories feature.

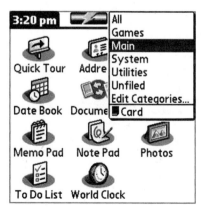

Figure 15.6 Default categories—Palm.

Adding a Category

Creating categories is the first step in getting your PDA organized. To begin this process, consider how you want to organize your device. That is, what categories would be most useful to you? Do you want to create categories according to specific activities or courses you are taking? Or do you want to organize it according to another method? The key is to create categories in a manner that makes sense to you and helps you streamline your work. Although thinking about this will be helpful before you proceed, any decision that you make will not be permanent, so you can experiment a bit until you find an organizational structure that best suits your style.

You can practice adding a category in the following exercise.

Test Drive . . . .

To create a new category, use the following simple steps outlined and illustrated in Figure 15.7.

1. Locate and tap on the ▼ on the upper right corner of your PDA screen, as shown in Figure 15.7A.
2. Select Edit Categories (see Figure 15.7B).
3. Select New and enter the new category, Calculators, using your preferred input method (see Figures 15.7C and D).
4. If you want to add additional categories, you can do so at this time. When finished, tap on OK and you will see that the new category has been added to the category list, as shown in Figure 15.7E. If you notice you have made a spelling error, highlight the misspelled word by tapping on it lightly and tapping on Rename. Make the spelling correction and tap on OK.
5. To finish, tap on OK again.

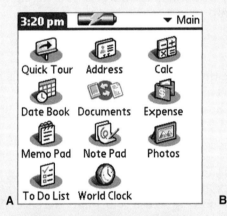

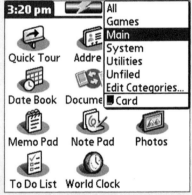

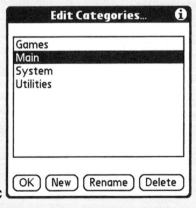

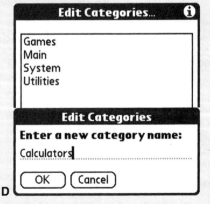

Figure 15.7 A–F Editing categories—Palm.

When you tap on the ▼ in the upper right corner of the screen, you will notice that there is now a new category called Calculators, as shown in Figure 15.7F.

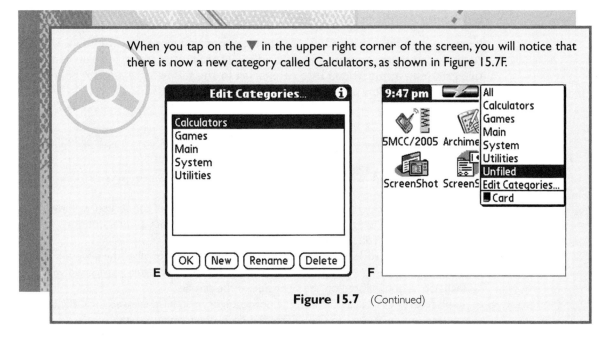

Figure 15.7 (Continued)

Deleting a Category

The process for deleting a category is also very simple. Use the following steps to delete a category. Note that if you delete a category that contains files or applications, you will not lose these items; they will instead be found in the broad Unfiled category.

1. Locate and tap on the ▼ in the upper right corner of your PDA screen, as shown in Figure 15.8A.
2. Select Edit Categories.
3. Highlight the category you wish to delete by tapping on it. Then tap on Delete and the selected category will disappear (see Figure 15.8B).

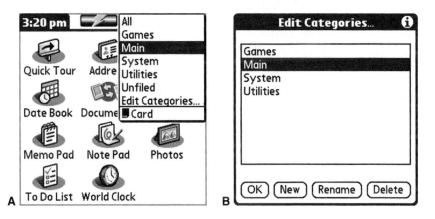

Figure 15.8 A–B Deleting categories—Palm.

Grouping Applications/Tools/References

Now that you have created all of the categories you want on your PDA, you are ready to put your programs, tools, and references into categories. You can practice grouping applications into categories in the following exercise. Follow the steps outlined below and illustrated in Figure 15.9.

Test Drive . . . .

1. To begin, tap on the time located in the upper left corner of the screen, as shown in Figure 15.9A. Doing so will reveal a drop-down menu with several options.
2. Select Category from the list shown in Figure 15.9B.
3. As shown in Figure 15.9C, this will provide you with a list of all of the programs and tools installed on your PDA. You will notice that the category associated with each application is listed on the right side of the screen.
4. To place the PDA calculator into the new category you have created for Calculators, tap on the ▼ next to Calc. From the drop-down menu, select Calculators (see Figure 15.9D).
5. You will notice that the application now has the new Calculators category associated with it (see Figure 15.9E).
6. Repeat this process with all other applications that you wish to organize into the categories you have created.
7. When finished, tap on Done.
8. To view each category, tap on the ▼ at the upper right corner of your PDA screen, as shown in Figure 15.9F.
9. Tap on Calculators on the drop-down menu, as shown in Figure 15.9G. In the next screen, depicted in Figure 15.9H, you will notice that the calculator program has been placed in the new folder.

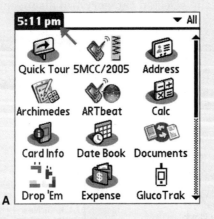 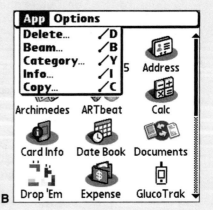

Figure 15.9 A–H Grouping applications/tools—Palm.

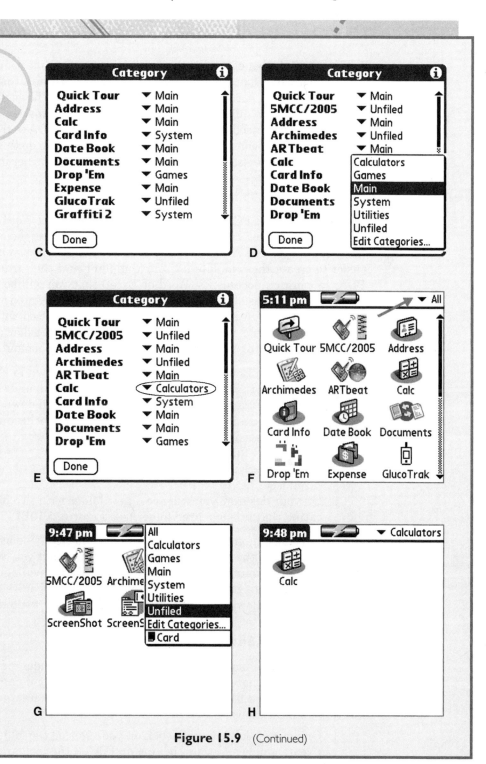

Figure 15.9 (Continued)

Creating Forms/Templates to "Lighten the Load"

Again, one of the benefits of having a PDA is to streamline some of the work you do. One method of streamlining is to create forms or templates, which can speed up your data entry, particularly the repetitious aspects. The goal is to create forms that can be used to quickly and accurately collect information while "on-the-go." However, you first need to set up a file system on your PDA so that all of your documents and forms can be easily located on your PDA. To do this, you need to use the same technique used to organize your applications earlier in the chapter.

Templates for Pocket PC/Windows CE

Because the Pocket PC/Windows CE devices have Pocket Word and Pocket Excel as standard features, creating templates and transferring them to your PDA is a fairly simple process. Although you can create templates on your PDA, it is often easier to create the template on your computer and then transfer it onto your PDA. To work on documents (Word or Excel) that you will be able to access on your PDA, you must first set up the sync option associated with this feature. To do this, your PDA must be connected and synchronized with your computer. From the ActiveSync window, follow the steps outlined below and illustrated in Figure 15.10 to share documents between your desktop computer and your PDA.

1. Click on Options located on the toolbar, as shown in Figure 15.10A.
2. Make sure that the box next to Files is checked, and click OK, as shown in Figure 15.10B. You may need to scroll down to see Files.
3. You will see a message notifying you that a synchronized file folder will be created on the desktop (see Figure 15.10C). Click OK to create the shared folder.
4. Your ActiveSync window will show that a shared file folder is synchronized (see Figure 15.10D).
5. On your desktop, you will see a new folder with two blue arrows indicating that it is a shared folder (see Figure 15.10E).

All of the documents on your PDA will automatically be available to you on your computer via the new shared folder. Anything that you wish to save to the shared folder on your desktop will automatically be available to you on your PDA. You can organize the folder just as you would organize any file folder on your PC. In the following exercises, you will learn how to do this.

Organizing Your Shared Folder

It is easier to make modifications to your shared file folder via your desktop. To do this, open the shared file folder on your desktop. By default, folders are already in the shared file folder (see Figure 15.11A). To create a new folder, follow these simple steps:

1. On your desktop, double-click on your shared file folder to open it. Create a new folder by clicking on File on the toolbar, highlighting New, and selecting Folder (see Figure 15.11B).

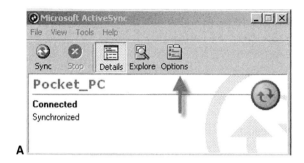

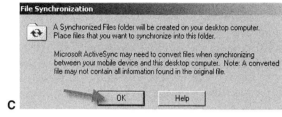

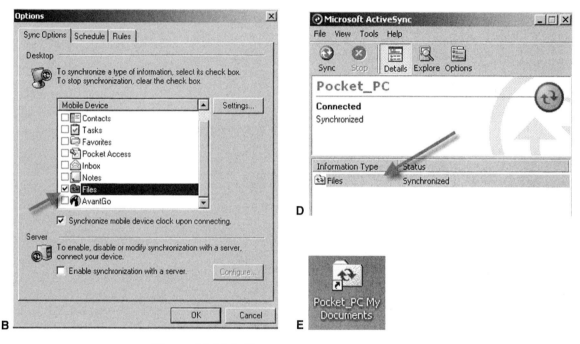

Figure 15.10 A–E   Creating a shared file—Pocket PC.

2. Ordinarily, you would give this new folder a name that is meaningful to you. For the purposes of this exercise, name the folder A & P Notes (abbreviation for Anatomy and Physiology). Refer to Figures 15.11C and D for clarification.

3. Next, to access this folder on your PDA, tap on Start → Programs → File Explorer. Refer to Figures 15.12A–C for clarification of this process.

Congratulations! You have taken the first step toward organizing your documents on your PDA.

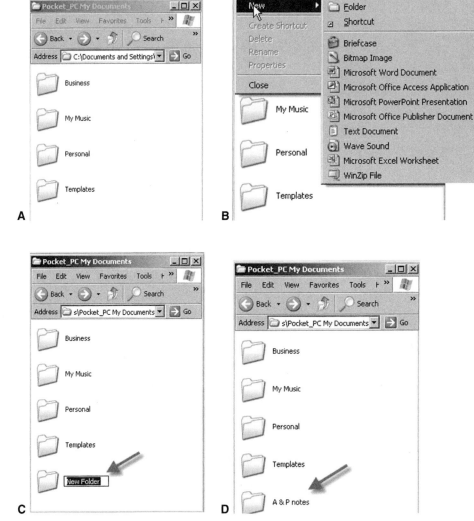

Figure 15.11 A–B Default shared folders—Pocket PC. **C–D** Creating a new shared folder—Pocket PC.

Speeding Up Your Note Taking

Creating templates will help you speed up your note taking and data entry. You can create a template from scratch, or you can use an existing template that someone else created. Existing templates can also be modified (tweaked) to meet your specific needs.

Many templates are available online, free of charge or for a nominal fee. Microsoft offers free templates that you can download from their Web site, http://office.microsoft.com/en-us/templates/default.aspx. Not all of these templates are

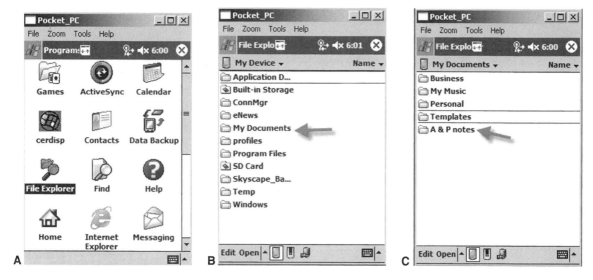

Figure 15.12 A–C   Accessing shared folder on the PDA—Pocket PC.

appropriate for the small PDA screen, but you may find one that you can adapt for your device.

If you find that you are frequently reentering the same information on many different documents, you may wish to create a template with the repetitious information in place. Then all you will need to do is use the template to complete a new document, saving yourself time in the process. In the following exercise, we will create a simple Word document template for your PDA.

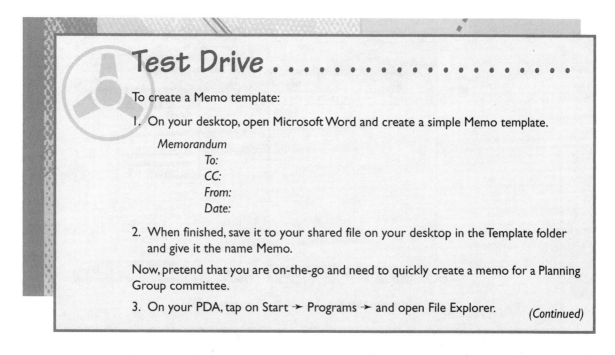

Test Drive . . . .

To create a Memo template:

1. On your desktop, open Microsoft Word and create a simple Memo template.

   Memorandum
   > *To:*
   > *CC:*
   > *From:*
   > *Date:*

2. When finished, save it to your shared file on your desktop in the Template folder and give it the name Memo.

Now, pretend that you are on-the-go and need to quickly create a memo for a Planning Group committee.

3. On your PDA, tap on Start ➤ Programs ➤ and open File Explorer.   *(Continued)*

4. Locate and open My Documents, as shown in Figure 15.13A.
5. Locate and open the Templates folder (see Figure 15.13B).
6. You will see, as shown in Figure 15.13C, that you have the Memo template in this folder.
7. Highlight this template (do not open it) and select Copy from the drop-down menu depicted in Figure 15.13D. *Hint:* Press and hold the stylus on the highlighted document to open the drop-down menu.

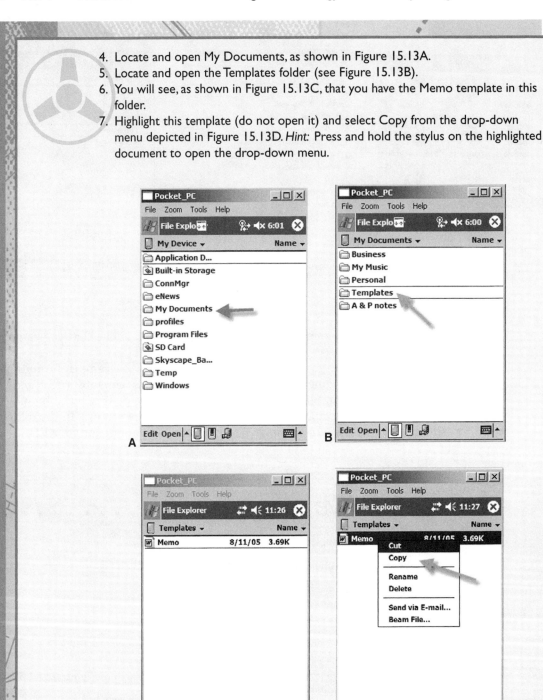

Figure 15.13 A–J   Creating and using templates—Pocket PC.

8. Next, navigate back to the My Documents folder by tapping on the ▼ located in the upper left corner next to Templates. From the drop-down menu depicted in Figure 15.13E select My Documents.

9. In the next screen, select and open the Business folder (see Figure 15.13F). Press and hold the stylus and select Paste to place the copy of Memo in this folder (see Figure 15.13G).

10. Highlight Memo (press and hold) and select Rename from the drop-down menu (see Figure 15.13H).

11. Rename the memo Planning Group (see Figure 15.13I).

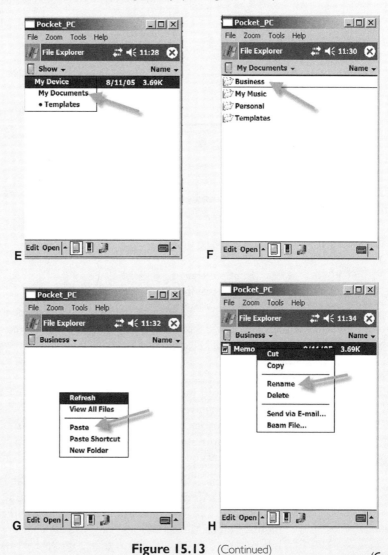

Figure 15.13 (Continued)

(Continued)

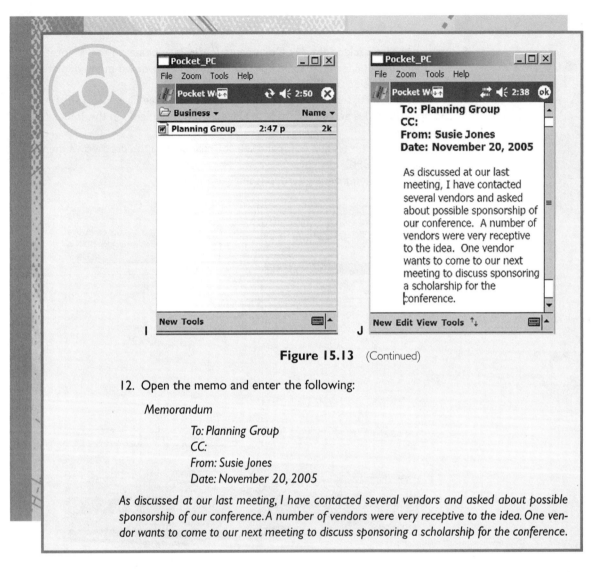

Figure 15.13 (Continued)

12. Open the memo and enter the following:

Memorandum

> *To: Planning Group*
> *CC:*
> *From: Susie Jones*
> *Date: November 20, 2005*

As discussed at our last meeting, I have contacted several vendors and asked about possible sponsorship of our conference. A number of vendors were very receptive to the idea. One vendor wants to come to our next meeting to discuss sponsoring a scholarship for the conference.

Your Memo should look something like Figure 15.13J. Congratulations! You have successfully created and used your first template!

There is also another method to accomplish the same thing. Both methods are similar, and determining which one to use is a matter of personal preference. This alternative method is detailed in the following steps:

1. Repeat steps 1 through 3 of the previous Test Drive.
2. On your PDA, tap on Start → Programs → and open Pocket Word.
3. Tapping on the ▼ in the upper left corner will reveal a drop-down menu. Select More Folders (tapping repeatedly) until Templates is visible on the drop-down menu (see Figure 15.14A).
4. Tap on the Templates folder to open it (see Figure 15.14B). You will see that you have the Memo template in this folder (see Figure 15.14C).

5. Highlight this template (do not open it) and select Create Copy from the drop-down menu, as shown in Figure 15.14D.
6. This will create a copy of the Memo called Memo(1), as shown in Figure 15.14E.
7. Highlight Memo(1) and select Rename/Move from the drop-down menu, as shown in Figure 15.14F.
8. In this window, rename the memo Planning Group, as shown in Figure 15.14G, and move it to your Business folder, as shown in Figure 15.14H.
9. If you have a storage card available, in the same window, you can elect to store this document on your Secure Digital (SD) card, as shown in Figure 15.14I. [Please note: the memo can also be placed on a Compact Flash (CF) card.]

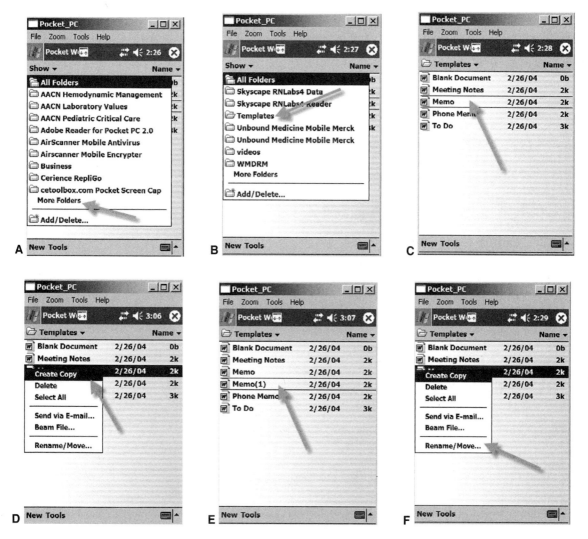

Figure 15.14 A–I Alternative method for creating and using templates—Pocket PC.

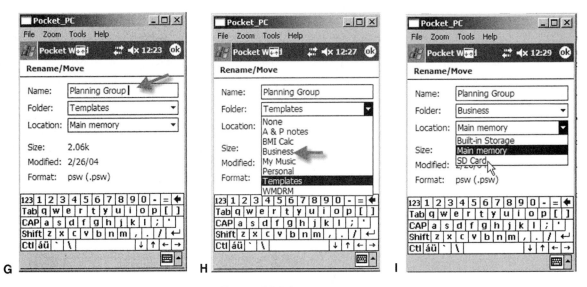

Figure 15.14 (Continued)

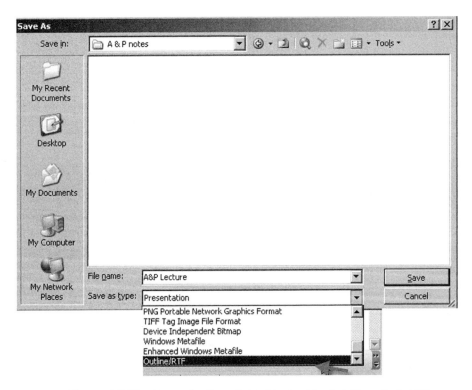

Figure 15.15 Converting PowerPoint slides to aid note taking—Pocket PC.

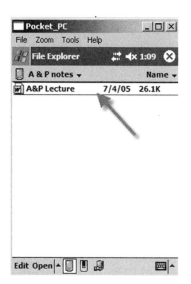

Figure 15.16 Accessing converted PowerPoint on your PDA—Pocket PC.

Converting PowerPoint Slides to Aid in Note Taking

Another time-saving technique is converting PowerPoint presentations into Word documents, which provides an outline structure to facilitate note taking in class. To do this you will need an obliging faculty member who is willing to give you the lecture PowerPoint slides in advance. Once you have the PowerPoint lecture, save it to your shared folder as an Outline/RTF, as shown in Figure 15.15. Note that some basic formatting may be necessary to ensure that the outline is easily viewable on your smaller PDA screen. At a minimum, you will need to reduce the font size to 10 so that it will be easier to read on your PDA. Selecting a simple font, such as Arial, will also improve readability of your document. To add class notes, open the document on your PDA, as shown in Figure 15.16, and begin entering your notes using your preferred input method.

Proprietary Applications

Sometimes the built-in functions of your PDA do not entirely meet your organizational needs. Many additional software applications are available either for purchase or as freeware or shareware (see Chapter 5). As you become more proficient using your PDA, you may wish to add more functionality to your PDA. The following sites are good starting points:

- Windows Mobile—http://www.microsoft.com/windowsmobile
- PocketPCSoftnet—http://www.ipaqsoft.net
- PocketGear—http://www.pocketgear.com
- Handango—http://www.handango.com

Templates for Palm

Organizing Your Notes

In Palm devices, Word does not come as a standard feature. If you wish to work with documents between your PDA and computer, you must purchase additional software. Several products are on the market, including Documents To Go by DataViz, QuickOffice Premier by QuickOffice, and PrintBoy by QuickOffice Bachman Software. These products will allow you to easily work with standard office documents including Word, Excel, and PowerPoint on your Palm device. The Palm Note Pad offers limited capability for carrying extensive notes and documents with you. If you need more, you might consider investing in additional software.

Even though Palm Note Pad has limited capabilities for extensive note taking, you may wish to use this feature to store snippets of information for easy access at the point-of-care. To organize your notes so that you can easily locate a particular note on your Palm device, follow the same instructions for creating categories for your PDA applications.

1. On your Palm PDA, open Note Pad.
2. Locate and tap on the ▼ on the upper right corner of the PDA screen, as shown in Figure 15.17A.

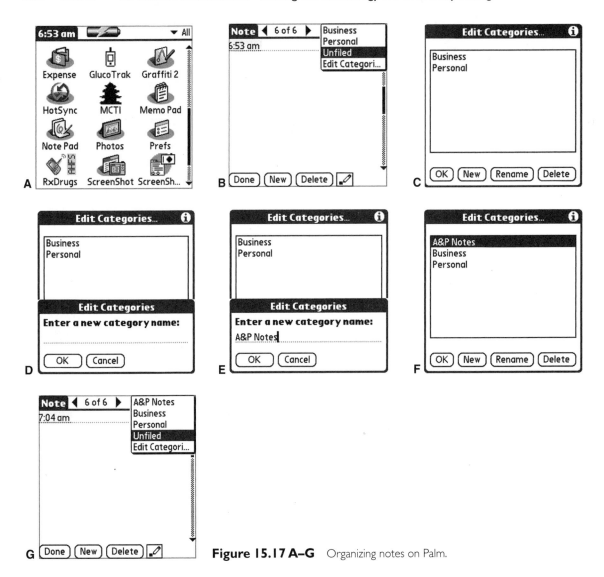

Figure 15.17 A–G Organizing notes on Palm.

3. Select Edit Categories from the drop-down menu, as shown in Figure 15.17B.
4. Select New and enter the new category, for example, A & P Notes, using your preferred input method, as shown in Figures 15.17C through E.
5. If you want to add additional categories, you can do so at this time. When finished, tap on OK and you will see that the new category has been added to the category list, as shown in Figure 15.17F. If you notice you have made a spelling error, just highlight the misspelled word by tapping on it lightly and tapping on Rename. Make the spelling correction and tap on OK.
6. To finish, tap on OK again.

Now when you are in Note Pad and tap on the ▼ in the upper right corner, you will notice that there is now a new category called A & P Notes, as shown in Figure 15.17G.

Proprietary Applications

As stated earlier in the chapter, there are several proprietary applications that allow you to expand your Palm device's functionality and work with standard office applications. If you plan to use your Palm device for more robust purposes, the following Web sites are good starting points:

- PalmSource—http://www.palmsource.com
- palmOne—http://www.palmone.com
- Handango—http://www.handango.com

Giving Presentations

You can give presentations using your PDA; however, both the Pocket PC and Palm devices require additional software to be installed before this is possible. Several products on the market allow you to transfer PowerPoint presentations to your PDA and then use the PDA to conduct a presentation. Imagine the convenience of hooking up your small handheld device to a projector—entirely bypassing the laptop. Using Margi, Lifeview FlyPresenter, Colorgraphic, PitchDuo, Pretec, and other presentation systems, you can display your presentations from your PDA to large groups, using a projector. This eliminates the need to bring along a laptop as well as having your presentation stored on a floppy disk or CD. What a wonderful feeling to have your PowerPoint presentation in your pocket!

No matter which presentation software you use, you must create the presentation on your computer before transferring it over to your PDA. Once you have transferred the presentation onto the PDA, you will not be able to make changes to your completed PowerPoint. You can create the PowerPoint using Microsoft PowerPoint on your desktop and then, using a simple plug-in application which comes with the presentation devices, you can easily transfer the files to your PDA during your next ActiveSync or HotSync.

Summary

We have reviewed some of the techniques you can use to customize your PDA to your personal preferences. Folders and categories organize your frequently used tools and applications for quick and easy access. The key objective is for you to streamline your work and let the technology "do the heavy lifting"!

Tips From the Experts

- When organizing your PDA, limit the number of tools or applications you place within a given folder or category to a maximum of 12 items. This will eliminate the need to scroll to access a particular item and, consequently, will speed things up for you.
- You can reassign the buttons on your PDA to applications or tools other than the default settings (Calendar, Contacts, etc.). This will allow you to quickly access a frequently used application or tool by simply pressing a button.

LEARNING ACTIVITIES

Pocket PC

1. Using the ActiveSync window on your PC, create a new folder on your Start Menu. Give it the name MS Office. Then move Pocket Word and Pocket Excel to the new folder. (Hint: you can move more than one item at a time by pressing the control key when selecting the desired items.)

2. If you have installed e-Books onto your PDA, create a new folder on your PDA, using your PDA only (do not use the ActiveSync interface). Create a new folder called either Books or References on your Start Menu. Move your e-Book(s) to the new folder. (Hint: you will need to move one e-Book at a time.)

Palm

1. On your PDA, create a new category and give it the name Help. Then move Quick Tour and Graffiti 2 to the new category.

2. If you have installed e-Books onto your PDA, create a new category on your PDA called either Books or References. Move your e-Book(s) to the category.

WebLink.   Visit http://thePoint.LWW.com/cornelius for supplemental information and activities.

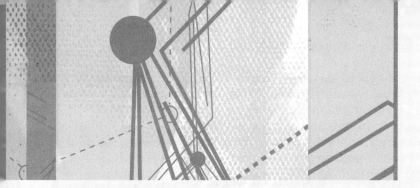

16

Clinical Decision-Making Tools

Frances H. Cornelius

Key Terms

Algorithm • A specific rule (or set of rules) or step-by-step procedure that details how to solve a problem or accomplish a goal

Clinical Decision Support (CDS) • A class of computerized information systems or software that uses database resources to assist users in decision-making activities, including patient care options, by providing structured (rules-based) information on diagnoses and treatments

Conditional logic • Programming strategy used in decision-making tools in which specific actions or responses will occur, depending on which conditions are met

e-Book • A book published in electronic form that can be downloaded to computers or handheld devices

e-Journal • An electronic format of a journal availalble via the Internet.

URL • Uniform Resource Locator—the "address" of a particular document/resource on the Internet that functions similarly to a house address; URLs begin with "http://" on the World Wide Web

nformation is critical to making sound decisions, and decision support information is essential to health care professionals. The process of accessing relevant and timely information is an essential component of decision making. For information to be useful, it must meet the following criteria: It must be the *right information* provided to the *right person* at the *right time* in the *right place* in the *right amount*. These criteria are referred to as the "Five Rights of Information" and are essential in effective decision making.

Because the amount of information available is overwhelming, and we as humans cannot reasonably expect to remember it all, an effective information retrieval system is essential to making the right information available when a person needs it. Ideally, this process of accessing information should occur with minimal effort and be provided in an amount that answers the question sufficiently without being overwhelming. In other words, the retrieved information should be "just enough, just in time." The PDA serves as a useful tool for health care providers, not only because of its functionality as a means of obtaining the right amount of information when needed, but also because of the mobility of the device. As PDAs become progressively more powerful with storage capacities of 4 GB and more, the possibilities for practice increase dramatically. PDAs are used in the clinical setting primarily for decision support and error reduction—checking drugs, dosages, and compatibilities (McGowen, 2003; Stolworthy & Suszka-Hildebrandt, 2002).

The number of health care providers using these powerful little devices is growing. Many health care professionals are beginning to realize that, by adopting handheld technology, they can provide high quality care that is likely to be more appropriate, effective, efficient, and safe because it is based on current information and resources; the benefit to patients is enormous.

As discussed in Chapter 1, handheld computers are being used increasingly to "extend the human mind's capacity to recall and process large numbers of relevant variables and to support information management, general administration and clinical practice" (Stolworthy & Suszka-Hildebrandt, 2002). These devices can provide the health care professional with **clinical decision support (CDS)** by providing a means to organize and present key information that guides practice. Clinical decision support in the clinical setting can improve the safety, quality, efficiency, cost-effectiveness, and outcomes of patient care. Clearly, in this situation, everyone wins—health care practitioners, health care organizations, and, more importantly, patients.

Many PDA-based tools and resources can be used at the point of care to guide decision making. For the most part, these resources can be organized into four categories: (1) electronic books (**e-Books**), (2) calculation tools (including basic calculators and more sophisticated **algorithms**), (3) evidence-based practice resources, and (4) differential diagnosis tools. This chapter presents a general overview of these resources.

References (e-Books)

Certainly, major resources that can support clinical decision making are electronic references (e-Books) that can be housed on your PDA. Virtually all the publishers of medical references have PDA versions of their books. Just as with traditional hard copy books, the quality of these references varies—some are excellent, whereas others fall short. Designing a functional e-Book is a complex process; it is not merely a case of converting an excellent reference to an electronic format. Because of the small screen and the way in which these powerful point-of-care references are used, the information must be presented in "bite-size" pieces so that the health care provider can easily obtain the needed information.

Because the design of the e-Book is an important consideration, it is advisable that you examine trial versions of e-Books before purchasing the references. Many publishers offer a trial version that contains limited content but provides a clear understanding of what the whole reference has to offer.

A good e-Book—one that is comprehensive and up-to-date—can help the health care provider with clinical decision making. Indeed, this is often the first resource accessed in the decision-making process. An e-Book is frequently used to check drug dosages or compatibilities, review the significance of specific lab findings, guide safe practice, and more.

Good starting points for obtaining PDA references include vendors, publishers, and educational institutions or professional organizations. Box 16.1 provides a list of vendors (a sample only, not an all-inclusive list) that have multiple references available from many different publishers and that have competitive prices.

| Box 16.1 | **VENDORS OFFERING E-BOOKS FOR THE PDA** |

CollectiveMed—http://www.collectivemed.com
> CollectiveMed has a vast library of e-books from multiple publishers and vendors as well as special pricing for e-Book Bundles.

Handheldmed—http://www.handheldmed.com
> Handheldmed offers good deals when you buy a customized book library (2- to 5-book package).

MobiPocket—http://www.mobipocket.com
> MobiPocket provides a large variety of electronic books and much more for mobile device users.

PDA Cortex: The Journal of Mobile Informatics—http://pdacortex.com
> PDA cortex is more than just a place to get information, resources, and lots of downloads on health care for physicians and nurses; it is an active network of PDA users—many who are transforming health care practice.

Pepid—http://pepid.com
> Pepid offers a subscriptions service for up-to-date e-Resources, but when the subscription expires, the entire resource is no longer available to you on your PDA.

Skyscape, Inc.—http://www.skyscape.com
> Skyscape has an extensive library of references from multiple publishers that are fully integrated through smARTlink technology, which links topics/content across multiple references.

Box 16.2	**EDUCATIONAL INSTITUTIONS AND ORGANIZATIONS OFFERING PDA REFERENCE/RESOURCE LISTS**

American Association of Critical Care Nurses (AACN)
http://aacn.pdaorder.com/welcome.xml

Nursing Library and Information Resources
http://info.med.yale.edu/library/nursing/reference/pda.html

Nursing Resources for the PDA
http://library.osfsaintfrancis.org/nursingpda.htm

University of Alberta
http://www.library.ualberta.ca/subject/nursing/pdahealth/index.cfm

American Medical Student Association
http://www.amsa.org

You can also buy your e-Book directly from a publisher. So, if you have a favorite reference, you may wish to contact that publisher to find out whether there is a PDA version available. Lippincott Williams & Wilkins offers various e-Books for the PDA, which you can find on their Web site, http://www.lww.com.

Educational institutions and professional organizations will also create extensive resource lists for their membership. These sites are often also a good place to locate standards of practice for specialties such as pediatrics, geriatrics, or others. Usually, these resources are developed to meet the specialty interests or needs of the membership, but often there are extensive general resource lists as well. Some examples of educational institutions and organizations offering such resource lists are given in Box 16.2.

An important consideration in selecting an e-Book is its look and feel. Is navigation smooth? Is it easy to get to the information quickly? And, of course, does it have the information you need? It pays to shop around to see what interface works best for you.

Calculation Tools

Calculation tools are also a very important clinical resource for decision support. At the very basic level, a standard calculator can be used to calculate a medication dose or an intravenous infusion rate. Using a standard calculator helps avoid common calculation errors, but only when the correct formula is used in the first place. In a busy practice environment, it is easy to make an error when one is in a hurry. Common errors usually involve basic math functions and decimal point placement. In health care, these errors have the potential to cause significant harm or even death.

Simple calculation tools, which are preprogrammed with commonly used formulas, provide a means to avoid these common calculation errors and supply

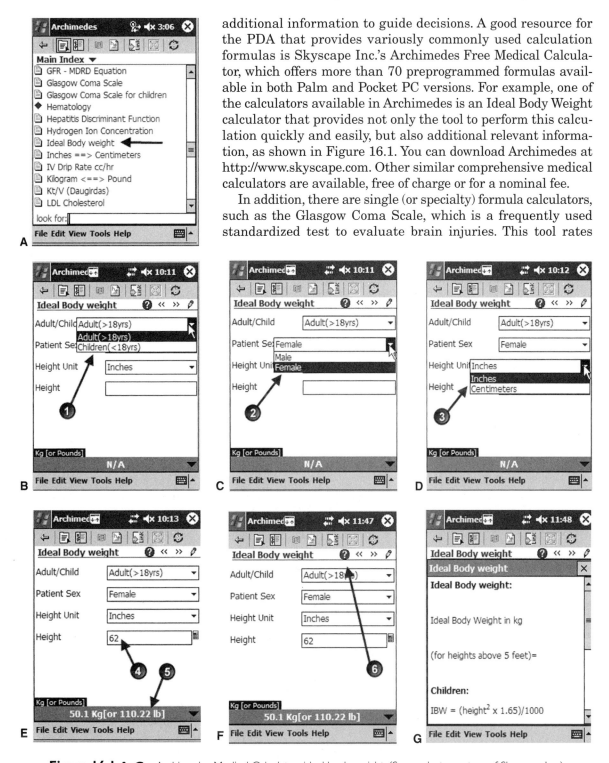

additional information to guide decisions. A good resource for the PDA that provides variously commonly used calculation formulas is Skyscape Inc.'s Archimedes Free Medical Calculator, which offers more than 70 preprogrammed formulas available in both Palm and Pocket PC versions. For example, one of the calculators available in Archimedes is an Ideal Body Weight calculator that provides not only the tool to perform this calculation quickly and easily, but also additional relevant information, as shown in Figure 16.1. You can download Archimedes at http://www.skyscape.com. Other similar comprehensive medical calculators are available, free of charge or for a nominal fee.

In addition, there are single (or specialty) formula calculators, such as the Glasgow Coma Scale, which is a frequently used standardized test to evaluate brain injuries. This tool rates

Figure 16.1 A–G Archimedes Medical Calculator: ideal body weight. (Screenshot courtesy of Skyscape, Inc.)

three categories of patient responses: (1) eye opening, (2) motor response, and (3) verbal response. The different levels of responses for the three categories indicate the degree of nervous system or brain impairment; total scores range from no impairment (score = 3) to high impairment (score = 15). As you can see in the example provided in Figure 16.2, the tool is very simple and straightforward. You can easily enter the levels of responses using the drop-down menus provided and then tapping Calculate to finish. Many versions of this tool are available, all of which function similarly. You can access the Glasgow Coma Scale from various sites; the simplest way to access a free version of the application is to do an Internet search for "Glasgow Coma Scale freeware for PDA."

Even more sophisticated calculators are available to assist in clinical decision making, and they operate using algorithms that use **conditional logic** and rely on a knowledge base of scientific evidence to help decision making and guide practice. In simple terms, an algorithm is a special calculator that uses a series of conditional statements or findings that, when present or absent, provide summary conclusions. For example, an algorithm can calculate the level of risk associated with certain lifestyle choices (i.e., smoking), using

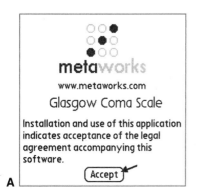

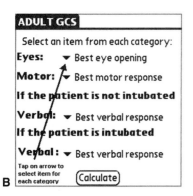
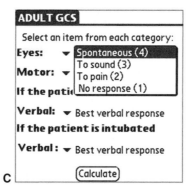
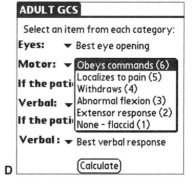

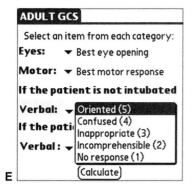
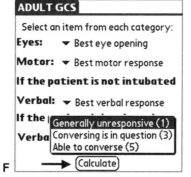
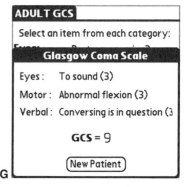

Figure 16.2 A–G Glasgow Coma Scale. (Reprinted with permission from Metaworks, Inc. Available at http://www.metaworks.com.)

research statistics associated with individual variables, such as age, race, blood pressure, and so on. Such a tool can identify the likelihood that this person would have a heart attack or stroke. It can be a very effective patient teaching tool when discussing lifestyle changes to promote health and reduce risk. In other instances, such a tool can calculate the risk benefit of a surgical versus nonsurgical treatment plan.

To clarify this, we will use the Coronary Vascular Disease (CVD) Risk Calculator provided by PDA Consults, Inc. Within this simple tool, the user enters the patient information depicted in Figure 16.3, which includes key data that are known through research to be significant variables influencing the risk of developing coronary vascular disease, such as sex, age, total cholesterol, history of smoking, and so on. Changing a variable (smoking) that can be controlled, as shown in the example depicted, will change the risk value for the better. Tools such as the CVD Risk Calculator can be excellent patient teaching tools by providing important information in a clear, concise manner.

Another example of a sophisticated calculation tool for the PDA is the National Heart, Lung, and Blood Institute's interactive treatment guideline tool for the treatment of obesity. This program is made available as part of the educational mission of the Obesity Education Initiative (OEI) of the National Institutes of Health (NIH) National Heart, Lung, and Blood Institute (NHLBI), so additional information regarding treatment guidelines is also available from this organization. This calculator, which includes a body mass index (BMI) classification table for adults, is available for both Pocket PC and Palm PDAs and accepts both English and metric system input. It is easy to use.

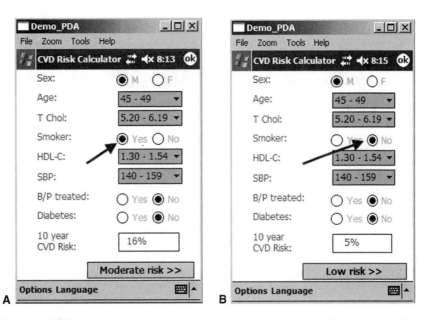

Figure 16.3 Calculating CVD risk: **A** Smoker. **B** Nonsmoker. (Coronary Vascular Disease (CVD) Risk Calculator courtesy of PDA Consults, Inc.)

For example, we will assume that you have a patient with the following characteristics:

Female
170 pounds
5 feet, 7 inches tall
Waist circumference = 27 inches
History of high blood pressure and diabetes
Family history of early cardiovascular disease (CVD)

The NHLBI OEI tool will provide specific treatment recommendations for this individual, based upon established practice standards for care. As you can see in Figure 16.4, the recommendation for this patient is lifestyle modification

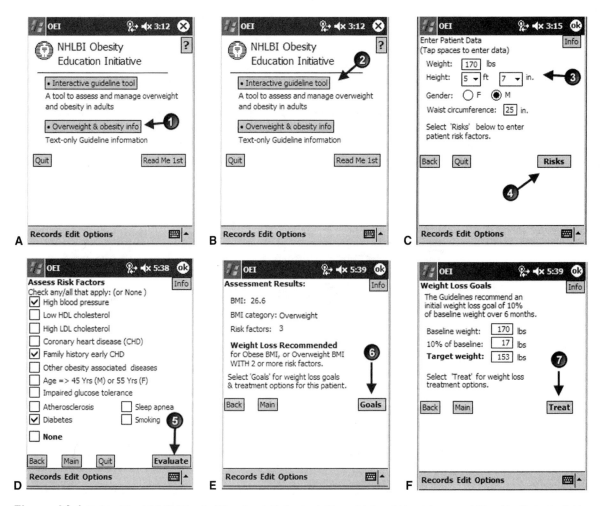

Figure 16.4 A–H   The NHLBI Obesity Education Initiative tool. (From National Heart, Lung, and Blood Institute. Available at http://hin.nhlbi.nih.gov/obgdpalm.htm.)

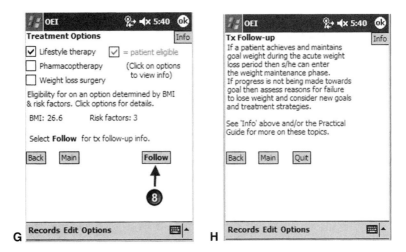

Figure 16.4 (Continued)

and a weight loss of 17 pounds (10% of baseline), along with recommendations for follow-up. To learn more about this initiative or to download it and install onto your PDA, go to the NHLBI Web site, http://hin.nhlbi.nih.gov/obgdpalm.htm.

In both examples provided, it is clear that these calculation tools would "do the heavy lifting" for the practitioner by presenting a considerable amount of statistical data from existing research in an organized manner, while incorporating certain parameters (i.e., unique individual variables/characteristics) or conditions (i.e., lifestyle, chronic illness, or treatment plan options) in the analysis. The end result is "good" information to assist decision making and to guide practice.

Evidence-Based Practice Resources

Evidence-based practice resources bring even more research into the clinical decision-making process. As mentioned earlier, it is very difficult to keep up with all of the new information and research findings that are generated on a daily basis. Clearly, this difficulty slows down the dissemination of important research findings and results in delayed benefit to patients. A number of resources can help a busy health care practitioner incorporate new evidence into practice more easily; these resources include (1) practice guidelines, (2) algorithms for decision support, (3) e-Journals, and (4) subscription news groups.

Practice Guidelines

The National Guideline Clearinghouse (NGC), a comprehensive database of evidence-based clinical practice guidelines and related documents, is a major resource for all practitioners. NGC is provided by the Agency for Healthcare

Research and Quality (AHRQ), which is within the U.S. Department of Health and Human Services. The purpose of NGC is to "provide physicians, nurses, and other health professionals, health care providers, health plans, integrated delivery systems, purchasers and others an accessible mechanism for obtaining objective, detailed information on clinical practice guidelines" (AHRQ, 2005). The NGC provides a PDA-friendly Web site that allows individuals access to a large database of clinical practice guidelines, with the specific purpose of facilitating the dissemination, implementation, and use of these guidelines in practice. The site has a robust search tool that quickly locates relevant material, using keywords, as depicted in Figure 16.5. The NGC is a free resource, and no registration is required. Visit http://www.guideline.gov to access the NGC.

The National Heart, Lung, and Blood Institute (NHLBI) of the NIH is also a good source for practice guidelines. One program in particular, the OEI, provides information about BMI from two major reports: the *Clinical Guidelines on the Identification, Evaluation, and Treatment of Overweight and Obesity in Adults: the Evidence Report* and the *Practical Guide to the Identification, Evaluation, and Treatment of Overweight and Obesity in Adults* and dovetails nicely with the interactive treatment guideline tool for the treatment of obesity described in the previous section.

Additional sources for practice guidelines are professional organizations. For example, the American College of Cardiology Foundation (ACCF) has collaborated with Skyscape, Inc., to adapt many of their clinical guidelines for download to a PDA, using the Palm OS and Pocket PC. These guidelines are provided at no charge, as part of an ongoing effort to use technology for training and education, at http://www.acc.org/clinical/palm_download.htm. Box 16.3 lists current guidelines offered.

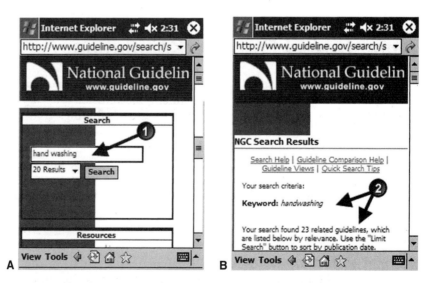

Figure 16.5 A–B The National Guideline Clearinghouse keyword search for guidelines on hand washing. (Available at http://www.guideline.gov/.)

| Box 16.3 | **CLINICAL GUIDELINES AVAILABLE FOR DOWNLOAD FROM THE ACCF** |

Arrhythmias

- Atrial fibrillation
- Pacemakers and antiarrhythmia devices

General Cardiology

- Echocardiography
- Heart failure in the adult
- Stable angina
- ST elevation myocardial infarction

- Unstable angina and non-segmented elevation myocardial infarction
- Valvular heart disease

Interventional/Surgery

- Coronary artery bypass graft surgery (includes preoperative risk calculator)
- Perioperative cardiovascular evaluation for noncardiac surgery (ACC, 2005)

Another resource is ebm2go (Evidence-Based Medicine to Go), provided by PDA Consults, Inc., a Canadian software development company that develops custom medical applications for PDAs. Ebm2go and ebmBooks were made possible through unrestricted grants from the company's supporting sponsors and are available at no charge, with the goal of disseminating evidence-based medicine as broadly as possible to benefit of patients. Ebm2go provides users the opportunity to access practice guidelines, such as chest x-rays for asymptomatic adults, as shown in Figure 16.6. In this example, it only takes a few taps with

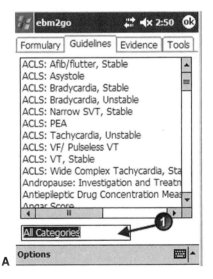

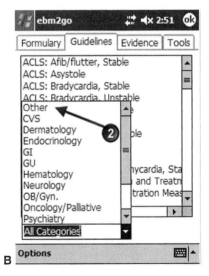

Figure 16.6 Ebm2go practice guidelines: **A** All categories of guidelines. **B** Select "other" category. (Screenshots courtesy of PDA Consults, Inc.)

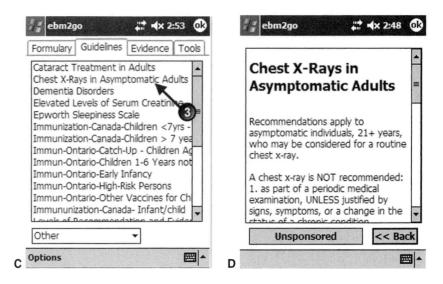

Figure 16.6 (Continued) **C** Select Chest X-Rays in Asymptomatic Adults. **D** View guidelines.

your stylus to get to the desired practice guideline. Visit http://www.ebm2go.com to access these resources.

Algorithms for Decision Support

Highly sophisticated algorithms can provide considerable assistance in clinical decision making. These complex calculators also use conditional logic and incorporate an extensive knowledge base of research and practice standards to guide practice. A good example of such decision support tools is TheraDoc Inc., a company that designs expert systems for clinical decision support. TheraDoc Inc. has two tools that provide decision support for treating infections and pain. These tools, Antibiotic Assistant and Pain Management Assistant, are available at no charge. To learn more and to see other products available, visit http://www.theradoc.com.

Now it is your turn to try using a decision support tool. Go to the TheraDoc Inc. Web site to download and install Antibiotic Assistant. Assume you are treating a 32-year-old woman for pneumonia. The following patient information is available to you:

She is breastfeeding her young son
Height: 58 inches
Weight: 120 pounds
Serum creatinine 1 mg/dL
Allergic to penicillin and reaction is immediate
She is being treated as an outpatient
The infection etiology is from an unknown organism

Test Drive. . . . .

Using the patient information provided, refer to Figure 16.7 as you follow these steps:

1. Open TheraDoc (Figure 16.7A).
2. Select the infection type, in this case, Pneumonia, and select Next (Figure 16.7B).
3. In the next screen, enter the information listed previously and select Next (Figure 16.7C).
4. Enter allergy information and select Next (Figure 16.7D).
5. Enter Treatment Location information and select Next (Figure 16.7E).
6. Select Unknown Organism and select Next (Figure 16.7F).
7. Select Next, because there are no Mitigating Factors (Figure 16.7G).
8. In the next screen, you will see the Treatment Recommendations (Figure 16.7H).
9. Tap on the arrow at the bottom of the screen and select Alternatives, to view the alternative treatment recommendations (Figure 16.7I).
10. In the next screen, you will see alternatives for First Line and Second Line Therapies (Figure 16.7J).

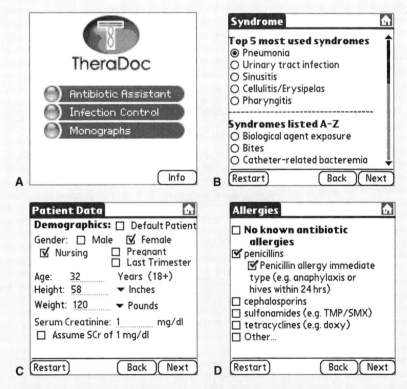

Figure 16.7 A–J Antibiotic Assistant treatment decision support tool. (Courtesy of TheraDoc, Inc., Salt Lake City, UT.)

(Continued)

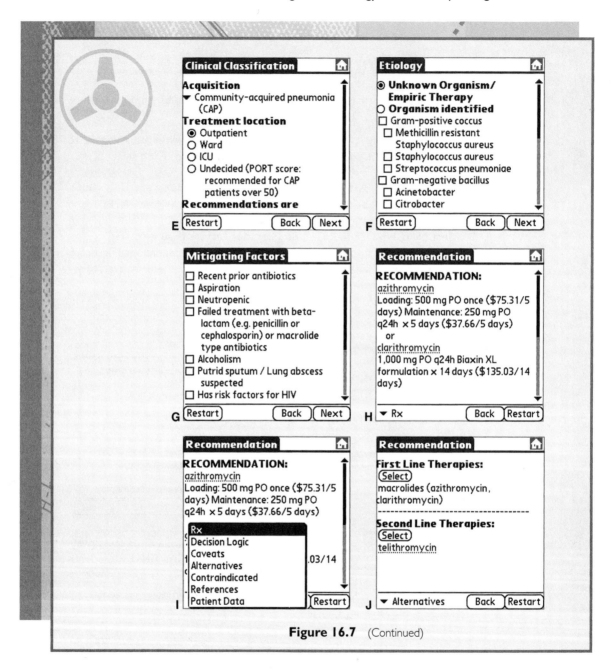

Figure 16.7   (Continued)

e-Journals

Various electronic journals (e-Journals) are available that can be accessed using the wireless capability of your PDA. Many institutions provide access to electronic databases, such as Medline or the Cumulative Index to Nursing and Allied Health Literature (CINAHL). Other sources include PubMed, Merck Medicus, and Journals-to-Go.

To access the electronic journal databases available in your institution, be sure that you are a recognized user for the resources because you will usually be required to enter a username and password when first entering. Using the wireless capabilities of your PDA, you can perform searches for current research literature on the topic of your interest. Using the skills you have developed in Chapter 15 for organizing your PDA by creating folders, you can save any articles that you want to keep on your PDA for later reference; this allows you to bring the relevant literature directly to the bedside for easy reference or teaching purposes.

Another terrific resource is the National Center for Biotechnology Information (NCBI), a division of the National Library of Medicine (NLM) at the NIH. This resource is provided at no charge and offers several information resources specifically designed for use on the PDA. These resources include PubMed and Entrez, a cross-database search engine, as well as many other comprehensive databases. To connect to these resources on your PDA, just enter the following Web address in the browser of your PDA: http://www.ncbi.nlm.nih.gov/Literature.

Test Drive. . . . .

Now try doing a search of the PubMed database using the keyword "SARS." Refer to Figure 16.8 as you follow these steps:

1. Turn on the wireless function and open the Internet browser on your PDA.
2. Enter the address, http://www.ncbi.nlm.nih.gov/Literature, in the URL window and tap on the green arrow in the upper right corner of your screen; this action should take you to the NCBI start page (Figure 16.8A).
3. Tap on the arrow next to the Search box and select PubMed (Figure 16.8B).
4. Enter SARS into the keyword search box and tap on Go (Figure 16.8C).
5. The next screen will show the extensive search results (Figure 16.8D).
6. Locate the article of interest and tap on the notepad icon (Figure 16.8E).
7. To read the full text article, tap on Full-Text Online (Figure 16.8F).
8. Scroll to view and read the entire article (Figure 16.8G).

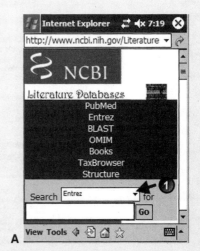

Figure 16.8 National Center for Biotechnology Information (NCBI) database search example: **A** Click on the drop-down menu for the list of literature databases. **B** Select PubMed. **C** Search for keyword SARS. **D** View search results. **E–G** Select and read full text article. (Available at http://www.ncbi.nlm.nih.gov/entrez/.)

(Continued)

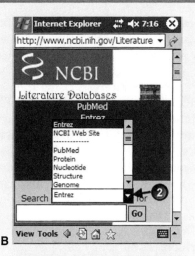

B

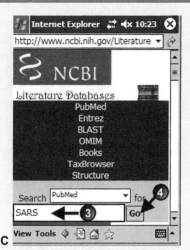

C

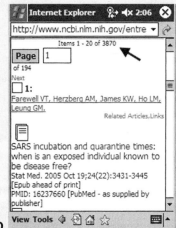

D

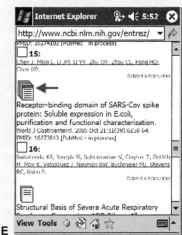

E

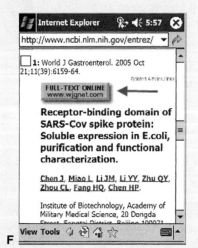

F

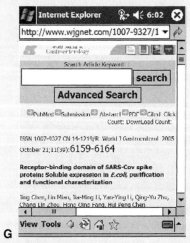

G

Figure 16.8 (Continued)

PubMed is an archive of life sciences journals that are provided free to everyone, and no registration is required. At PubMed you can access over 300,000 full text articles from over 150 journals. Another way to access PubMed is via Web site, http://pubmedhh.nlm.nih.gov/nlm/. This site is also designed specifically for the PDA, providing mobile users a very nice interface to search this rich database and similar functionalities offered by the NCBI site.

One useful feature offered by this resource is the capability to access the resources off-line. You can search off-line by using a product such as AvantGo (http://www.avantgo.com). AvantGo allows Internet content to be captured and loaded to a PDA that has no Internet access by syncing with a computer that does. AvantGo is discussed in more detail later in the chapter. You can get more information regarding PubMed and available options at the following link: http://www.ncbi.nlm.nih.gov.

Yet another excellent resource available from the NLM is MD (Medline Database) on Tap. MD on Tap is an application that allows you to retrieve Medline citations on your PDA, using a wireless connection to the Internet, and is available for both Palm and Pocket PC PDAs. This is an ongoing NLM project striving to develop effective PDA interfaces and design features that facilitate access to online information by health care professionals at the point of service. Features of MD on Tap include:

- An auto-spell check option
- Several search limit options
- History of previous queries
- Saving selected citations to the Memo Pad
- Two clustered results options
- Link-out to full-text Web sites
- Selecting from two search engines
- Automatic saving of user preferences (NLM, 2005)

Visit http://mdot.nlm.nih.gov/proj/mdot/mdot.php to learn more about this tool or to download it onto your PDA.

Finally, a very important resource from NLM is the Wireless Information System for Emergency Responders (WISER), a system designed to assist first responders in hazardous material incidents. WISER is available for PDA (both Palm and Pocket PC) and provides an extensive range of information on hazardous substances (over 390 known hazardous substances), including substance identification support, physical characteristics of substances, human health information, as well as containment and suppression advice. WISER is a very rich resource for individuals working in areas in which they may be asked to assist as a first responder in emergency situations (see Figure 16.9). More information and the download link for WISER can be obtained at http://www.nextcentury.com/HostedProjects/WISER.

Mobile Merck*Medicus,* http://www.merckmedicus.com, is a very rich resource for clinical decision-making tools. This resource is made available to health care professionals at no charge. You will find extensive online and PDA-enabled information, tools, and resources, which can be downloaded and updated each

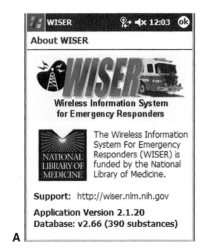
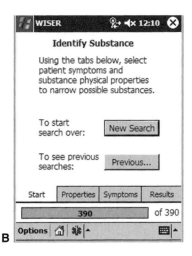

Figure 16.9 A–B Wireless Information System for Emergency Responders (WISER) system. (Available at http://wiser.nlm.nih.gov/.)

time you synchronize your PDA. The available information is from the following resources:

- The Merck Manual, 17th Edition
- Pocket Guide to Diagnostic Tests
- Reuters Medical News
- MEDLINE Journal Abstracts
- Merck*Medicus* and MEDLINE Search

A particularly useful component of this resource is the Merk*Medicus* and Medline search tool, which allows you to "capture the questions" that often arise in the clinical setting and will provide a search response to you the next time you sync your PDA. For example, assume that you are caring for a patient who asks you, "What are the latest treatment options available to me?" You can use the Merck*Medicus* or Medline search tool to enter the keywords associated with the diagnosis and new treatment modalities—capturing the question then and there—and later, after you sync, you can view the results of your query. This not only saves you time but also eliminates the risk of forgetting to follow up and do the literature search.

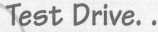

Test Drive. . . . .

To conduct a search of Merck*Medicus*, refer to Figure 16.10 and follow these steps:

1. Open the Merck*Medicus* application and select Search (Figure 16.10A).
2. Choose which database you wish to search. For this example, select the Merck*Medicus* database (Figure 16.10B).

3. In the Keyword(s) textbox, type in the topic of interest. In this example, the topic is asthma (Figure 16.10C).
4. Tap on Submit and you will receive the following message: "Your search will be posted to your Web Library on next Sync" (Figure 16.10D).
5. Tap on OK to finish. Your query will be submitted upon synchronization, and you will be able to view the search response in your personal Merck*Medicus* library on the Web, at http://www.merckmedicus.com.

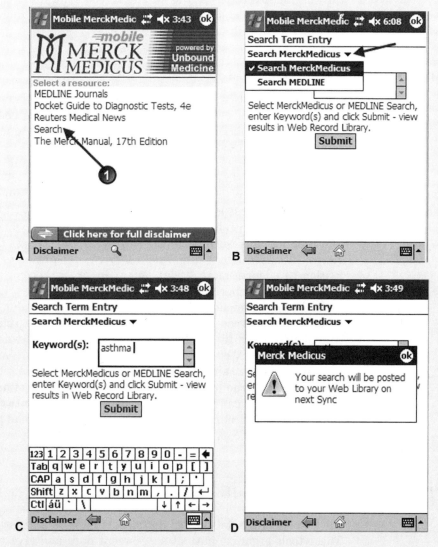

Figure 16.10 A–D Literature search using Mobile Merck*Medicus*. (Available at http://www.merckmedicus.com/pp/us/hcp/hcp_home.jsp.)

This mobile tool clearly saves time first by capturing the question in the clinical setting (or mobile environment) and then by providing the "answers" later when you are seated in front of the computer and are able to review new information at a more leisurely pace.

JournalToGo is a free resource that also allows health care professionals to stay current on new literature and health care news. You can sign up for this service and receive information from select topic areas of interest as well as peer-reviewed journal abstracts from the NLM and news articles from Reuters. You can read abstracts and news articles while you are off-line and on-the-go. If you read an abstract that piques your interest, you can bookmark the abstract for retrieval the next time you sync your PDA. JournalToGo provides upgraded subscription services for a fee. For more information, go to http://www.journaltogo.com.

Subscription News Groups

Subscription news services for individual users are also a good way for you to stay up-to-date and bring current information to the bedside. Resources like AvantGo and MobiPocket provide some services at no charge but charge for some advanced functionalities or subscriptions.

AvantGo is a PDA product that works with all mobile devices currently on the market. Users can access AvantGo content in an off-line mode as well as online. Perusing Web content in the off-line mode is convenient because wireless Internet access is not always readily available. AvantGo provides a means to stay current with breaking news. Within AvantGo, you can subscribe to various publications such as *AccuWeather, CNET News, USA Today, Reuters, Yahoo, New York Times,* and *Business Week,* in addition to health-related information. To learn more about AvantGo or to become a subscriber, go to http://www.ianywhere.com/avantgo.

As discussed earlier, MobiPocket is an e-Book vendor, and it also provides other PDA resources, including a means for you to keep current with the news. A neat feature is that MobiPocket supports AvantGo channels and mobile-device optimized Web sites; it also enables you to create your own eNews channels from any Web site you access frequently. For example, if you like to keep up-to-date with the latest Centers for Disease Control and Prevention alerts and updates, you can use MobiPocket's eNews Creator to create your own news channel. To learn more about MobiPocket or to download products, go to http://www.mobipocket.com.

Differential Diagnosis Tools

Another resource for clinical decision making is a differential diagnosis tool. These tools organize patient assessment data and give you suggestions for a possible diagnosis. Usually, lists of potential diagnoses are provided to point you in the right direction, but the final diagnosis must be made by the practitioner. These tools just serve to ensure that you are considering all possibilities and not to make the final definitive diagnosis. A number of these differential diagnosis tools are available to provide this functionality; some are free, whereas others are provided for a fee.

Diagnosaurus is a free differential diagnosis tool available in both Palm and Pocket PC formats, providing a list of potential diagnoses when the user selects the presenting symptoms. For example, when selecting the symptom "Periorbital edema or swelling," the list of potential diagnoses are displayed, as depicted in Figure 16.11. For more information about this tool, go to http://books.mcgraw-hill.com/medical/diagnosaurus.

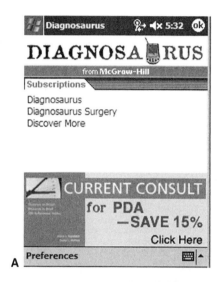
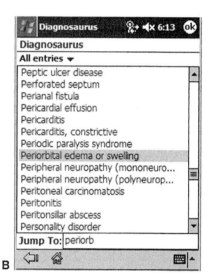
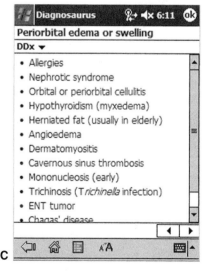

Figure 16.11 **A** Diagnosaurus main screen. **B** Screen to select symptoms. **C** List of potential diagnoses. (Courtesy of McGraw-Hill.)

Another example of a differential diagnosis tool is Psychiatric Diagnosis + Tools, which can be used to help perform differential diagnoses and risk assessments for psychiatric patients. As with Diagnosaurus, this tool is designed to provide suggestions to the practitioner and to assist in the process of identifying all possible diagnoses (see Figure 16.12). This application is distributed through third-party vendors, so for more information or to locate this application for download, visit http://www.softpsych.com or do an Internet search for "Psychiatric Diagnosis + Tools."

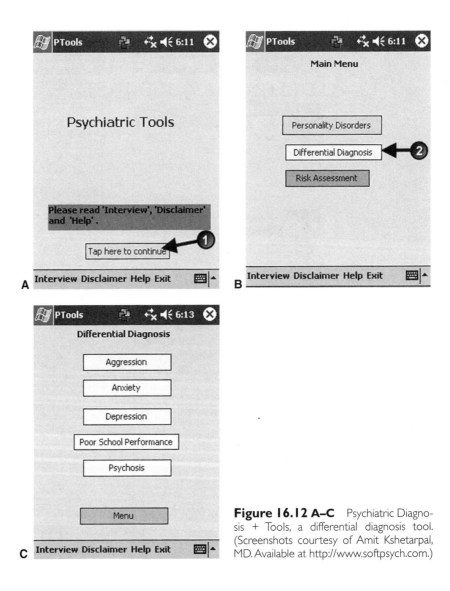

Figure 16.12 A–C Psychiatric Diagnosis + Tools, a differential diagnosis tool. (Screenshots courtesy of Amit Kshetarpal, MD. Available at http://www.softpsych.com.)

Summary

You have learned about the concept of clinical decision support (CDS) and various resources available to support clinical decision making. CDS tools presented in this chapter include references (e-Books), applications that use sophisticated algorithms, and Web-based resources that are uniquely designed to support the practitioner in a mobile environment. Although the major types of CDS tools and supports were discussed, all available resources could not be presented in this chapter. New tools and applications are emerging, and health care professionals like you will likely be the driving force for innovation in mobile technology. The key component for innovation is, of course, necessity, and such innovation is only limited by our imagination.

Tips From the Experts

- Take advantage of opportunities to "test drive" an e-Book, if the publisher offers a free trial version; it will give you the opportunity to determine whether the reference meets your needs before you purchase it.
- To optimize the Web browser view on your PDA, be sure to change the View to present the screen in one column.
- The **URL** may change from time to time for certain Web content, so if a link that is provided in the text no longer takes you to the item described, just do an Internet search for the name of the item or product and you should be able to locate its new home in cyberspace. Another strategy is to go to the "stem" of the original URL (i.e., if the link is http://www.ncbi.nlm.nih.gov/genomes/FLU/FLU.html, delete the tail, and go to http://www.ncbi.nlm.nih.gov and see whether you can locate the item from the organization's home page.
- Many other excellent resources offer similar functionalities as the tools described in this chapter. A good way to locate additional medical calculators for your PDA is to do an Internet search for "Medical Calculators for PDA" or "Decision Support for PDA." This strategy will also work for other resources or tools.

LEARNING ACTIVITIES

1. Download and install Skyscape Inc.'s Archimedes onto your PDA. Go to http://skyscape.com and use Skyscape's search engine to locate and install the free calculator. If you have an SD or CF memory card, install the calculator to the memory card.

2. After you have installed Archimedes onto your PDA, do the following calculations:

   a. What is the BMI for a man who is 6'5" tall and weighs 224 pounds?

   b. What is the basal metabolic rate (BMR) for a 9-year-old girl who is 4'3" tall and weighs 89 pounds?

   c. Suppose the 9-year-old girl in the previous question has minor surgery. What will be the calculated caloric requirement for her?

3. If you have a wireless PDA and are in a wireless environment, access the NGC using the following link: http://www.guideline.gov. Perform a keyword search for hand washing. Locate the most recently published guideline for hand washing.

4. If you have a wireless PDA and are in a wireless environment, access PubMed using the following link: http://pubmedhh.nlm.nih.gov/nlm/. Perform a keyword search on one of the following topics:

   a. Asthma

   b. Diabetes

5. Create your own algorithm, using at least three conditional variables.

WebLink. | Visit http://thePoint.LWW.com/cornelius for supplemental information and activities.

References

Agency for Healthcare Research and Quality. (2005). National Guideline Clearinghouse: About NGC. Retrieved October 12, 2005, from http://www.guideline.gov/about/about.aspx.

American College of Cardiology Foundation. (August 31, 2005). AACF Clinical guidelines. Retrieved on October 12, 2005 from http://www..acc.org/clinical/palm_downloadpcpocket.htm.

McGowen, K. (November 1, 2003). Trends in mobile computing in healthcare. PDA cortex. Retrieved November 4, 2004, from http://www.pdacortex.com/Trends_Mobile_Computing_Healthcare.htm.

National Library of Medicine. (2005). Medline Database on Tap. Retrieved October 23, 2005, from http://mdot.nlm.nih.gov/proj/mdot/mdot.php.

Stolworthy, Y., & Suszka-Hildebrandt, S. (2002). Mobile information technology at the point-of-care. PDA cortex. Retrieved June 2, 2003, from http://www.pdacortex.com/mitatpoc.htm.

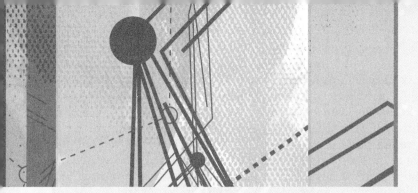

17

Media: Players, Cameras, and More

MaryCate Gordon • Mary Gallagher Gordon

Key Terms

JPEG (Joint Photographic Experts Group) • A type of picture image (filename.jpeg) required for viewing pictures and images in IPAQ Image Zone; the default image viewing program for Pocket PC. JPEG is a compression method standardized by ISO

Media files • The nature or type of media file; this is found after the title of the file (e.g., song.mp3 is an MP3 media file). Plenty of variations of media files exist, but only Windows Media and MP3 files work in the default Pocket PC media player

Skin • External appearance of your media player; the theme for your media player

Theme • Determines the color scheme and background picture of the PDA and allows the user to personalize the PDA to his or her specific tastes

Windows Media Player • The default media player that comes as a standard feature for Pocket PCs

Many auxiliary default features can help enhance your PDA experience. Themes, picture viewing, and media players are standard features on most PDAs that can be used to help you personalize and enjoy the many capabilities of your PDA. Themes allow you to customize the color scheme, background picture, and other features of your PDA to your liking. Picture viewers allow you to sync pictures to your PDA and offer various ways to view and share your pictures. Media players also allow you to sync media files (both audio and video) to your PDA, so you can watch and listen on-the-go. This chapter details the many features of themes, image viewers, and media players on both Pocket PC and Palm devices.

A helpful hint regarding media files (both movies and music) is to remember that they take up a lot of memory space. Consider this fact before syncing them to your PDA. Enhancing the memory of your device with a memory card might be a smart investment, if you are planning to use your PDA as a significant media playing device.

Media Players

Media Players for Pocket PC

Your Pocket PC has the default capability to store and play both audio and video media files. To move music files from desktop to PDA, follow these steps:

1. Create a folder called Media in the shared folder 🗐 on your desktop; place the music or video files that you want to move over to your PDA in that folder; place your PDA into the cradle to sync with your computer.
2. The files will move automatically over to the PDA.
3. The files can now be found in the folder in which you placed them or through the default media player.
4. From the folder, click on the file that you want and it will automatically open the player and commence playing the file.

The default media player on the Pocket PC is Windows Media Player, which can be found from the Start menu under Programs (see Figure 17.1). Because Windows Media is the default player, the music files moved from the computer to the PDA must be either Windows Media files or MP3 files. To determine what type of media file you have, do the following:

1. Locate the media file and right-click on it.
2. Select Properties from the drop-down menu, as seen in Figure 17.2.
3. Under Properties, the current Type of File is named and can be changed to fit the standards of the PDA to play.
4. Change the nature of the file to a Windows Media (.wma) or MP3 (.mp3) file before syncing to ensure that it will play once synced to the PDA.

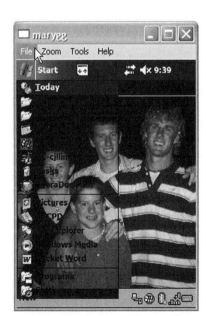

Figure 17.1 You can access Windows Media Player, the default media player for Pocket PC, under Programs on the Start menu.

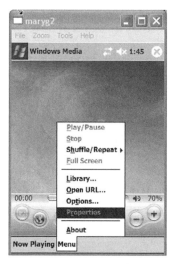

Figure 17.2 To determine what type of media file you have, right-click on the file and select the Properties option from the drop-down menu.

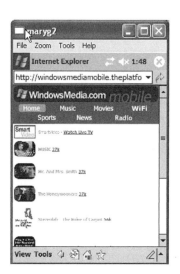

Figure 17.3 Connection to the Internet and a default Windows Media Web site called Windows Media.com.

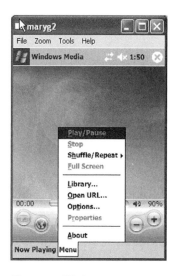

Figure 17.4 Organization of your playlists under the Organize Playlists option in the menu section at the bottom of the screen.

Media files can be configured to Windows Media files in the same way as the music files, if you desire to change the file type. Sync the desired media file to your PDA, and try following the steps described in the following paragraphs.

Open the file either in Windows Media Player or through the file folder from which you moved it. Again, movie clips and other media files must be Windows Media files to play on the default Windows Media Player.

Once you access a file in Windows Media Player, there is a title bar that labels the media file being played at the current time (a default 9-second clip for Windows Media Player is the only media file available until syncing occurs). To the left of this title bar is a button with a picture of a world globe and a music note, which, when selected, connects you to the Internet and a default Windows Media Web site shown in Figure 17.3 called WindowsMedia.com. To the right of the title bar is a button containing a square with an arrow that, when selected, fits the video file to full screen.

A screen for movie clip media files is shown; the screen in the default mode says Windows Media Player while playing audio files (see Figure 17.4). Another information bar is found under this video screen, listing the number on the playlist of the song that is playing, whether the file is playing, paused, or stopped, and the time elapsed. This tool bar allows you to easily identify the media file that is playing and further control what you are viewing. Under this information bar is a tracking bar that shows what point in the file is currently cued up and allows for quick fast-forwarding and rewinding (merely place your stylus on the small green and gray bar and drag left to rewind and right to fast forward).

The Tools menu includes an About section detailing the basics about the Windows Media Player; it also has a drop-down menu labeled Settings that includes Audio and Video, Network, Buttons, and Skin Chooser. Under the

Audio and Video selection are options for audio (e.g., continue or pause play-back) and video (e.g., fit videos to full screen, shrink to fit in window, and 180 degree rotation). Network allows you to choose Internet connection speed and protocol. Buttons allow you to choose the buttons you want in your button panel (with Play/Pause, etc., coming as the default buttons) and then map them as to how you want them to pan out in your Windows Media Player. The Skin Chooser allows you to choose a different **skin** (appearance) of your media player to tailor it toward your personal taste and interests.

After the Settings drop-down menu, the Tools section also includes a Prop-erties option, allowing you to see the properties of the currently selected or playing media file. Also included under the Tools menu is an option allowing you to add the currently selected media to your Web Favorites, a Repeat option to repeat the currently playing media, and a Shuffle option allowing you to generate a random playing order from your selected playlist, rather than have them play in the consecutive order in which they are listed.

Media Players for Palm

Palm devices may not come with preinstalled media players. RealPlayer, however, now offers a free media player for Palm (see Figure 17.5A), which can be accessed via the following Web link: https://www.real.com/realcom/palm VersionRedirect?palmVersion=1.6.1. In addition, there are many other software programs available that can be purchased and installed to allow media viewing on a Palm device. Many varieties are available of this type of software, such as MMplayer, Ptunes, or Kinoma Player3. It is a good idea to shop around to com-pare prices and to see what each application offers to determine what is best for you. Good starting points for looking for applications include the following:

- PalmOne—http://www.palmone.com
- PalmSource—http://palmsource.com
- Tucows—http://www.tucows.com

The RealPlayer shown in Figure 17.5A is a typical and useful panel con-taining the play/pause, stop, and skip (back and forward) buttons, a mute but-ton, and volume control. Under this panel are the Playlist and Tools menus. Under the Playlist menu, various playlists can be configured. Using the Orga-nize Playlist feature, you can select music from your Local Content and Web Favorite files to customize a playlist; this option also allows you to rename and delete old files, as well as create new media files. Organize your playlists in any way that suits you under the Organize Playlists option in the menu section at the bottom of the screen (see Figure 17.5B).

The media players for Palm will allow you to transfer your personal music collection onto an expansion card and listen via headsets. You would also have the option to purchase music and load onto the Palm.

Podcasting

What is a podcast? A podcast is the distribution of audio or video files over the Internet. The term *podcasting* implies that you need an iPod, but that is not

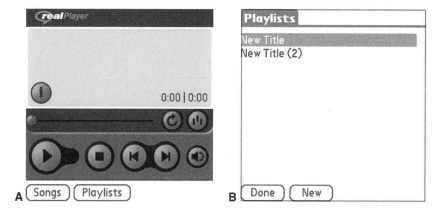

Figure 17.5 **A** RealPlayer for Palm. **B** Playlist menu: Create playlists from your music files and organize your playlists.

always the case. If you download the proper software to your particular PDA, either a Palm or Pocket PC, you will have the ability to download your favorite podcast. Podcasting allows you to sign up for an audio or video program that is published via the Internet and downloaded to your PDA. Many of the podcasting software on the market will allow you to automatically sync to your PDA the new issue of the podcast programs to which you are subscribed, allowing you to listen to your favorite radio show whenever you want. Educators are also looking at podcasting as a teaching tool. As time goes on, podcasting will likely evolve and become part of everyday life, much like e-mail and cable television.

Pictures and Images

Both Pocket PC/Windows CE and Palm devices can offer users the capacity of a mobile photo album, easily transporting and storing your favorite photos. The Pocket PC/Windows CE devices have a default picture viewer; most Palm devices do not. Another option is to have a PDA with a camera. The idea of having a camera within your handheld device, rather than having to keep track of two pieces of equipment, may be enticing to some. You would also have the camera at the point of need, if you are a person who is always keeping your PDA in the palm of your hand. Two options are available: You may have the camera built in to the device when you purchase it, or you may have the camera as an add-on; the choice is yours.

Pictures and Images for Pocket PC

For Pocket PC devices, picture transfer requires the same syncing method as the media files and works best with **JPEG** images (because these are the default format utilized on the PDA program). The default picture viewer for Pocket PC is called Pictures, The format of any image can be changed by going to its properties and transferring it to a JPEG image. The picture can be viewed by navigating to the Picture program and opening up the synced picture or by directly opening the file or folder that you synced from your computer. Try opening a picture directly from the synced folder in the following exercise:

Test Drive . . . .

1. Go to the Start menu.
2. Select Programs.
3. Select Pictures.
4. The picture is shown, followed by the name of the picture and its size, the date and time it was synced to the PDA, along with the pixel size of the image. Next, you will see a thumbnail gallery of the available images, a scrollbar to navigate through the thumbnails on the right side, and, last, at the bottom of the screen, a menu with File, Edit, and View Options.

Organizing and Naming

Your pictures are in the folder. If you did not give the picture a meaningful name, you can do so by following these steps:

1. Press Start in the top left corner of the pocket PC.
2. Tap on Program.
3. Tap on Pictures.
4. Tap on the picture you would like to change from the thumbnail gallery, as shown in Figure 17.6A.
5. At the bottom of the screen, tap on the Tools menu. You will see the option to "Save picture as," as shown in Figure 17.6B.
6. Now you can rename the picture and select where you would like the picture to be stored, as shown in Figure 17.6C. (Remember, the more information on the storage card, the quicker the PDA will function.)
7. Once you have named and stored the picture where you want it, press OK.

You can follow these steps to name each picture in your folder.

Editing

Options are available to change the view of individual pictures in the PDA; these options are cropping, brightness, closer view, and rotating to name a few. These tools are located in the picture folder and under each picture. Tap on an individual picture and look at the bottom of the screen for the tools available on your PDA.

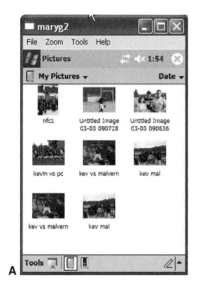 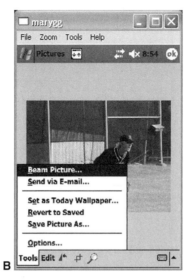 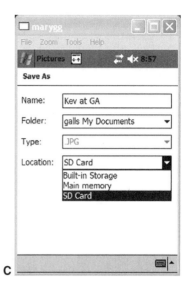

A   **B**   **C**

Figure 17.6   **A** Tap on the picture you would like to change from the thumbnail gallery. **B** By tapping on the Tools menu, you will see the option "Save picture as." **C** Rename the picture and select where you would like the picture to be stored.

Editing can also be done on the desktop using the application you loaded to store your pictures on the main computer (see Figure 17.7).

Slide Shows

If you want to create a slide show of pictures on your PDA, this can be done by more than one option. Many PDAs have what looks like an old-fashioned movie screen projector at the bottom of the picture folder; tap on that image and you will begin the slide show of the pictures stored in your folder.

To program the slide show, do the following:

1. Tap on the Start menu.
2. Tap on Program.
3. Tap on Pictures.
4. Tap on Tools at the bottom of the picture folder and select Options (see Figure 17.8A).
5. A button for the slide show is shown at the bottom of the screen (see Figure 17.8B).
6. Once you tap on the slide show button, you will have options to personalize the slide show for your PDA (see Figure 17.8C).

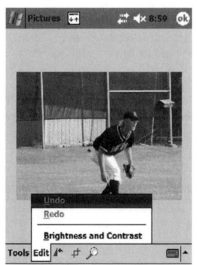

Figure 17.7   Tools and Edit options for individual pictures on the PDA.

The picture viewing program is a great way to view photos on your PDA, and it has many great features to enhance your photo viewing and sharing experience!

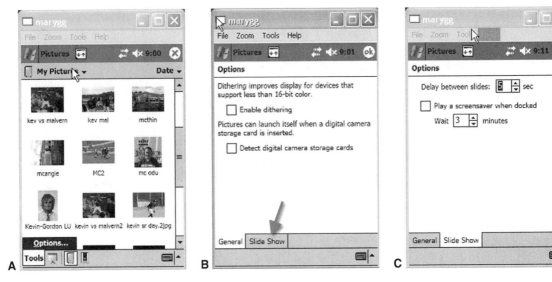

Figure 17.8 Using the slide show for pictures: **A** Tap on Options. **B** Tap on the Slide Show button at the bottom of the screen. **C** Select options to personalize your slide show.

Pictures and Images for Palm

As stated previously, most Palm PDAs do not come with a default image viewer. Software that can be downloaded to allow image viewing on a Palm is available, some free and some at a nominal cost. Many varieties of this type of software exist, so compare prices and see what each offers to determine what is best for you.

The exception is found in Palm devices that have a built-in camera. These devices offer default image viewing software that allows the user to sort, view, and delete photos. A Palm device may come with a camera; where the lens is located will vary and improve with newer devices. Some models have a sled where you slide the Palm up and expose the lens, whereas on others the lens is located on the back. By pointing the Palm device's lens toward the subject of your picture and pressing the button, you can take a picture as you would with a normal camera; the pictures will be stored in the photo section of the Palm device.

To find the photo section of the Palm, do the following:

1. Tap on the Home icon.
2. Scroll down and tap on Photos (see Figure 17.9).
3. In the Photos folder you will find the pictures you just took.

Organizing and Naming

Once you have begun to take pictures, you will want to organize them so that you can find them quickly and easily. To organize your pictures, follow these steps:

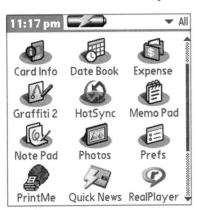

Figure 17.9 Accessing the photo option on a Palm device.

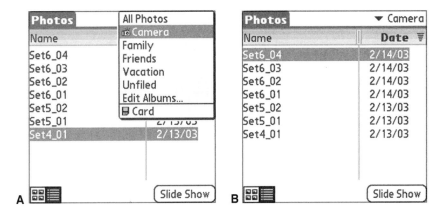

Figure 17.10 **A** In the photo section, you can edit the categories used to organize your photos or use the categories already listed. **B** Photos can be named by category.

1. Tap on the Home icon.
2. Tap on Photos.
3. In the top right corner, tap and you will see various categories listed in the drop-down box; you can edit these categories or use the ones listed (see Figure 17.10A).
4. Highlight a category, such as Vacation, and then go to the bottom of the screen and tap on Organize.
5. Once you tap on Organize, all of the pictures will appear. Tap on those that were from your vacation, and they will be sent to the vacation album.
6. You name them by category, but you cannot individually name each picture, as shown in Figure 17.10B.

Slide Shows

A slide show will be an option, found in the bottom right of the photo category (see Figure 17.11). Press on the slide show and the category that you had highlighted will begin in a slide show. If you want to see all of your pictures in the show, press All in the top right corner of the photo category.

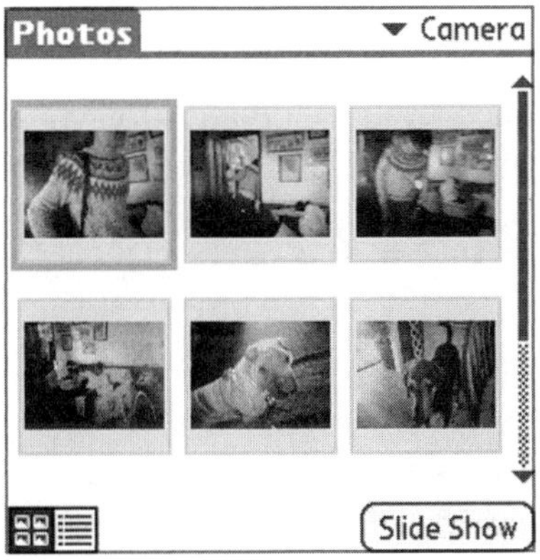

Themes

Themes are a way to personalize PDAs so that they are visually pleasing to each individual. Themes allow for changes in the background picture, Start menu, and color in various menus and dialogue boxes. Many theme programs can be downloaded (often for free) online to personalize your PDA for both Palm and Pocket PC devices. Many of these programs allow the individual to either choose from preset themes or

Figure 17.11 The Slide Show button can be found in the bottom right corner of the screen.

create his or her own themes. As a bonus, once themes are created, they can be beamed to others for use as well.

To change the theme on a Pocket PC device, try the following exercise:

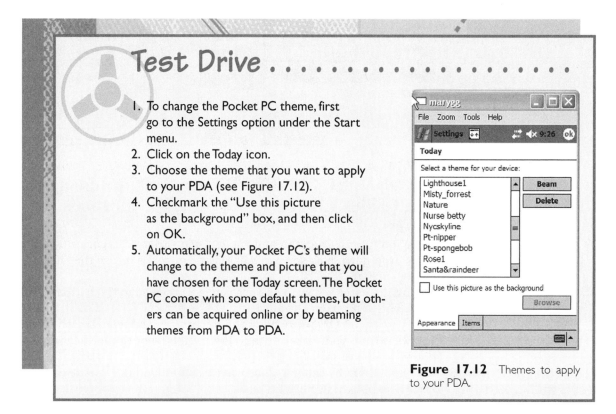

Test Drive . . . .

1. To change the Pocket PC theme, first go to the Settings option under the Start menu.
2. Click on the Today icon.
3. Choose the theme that you want to apply to your PDA (see Figure 17.12).
4. Checkmark the "Use this picture as the background" box, and then click on OK.
5. Automatically, your Pocket PC's theme will change to the theme and picture that you have chosen for the Today screen. The Pocket PC comes with some default themes, but others can be acquired online or by beaming themes from PDA to PDA.

Figure 17.12 Themes to apply to your PDA.

Your Palm OS themes can also be easily changed. Try changing the theme on your Palm device in the following exercise:

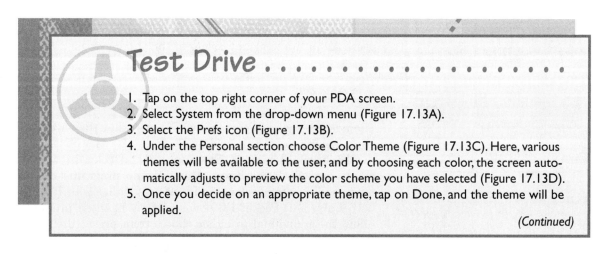

Test Drive . . . .

1. Tap on the top right corner of your PDA screen.
2. Select System from the drop-down menu (Figure 17.13A).
3. Select the Prefs icon (Figure 17.13B).
4. Under the Personal section choose Color Theme (Figure 17.13C). Here, various themes will be available to the user, and by choosing each color, the screen automatically adjusts to preview the color scheme you have selected (Figure 17.13D).
5. Once you decide on an appropriate theme, tap on Done, and the theme will be applied.

(Continued)

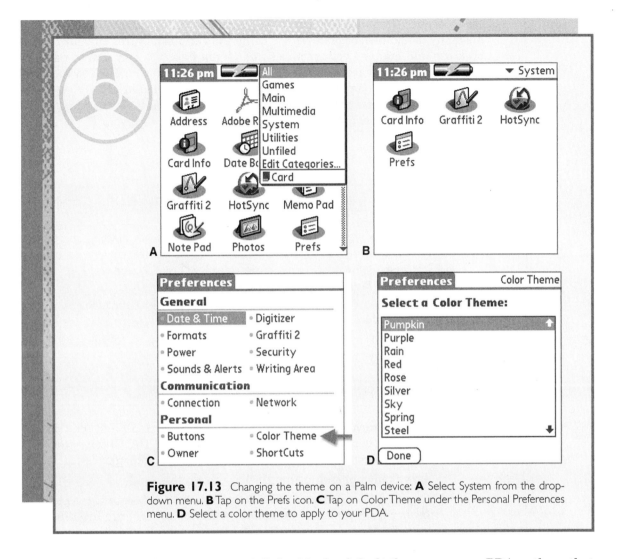

Figure 17.13 Changing the theme on a Palm device: **A** Select System from the drop-down menu. **B** Tap on the Prefs icon. **C** Tap on Color Theme under the Personal Preferences menu. **D** Select a color theme to apply to your PDA.

If you are not satisfied with the default themes on your PDA or those that have been beamed to you, you can download a theme generator, which will help you create new themes to use on your PDA. To acquire a theme generator, find a suitable program online that is compatible with your PDA. Download the program and follow the easy instructions for choosing or creating your theme. Once the theme is created, it can be applied to the PDA, and the appropriate changes will be made, including background picture, color scheme, and other designated changes.

Summary

PDAs can be a great way to take your most important and favorite media files and pictures along with you. Just make sure you are saving them to a memory card, because the internal memory of your PDA will not likely be able to handle many media files or pictures. By using the various features on your PDA to organize and manage your pictures and media files, you can share and show your files as you please. Themes allow you to customize your PDA to your aesthetic liking, personalizing your background picture and the PDA's color scheme to your specifications. Plenty of software are available that adds to the PDA media experience and allows you to do even more with your PDA's media, imaging, and thematic capabilities.

Tips From the Experts

- Be sure to know how much room you have on your device before you begin the process of downloading music, pictures, or podcasting.
- Place as much information as you can on the SD or CF card to keep your device running faster.
- Be sure that the music you load is licensed and that you are following the correct procedures for downloading.

LEARNING ACTIVITIES

1. Do an Internet search for free themes for your PDA and then download the themes and transfer them onto your PDA. Change the theme on your PDA to one of the new ones you downloaded.

2. Download a useful media file for your professional use.

3. Create a folder on your PDA called My Photos. Locate three pictures (either from your personal photo collection or from the Internet) and transfer them onto your PDA. Bonus activity: Try to place your pictures in a slide show on your PDA.

 Visit http://thePoint.LWW.com/cornelius for supplemental information and activities.

18

Accessories to Expand Functionality

Frances H. Cornelius

Key Terms

Bar code • A group of lines of varying width printed on the label of a product; the common term for Universal Product Code

Bar code scanner • A data capturing device that "reads" bar codes and then communicates the data to computer systems

Ethernet • A local area network (LAN) connecting several computers; it allows computers to transfer data over a communications cable

GPS (Global Positioning System) • A system of satellites and receiving devices used to compute, with great accuracy, positions on Earth; GPS is used in navigation

LAN (Local Area Network) • See *Ethernet*

Trilateration • A geolocation technique used by a GPS, which involves calculation of the distance of a specific location from four or more Earth-orbiting satellites

WAN (Wide Area Network) • A network that interconnects geographically distributed computers or LANs, such as across two campuses or libraries located across town

WLAN (Wireless Local Area Network) • A wireless network that uses radio frequency technology to transmit network messages through the air for relatively short distances, interconnecting devices in an office building or a college campus

Many accessories are available from various vendors that can further expand the functionality of your PDA. These PDA extenders include accompanying software that is easily installed onto your PDA (see Chapter 5). This chapter focuses on specific accessories that have particular use for the health care practitioner. Accessories that are discussed in detail in this chapter include bar code scanners, GPS, power accessories, and connectivity accessories such as modems.

Bar Code Scanners

Bar code scanners are commonplace in contemporary commercial industry. Bar codes are used to manage product inventory, track shipments, and more. A bar code consists of a series of lines and spaces that can be interpreted by a scanner as a unique product or item identifier. As you can see by the example in Figure 18.1, the UPC symbol printed on a package or item has two parts:

- The machine-readable bar code
- The human-readable 12-digit UPC number

For some time, the health care industry had looked at the use of bar coding as a means of tracking medication administration to provide additional patient safety. In February 2004, the Food and Drug Administration (FDA) published a final rule, *Bar Code Label Requirements for Human Drug Products and Biological Products*, which requires bar codes on certain over-the-counter drugs, on most prescription drugs, as well as on blood and blood components intended for transfusion (see Boxes 18.1 and 18.2). The anticipation is that the introduction of bar code will reduce medication administration errors by 50% or greater. The FDA estimated that the "bar code rule, once implemented, will result in more than 500,000 fewer adverse events over the next 20 years" (2004). Under the new ruling, all new drugs must have bar codes within 60 days of FDA approval, and all previously approved drugs are required to have bar codes by 2006. You can find additional information on this ruling at the FDA Web site, http://www.fda.gov/oc/initiatives/barcode-sadr.

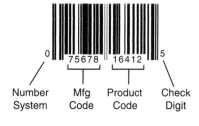

Figure 18.1 Sample bar code. (Courtesy of http://www.cummingsdesign.com.)

| Box 18.1 | **HEALTH AND HUMAN SERVICES ISSUES PRESS RELEASE— BAR CODES** |

February 25, 2004

HHS Announces New Requirements for Bar Codes on Drugs and Blood to Reduce Risks of Medication Errors

HHS Secretary Tommy G. Thompson today announced that the Food and Drug Administration is issuing a final rule requiring bar codes on the labels of thousands of human drugs and biological products. The measure will help protect patients from preventable medication errors and reduce the cost of health care and represents a major step forward in the department's efforts to harness information technology to promote higher quality care.

"Bar codes can help doctors, nurses and hospital (*sic*) make sure that they give their patients the right drugs at the appropriate dosage," Secretary Thompson said. "By giving health-care providers a way to check medications and dosages quickly, we create an opportunity to reduce the risks of medication errors that can seriously harm patients."

"We're encouraging widespread use of technologies that can help health care providers avoid hundreds of thousands of medication errors," FDA Commissioner Mark B. McClellan, M.D., Ph.D., said. "Bar coding systems have proved their dependability and effectiveness by ensuring the accuracy of a myriad of actions in commerce and industry. We're now advancing the adoption of these systems in settings where they can help save lives."

The FDA rule calls for the inclusion of linear bar codes—such as are used on millions of packages of consumer goods—on most prescription drugs and on certain over-the-counter drugs that are commonly used in hospitals and dispensed pursuant to an order. Each bar code for a drug will have to contain, at a minimum, the drug's National Drug Code number. This information will be encoded within the bar code on the label of the product. Companies also may include information about lot number and product expiration dates.

In addition, the rule requires the use of machine-readable information on container labels of blood and blood components intended for transfusion. These labels, which are already used by most blood establishments, contain FDA-approved, machine-readable symbols identifying the collecting facility, the lot number relating to the donor, the product code, and the donor's blood group and type.

The bar-code rule is designed to support and encourage widespread adoption of advanced information systems that, in some hospitals, have reduced medication error rates by as much as 85 percent. In these institutions, patients are provided with identification bracelets that bear a bar code, which identifies the patient. The health care professional then scans the patient's bar code and scans the drug's bar code. The information system then compares the patient's drug regimen information to the drug to verify that the right patient is getting the right drug, at the right time, and at the right dose and route of administration. In a study conducted at a Veterans Affairs Medical Center employing such a bar-code scanning system, 5.7 million doses of medication were administered to patients with no medication errors.

FDA estimates that the bar-code rule, when fully implemented, will help prevent nearly 500,000 adverse events and transfusion errors over 20 years. The economic

(Continued)

benefit of reducing health care costs, reducing patient pain and suffering, and reducing lost work time due to adverse events is estimated to be $93 billion over the same period.

FDA first proposed bar-code requirements in March 2003. Comments from hospitals, health care professionals, trade and professional associations and others showed widespread support for the approach to improving patient safety and promoting higher quality care.

The final rule applies to most drug manufacturers, repackers, relabelers, private label distributors and blood establishments. New medications covered by the rule will have to include bar codes within 60 days of their approval; most previously approved medicines and all blood and blood products will have to comply with the new requirements within two years.

Source: FDA. (February 25, 2004). HHS announces new requirements for bar codes on drugs and blood to reduce risks of medication errors. Retrieved January 15, 2005, from http://www.fda.gov/bbs/topics/news/2004/hhs_022504.html.

Box 18.2   OVERVIEW—FDA BAR CODE REGULATION

February 25, 2004

Today's Action

In an effort to improve patient safety in the hospital setting by reducing medication errors, the Food and Drug Administration (FDA) has published a final rule titled, *Bar Code Label Requirements for Human Drug Products and Biological Products.*

THE FINAL RULE

FDA is issuing a final rule that requires "bar codes" on most prescription drugs and on certain over-the-counter drugs. Bar codes are symbols consisting of horizontal lines and spaces and are commonly seen on most consumer goods. In retail settings, bar codes identify the specific product and allow software to link the product to price and other sales- and inventory-related information. FDA's bar code rule uses bar codes to address an important public health concern—medication errors associated with drug products.

HOW WOULD IT WORK

The final rule requires linear bar codes on most prescription drugs and on over-the-counter drugs commonly used in hospitals and dispensed pursuant to an order. The bar code must, at a minimum, contain the drug's National Drug Code (NDC) number, which uniquely identifies the drug.

For blood and blood components intended for transfusion, the final rule requires the use of machine-readable information in a format approved for use by FDA. The machine-readable information must include, at a minimum, the facility identifier, the lot number relating to the donor, the product code, and the donor's ABO and Rh.

Bar codes on drugs would help prevent medication errors when used with a bar code

(Continued)

scanning system and computerized database. This system would work as follows:

- A patient is admitted to the hospital. The hospital gives the patient a bar-coded identification bracelet to link the patient to his or her computerized medical record.
- As required by the rule, most prescription drugs and certain over-the-counter drugs would have a bar code on their labels. The bar code would reflect the drug's NDC number.
- The hospital would have bar code scanners or readers that are linked to the hospital's computer system of electronic medical records.
- Before a healthcare worker administers a drug to the patient, the healthcare worker scans the patient's bar code. This allows the computer to pull up the patient's computerized medical record.
- The healthcare worker then scans the drug(s) that the hospital pharmacy has provided to be administered to the patient. This scan informs the computer which drug is being administered.
- The computer then compares the patient's medical record to the drug(s) being administered to ensure that they match. If there is a problem, the computer sends an error message, and the healthcare worker investigates the problem.
- The problem could be one of many things:
  - Wrong patient
  - Wrong dose of drug
  - Wrong drug
  - Wrong time to administer the drug
  - The patient's chart has been updated and the prescribed medication has changed

So, for example, a bar code system could prevent a child from receiving an adult dosage of a drug and prevent a patient from mistakenly receiving a duplicate dose of a drug he or she had already received. A bar code system can also allow the computer to record the time that the patient receives the drug, ensuring more accurate medical records.

IMPROVING PATIENT SAFETY

The Institute of Medicine and other expert bodies have concluded that medical errors have substantial costs in lives, injuries, and wasted health care resources, and that drug-related adverse events are a major component of those errors.

FDA estimates that the bar code rule, once implemented, will result in more than 500,000 fewer adverse events over the next 20 years. Thus, FDA estimates a 50% reduction in medication errors that would otherwise occur when drugs are dispensed or administered, even though some hospitals that currently have bar code systems in place report a higher error reduction from bar code usage.

OTHER BENEFITS

Patients would avoid pain, suffering, and extensions of hospital stays with an estimated value of $93 billion over the next 20 years. In addition, hospitals are expected to avoid litigation associated with preventable adverse events, reduce malpractice liability insurance premiums, and increase receipts from more accurate billing procedures.

Also, the bar coding system could help with inventory control for drug manufacturers, wholesalers and pharmacists, as well as efficiencies in ordering and billing.

Source: FDA. (February 25, 2004). FDA issues bar code regulation. Retrieved January 15, 2005, from http://www.fda.gov/oc/initiatives/barcode-sadr/fs-barcode.html.

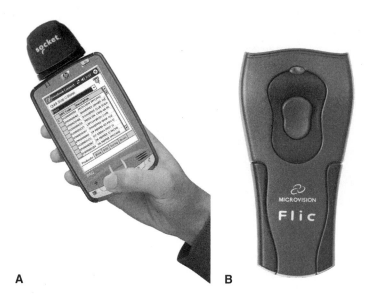

Figure 18.2 Examples of bar code scanners: **A** Socket scan card with CF slot. (Courtesy of Socket, Inc.) **B** Microvision Flic Bluetooth bar code scanner. (Courtesy of Microvision, Inc.)

A

B

Bar coding is seen by many not only as a means to reduce medication administration errors and increase patient safety, but also as a means to streamline a very important and time-consuming nursing procedure. Bar coding can reduce the time spent double checking the most current medication order as well as the time spent in documentation, allowing more time for the nurse to focus on monitoring, assessment, and patient teaching.

As shown in Figure 18.2A and B, bar code scanners for PDAs are available in several designs and can be attached, using the PDA's compact flash (CF) slot or via Bluetooth (see Chapter 6). A wide range of data collection software can be installed onto your PDA, which will allow you to easily scan a bar code for immediate data entry; the data can be stored on your PDA, transmitted to a local or network database by syncing or wireless connection.

Global Positioning System Receivers

When most people talk about a **GPS (Global Positioning System)**, they are really talking about a receiver. The actual GPS is a network of 27 Earth-orbiting satellites that was initially developed by the United States military as a military navigation system (see Figure 18.3A–C). The network is really operating with 24 satellites, with 3 extra for backup in the event that one of the satellites fails. This remarkable system is now open to everyone. The GPS receiver is the device that allows individuals to tap into the system.

Using high-frequency, low-power radio wave frequencies, a GPS receiver locates four or more of these satellites and records the distance to each satellite; the device then uses this information to precisely calculate its own location. This operation is based on a simple mathematical principle called **trilateration**, a geolocation technique used by a GPS, which involves calculation of the distance of a specific location from four or more Earth-orbiting satellites. To make this

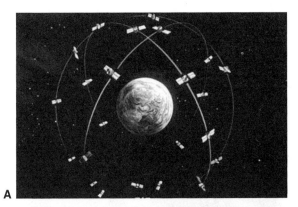

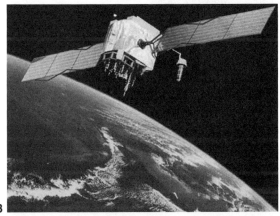

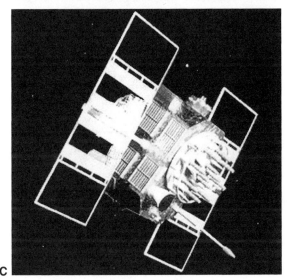

Figure 18.3 GPS: **A** Artist's concept of the GPS system. (Courtesy of US Department of Defense.) **B** Satellite. (Courtesy of US Army.) **C** Satellite-Navstar. (Used with permission from NASA.) (Images modified by J. Angat.)

calculation, the GPS receiver needs two pieces of information:

- The location of at least three satellites
- The distance between you and each of the satellites

The GPS receiver performs an analysis of the radio signals from the GPS satellites and displays its exact location. Higher-end GPS units have multiple receivers, so they can pick up signals from several satellites simultaneously and speed up the calculation process.

Now that you understand how the GPS works, we will discuss how data from this system can be put to use. To review, the GPS receiver takes the data, makes a calculation, and displays your exact location on Earth: latitude, longitude, and altitude. Clearly, to most users, displaying this "raw data" is not helpful; so, to make the navigation system more user-friendly, most receivers integrate the raw data into map programs or files stored in the device memory. Most GPS receivers can do more than identify your location on a map at any given time (see Figure 18.4). Other capabilities include:

- Tracing your path on the map as you travel (recording and showing your movement)
- Recording how long you have been traveling
- Displaying your current speed and average speed
- Estimating your time of arrival at a particular location

Many different GPS receivers for your PDA are available on the market. GPS receivers can be added to your PDA using a CFslot, secure digital input/output (SDIO) slot, or a special cradle that can be mounted on an automobile dashboard (see Figure 18.5A–C). Application of this technology for health care may include community-based practice

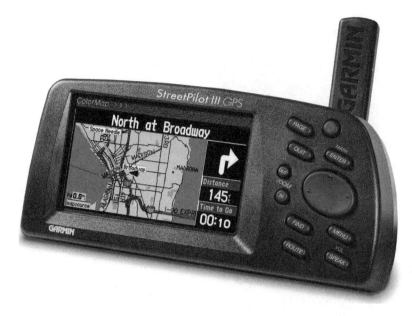

Figure 18.4 StreetPilot map display. (Courtesy of Garmin International Ltd.)

settings in which home visiting/traveling is necessary as well as in emergency medical services. The use of a GPS in emergency vehicles would help emergency personnel locate and arrive at the site of an emergency situation more quickly, saving precious minutes.

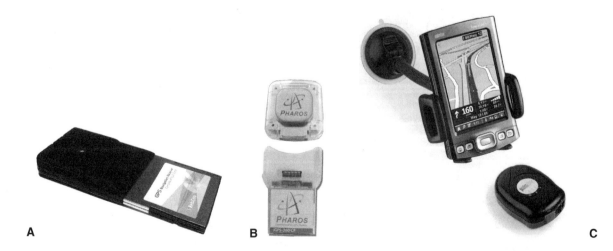

A   **B**   **C**

Figure 18.5 **A** Ambicom GPS Navigator CF. **B** Pharos SDIO GPS. (Courtesy of Pharos GPS; http://www.pharosgps.com.) **C** Palm GPS car kit. (Courtesy of Palm, Inc.)

Power Accessories

Although your PDA has a battery with a long life and, typically, enough power to get you through the day, having power accessories as a backup is a good idea. Some activities on your PDA, such as wireless or Bluetooth, require more power and therefore may more quickly drain your battery. A range of accessories are available that will meet your power needs in various settings. It is wise to consider where you will likely be using your PDA (i.e., hospital, home care, and so forth) and to invest in an accessory that will help you quickly get "back up and running" no matter where you are!

Mobile chargers can be invaluable for the busy, on-the-go health care professional. For the most part, mobile chargers come in three major versions that can use an alkaline battery, a car cigarette lighter adapter, or a solar panel. Most of these chargers are specifically designed for use with a particular device; however, there are some universal mobile chargers; these universal chargers come with various adapters to fit your PDA.

Mobile Battery Chargers

These handy accessories are also called emergency power chargers because they can instantly recharge PDAs (and cellular phones) with common 9V alkaline battery at anytime, anywhere, when no other source of power is available (see examples in Figure 18.6A and B). The emergency power charger is specially designed to quickly recharge the PDA without risk of overcharging or short-circuiting the device—just what you need to get "back up and running!"

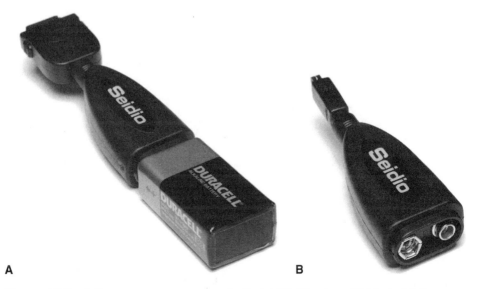

A   **B**

Figure 18.6   A Emergency power accessory for Pocket PC. (Courtesy of Seidio, Inc.) **B** Emergency power charger for Treo 650/Tungsten T5/Lifedrive. (Courtesy of Seidio, Inc.)

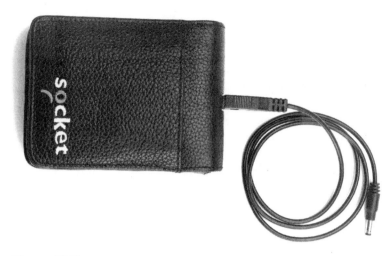

Lithium ion battery packs function similarly but provide considerably more power and will extend your PDA battery life up to five times longer. Power packs are light and portable, as shown in Figure 18.7. A power pack can be charged using a car lighter adaptor and will store power. You can use it to charge your PDA, as described previously, or keep it connected to provide an extended power source. These power packs are a bit pricier but provide a reliable power source for the highly mobile professional.

Figure 18.7 Socket mobile power pack. (Courtesy of Socket, Inc.)

Car Adapters

For health care professionals who work in the field and spend a good deal of time on the road, car adapters can be indispensable. It is very handy to be able to tap into the available power source generated by your car's engine. Using a car adapter provides a secure, convenient means to recharging your PDA while you are traveling between stops so that your device will be fully operational when you arrive at your destination. Figure 18.8A and B shows some examples of car adapters for different types of PDAs.

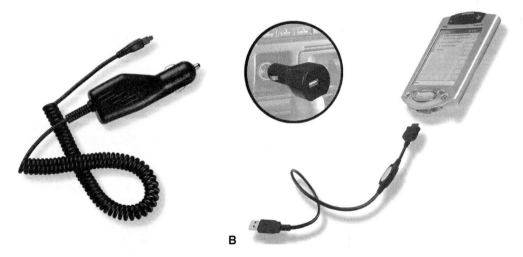

A　　　　　　　　　　　　　　　**B**

Figure 18.8 **A** Palm car charger. (Courtesy of Palm, Inc.) **B** Universal Sync car adapter. (Courtesy of Belkin Corporation.)

Solar Panels

Simply stated, solar charging devices use semiconductors to absorb light to generate energy that can be used to charge electronic devices. A solar panel can charge your cellular phone, PDA, notebook computer, GPS, MP3, and more in about 3 to 6 hours. It takes less time to charge when outdoors in direct sunlight and slightly more time when indoors. A solar panel can be placed on your car's dashboard to charge your device when traveling. Indoors, it can be placed near a window or under a lamp light to charge your device. Solar panels for your PDA come in various sizes and forms, ranging from clutchbag size units to those that are flexible and can be rolled up into small bundles. Various available solar panels are depicted in Figure 18.9A–C.

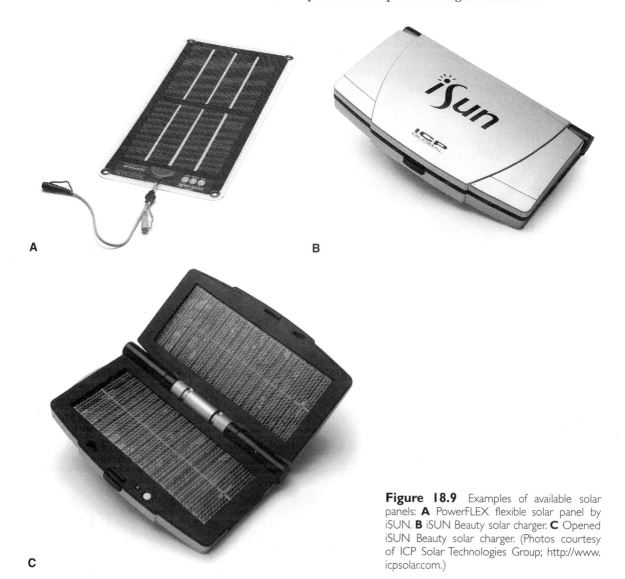

A

B

C

Figure 18.9 Examples of available solar panels: **A** PowerFLEX flexible solar panel by iSUN. **B** iSUN Beauty solar charger. **C** Opened iSUN Beauty solar charger. (Photos courtesy of ICP Solar Technologies Group; http://www. icpsolar.com.)

Connectivity Accessories

If your PDA does not have a built-in wireless card but has an available SD or CF slot, you can purchase accessories that will provide you with Internet connectivity. Available options include a 56K modem, an Ethernet (LAN) card, or an external wireless card. All three accessories will provide you with reliable access to the Internet. In addition, all three accessories are available in SD or CF, so no matter which expansion slot you have available, you will be able to expand your PDA's functionality.

Modems

Modems were first introduced in the 1960s as a means to transmit data from one computer to another over a phone line. The word *modem* is really an abbreviation of the words modulator-demodulator. A typical modem is a device that allows information to be transmitted over a phone line. Simply stated, the modem that is sending the digital data modulates (translates) the data into a signal that can be transmitted over the phone line. The receiving modem demodulates the signal back to its original form. Wireless modems use a similar process but convert the digital data into radio signals for transmission and then back again into their original form when the data arrive at the destination. A similar process occurs when transmitting data over a cable line, but cable systems use fiber optics to transmit data at much higher speeds than are available with standard modems.

Various modems are available on the market that will provide a means to connect your PDA to the Internet; they are available for both Pocket PC/Windows CE and Palm operating systems. Most insert easily into an available CF or SD slot (see Figure 18.10A and B). Some modems have a port to plug in a phone or network cable (LAN or WAN), whereas others are wireless, requiring you to connect a base receiver to your telephone. If you do not have an available SD or CF slot, some modems use a sled-like mechanism to connect, similar to

Figure 18.10 A CF 56K modem. **B** SDIO 56K modem. (Courtesy of Socket, Inc.)

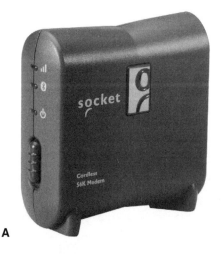

A

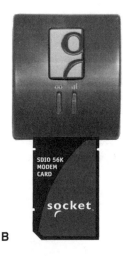

B

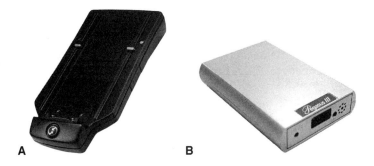

Figure 18.11 **A** Palm 56K modem. (Courtesy of Palm, Inc.) **B** Pegasus III Infrared 56K data-fax modem. (Courtesy of ENR Technologies.)

placing your PDA in its cradle (see Figure 18.11A); others use infrared to connect, as shown in Figure 18.11B. The wireless modems function much like a cordless phone using a radio signal to complete the connection.

Wireless (Wi-Fi) Cards

As was mentioned in Chapter 1, Wi-Fi is an abbreviation of the term "wireless fidelity," which is a high-frequency wireless local area network (WLAN) that uses high-frequency radio signals to transmit and receive data over an area of about 200 feet. Many newer PDAs come equipped with a built-in Wi-Fi card, but if your PDA does not have Wi-Fi built-in, you can purchase a Wi-Fi card. As with the external modems, Wi-Fi cards are available in both CF and SD format (see Figure 18.12A and B).

Setting up a Wi-Fi card is a simple process, involving easy installation of the associated driver after sliding the card into your available CF or SD slot. Once that procedure is completed, you can look for Wi-Fi hotspots and surf the Internet to your heart's content.

What is a hotspot? A *hotspot* is a connection point for a Wi-Fi network that is supported by a small box (hub) that is hardwired into the Internet. The hub contains an 802.11 radio that can simultaneously communicate with about 100 or so Wi-Fi enabled devices, such as your PDA. Many Wi-Fi hotspots are now available in public places, for instance, restaurants, hotels, libraries, and airports.

Figure 18.12 Wi-Fi cards: **A** AmbiCom wireless SD card. **B** ASUS wireless CF card. (Courtesy of ASUS Computer International.)

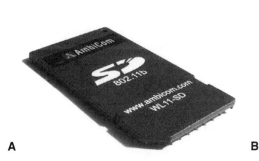

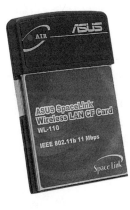

PDA Data Cables

PDA data cables allow you to connect to the Internet using your cellular phone. These cables plug directly into the PDA and then directly into the cell phone and do not require a modem. PDA data cables are currently available for most PDAs and a large variety of cell phones; this is a very reasonable alternative for those individuals who need Internet access but are frequently not in areas that provide access to a LAN, WAN, or WLAN. Clearly, this would be invaluable for the health care professional working in the community.

Summary

We have discussed several PDA accessories that can support and enhance the work you need to do as a health care professional. Accessories such as the bar code scanner and the GPS receiver can help the health care professional provide safe and efficient care, improving safe medication administration as well as ensuring timely arrival at the scene of an emergency. The accessories reviewed are only a small sampling of what is available on the market; many more are available that may be of interest to you. As technology improves, even more accessories will become available to consumers. As your skill level and needs change, we encourage you to explore available resources in more depth.

Tips *From the Experts*

- If you think that, in the future, you might want to expand your PDA's functionality, be sure to get a PDA that has two expansion slots (SDIO and CF); this way, you will not have to sacrifice additional memory for additional functionality.
- Before installing the driver for any new accessory, be sure to do a backup; this way, if the new accessory does not perform as expected or creates operating system errors, you can do a "hard reset" and "restore" to quickly get "back up and running."
- As a rule, you want to install all new drivers, applications, and tools onto your SD or CF card because this helps you keep maximum memory available for running applications.
- Usually, applications such as external keyboards or antivirus programs will not perform properly if installed on a memory card. If you have installed these programs onto a memory card and find that the programs do not work, simply remove the program and reinstall onto the main memory of your PDA. (If you followed the first tip, doing a "restore" from your backup will accomplish the same thing.)

LEARNING ACTIVITIES

1. Describe how bar coding works. How does this technology help improve safety for patients?

2. In your own words, define GPS. What is the benefit of this technology to the health care provider?

3. Compare and contrast connectivity accessories. What are the benefits and limitations associated with each?

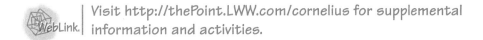

Visit http://thePoint.LWW.com/cornelius for supplemental information and activities.

References

FDA. (February 25, 2004). FDA issues bar code regulation. Retrieved January 15, 2005, from http://www.fda.gov/oc/initiatives/barcode-sadr/fs-barcode.html.

FDA. (February 25, 2004). HHS announces new requirements for bar codes on drugs and blood to reduce risks of medication errors. Retrieved January 15, 2005, from http://www.fda.gov/bbs/topics/news/2004/hhs_022504.html.

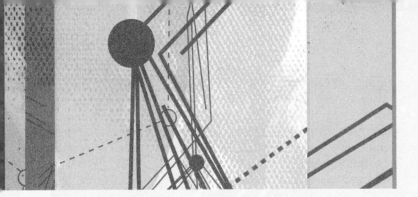

19

Troubleshooting Your PDA

Frances H. Cornelius • Mary Gallagher Gordon

Key Terms

Boot-loop error • An error message that continues to emerge even after a soft reset. This error occurs because a problem third-party application is looping

Fatal error • An event that occurs for any number of reasons while operating a computer or PDA and often causes the system to shut down or "crash," resulting in the loss of any unsaved work

Hard reset • A system reset that effectively stops all currently running programs, removes all third-party applications or tools, and returns the device to original factory settings; this is used only when the system has crashed so badly that soft reset or "reboot" does not work

Soft reset • The same as rebooting a computer; a soft reset stops all currently running programs but does not result in any loss of third-party installed applications or tools

Warm reset • A system reset that tells your device to stop what it is doing, allowing it to reboot normally and bypass any problematic system extensions (boot-loop error)

Sometimes things just do not work, even though you follow the directions. This chapter provides some tips to try and correct some of the most frequently occurring problems experienced by PDA users. You may also want to visit the official Web site of the device you purchased and go to the frequently asked questions for device issues. Links to these sites can be found at the end of this chapter.

A common saying by many is that when you find that something does not work, the first step is to read the directions. Although it is true that the operation of most devices is somewhat intuitive and often we can get things to work without reading the directions, this is not always the case when managing a PDA. Often nuances and subtleties exist that will make using your device easier and trouble-free. Being proactive and reading the directions is really a good idea. If you have misplaced your owner's manual, you will be able to access this information online at the manufacturer's Web site.

This chapter reviews some of the common problems that users may experience but that are not fully comprehensive. You are advised to refer to your owner's manual for a more extensive list of problems to guide your troubleshooting efforts. If the owner's manual does not help, you may find the answer posted online on a user support site hosted either by the manufacturer or by a special interest group. An Internet search may also help you locate an answer.

Problems With Pocket PC/Windows CE

Device Not Operating Properly

The most common "fix" for problems associated with your PDA is a soft reset. A soft reset is the equivalent of rebooting your computer; this action is often sufficient for resolving any problems, such as freezing or improperly functioning tools or applications. Sometimes these problems will occur because too many applications are running simultaneously. Your device has a limited amount of RAM (random-access memory) available. When you run several applications at the same time, the device may run out of memory and respond very slowly or even freeze. So, before you try anything else, perform a soft reset. In most cases, this simple action is sufficient for resolving the problem. Usually, a soft reset involves inserting your stylus into the reset button, a small opening on your PDA. To perform a soft reset, you should consult your owner's manual to determine where the reset button is for your particular device.

Problems With Setup

A frequent problem experienced by novice PDA users is failure to properly install the software accompanying your new device. It is important to follow the directions closely for this process to avoid unnecessary problems and possible permanent damage to your PDA. Your device should have come with an installation CD that contains Microsoft ActiveSync for your PC. If you have misplaced that CD, you can go to the Microsoft Web site (http://www.microsoft.com) and download the latest version of ActiveSync that is compatible with your device and computer.

Microsoft periodically updates and rebuilds ActiveSync to improve the synchronization between your computer and device. If you feel these updates pertain to your version of ActiveSync, go to the Microsoft Web site and find out whether there is a more current version of ActiveSync available for you. If there is a more recent version and it is compatible with your device and computer, you will want to first remove the old ActiveSync from your computer. It is important to note, however, that if you remove ActiveSync, you will also remove your partnerships and will have to reestablish them again the next time you connect your PDA to your PC. Before you begin this process, disconnect your PDA from the cradle; it is okay to leave the cradle connected to your PC, but you *must not leave your PDA in the cradle*. If you do, it may damage your PDA.

To remove an older version of ActiveSync from your computer, follow these steps:

1. Go to the start button on your computer and select Control Panel.
2. Select Add/Remove Programs.
3. Scroll to Microsoft ActiveSync and click on Remove.
4. After the program has been successfully removed, restart the computer.

Now go to the Microsoft Web site for downloads, http://microsoft.com/downloads. Locate and download the most recent version of ActiveSync that is compatible with both your device and computer. During the installation process, you will receive a cue to reconnect your PDA to the computer by placing it back into the cradle and establishing a partnership. Follow the cues to complete the setup.

Persistent Problems Connecting via ActiveSync

If you continue to have problems connecting with ActiveSync, you should delete ActiveSync from your computer using the instructions listed in the previous section and go to the Microsoft Web page (http://www.microsoft.com) to download and install the most recent version of ActiveSync. Microsoft distributes updates for the ActiveSync program on a regular basis. In most cases, this updated version will resolve any problems you are experiencing and correct any "bugs." Often, the newer version adds increasing functionality and stability to the syncing process. Therefore, you should check the Microsoft Web site for updates on a regular basis. If you decide to update, be sure to first remove ActiveSync from your PC using the steps outlined earlier in this chapter.

Device ID Already in Use

On occasion, when you attempt to connect your device, you may see the message, "the device name is in use." In this event, you have two options to get your device connected. The first option (and the preferred option) is to delete the partnership and start anew. To do this, follow these steps:

1. Remove your device from the cradle.
2. Via the ActiveSync window on your desktop, select File.

3. From the drop-down menu, select Delete partnership.
4. You will see the following message: "Deleting the selected partnership deletes all device-specific information on this computer. However, any existing back-up files for this partnership will not be deleted. Are you sure you want to delete this partnership?"
5. Select Yes to delete the partnership.
6. The next message you will see is, "Would you like to delete the synchronized files folder?" At this juncture, you can either select Yes to delete the folder or No to save the folder. It does not matter what you choose. It may be more reassuring to you if you don't delete this.
7. Now you can reconnect your device and follow the cues to establish a standard partnership, and your old device name will be accepted.

The second option available is for you to select a new name for your device that has meaning to you. This action, however, is not preferred unless you really do want to change your device name. If you do select a new name for your device, you will have to "clean up" your desktop after you have set up this new partnership. To clean your desktop, you must remove all remnants of the previous name by deleting the old partnership, using the seven steps previously described. When you get to step number 6, select Yes to delete the synchronized files folder.

Problems With Charging the PDA

If you find that your PDA is not holding its charge, first be sure that the connections are secure when charging. If you are charging the device using the cradle, be sure that you have placed the device *securely* in the cradle and that it is plugged into an electrical outlet. If you are using the adaptor to charge your device directly, check to ensure that the connections are secure. You may also want to check to see whether there is debris in the area where your device connects to the cradle. In addition, examine your cradle and cables; are there any broken areas? This may be the cause of the problem. If the PDA is still not charging, do a soft reset and place the device back into the cradle. For the most part, these simple measures will resolve any charging difficulties.

Calendar "Losing" Older Appointments

If you had been using Microsoft Outlook before the purchase of your PDA, you may have a lot of information on your calendar. The calendar feature on the device defaults to syncing only the last 2 weeks of your calendar from the desktop. If you would like to have all of the information transferred over to the PDA, do the following:

1. Open ActiveSync.
2. Select Options on the toolbar at the top of the window.
3. Under the Sync Options tab, highlight Calendar.

4. Tap on the Settings button.
5. Select the option, Sync all appointments.
6. Select OK to save the new settings.

It will take a few minutes to sync if this is the first time and if you have a lot of information to transfer.

Modifying PC-PDA Partnerships

Many Pocket PC devices will accept only two partnerships with computers—one primary partnership and one secondary partnership. Therefore, if you have used ActiveSync to connect with two computers and you want to have a standard partnership with a third computer, you will have to delete one of the two earlier partnerships before you can sync with a third. This will allow you to establish a partnership between your device and the new computer. To delete an earlier partnership, select that partnership when prompted during the setup process as you are establishing a new partnership between your device and new PC.

Problems With Stylus Accuracy

On occasion, you may notice that your stylus taps are no longer accurate. Screen alignment becomes an issue when you press on one key and a different letter or numeral appears. To resolve this problem, you must realign your PDA by following these steps:

1. Go to Start.
2. Select Settings.
3. Select the System tab at the bottom of the screen.
4. Locate and select Screen.
5. Follow the instructions to realign the screen.

Removing a Problematic Program

If you find that a program you have installed is not functioning properly and you have decided to remove a program, follow these steps:

1. Go to Start.
2. Select Settings.
3. Select the System tab at the bottom of the screen.
4. Locate and select the Remove Program icon.
5. Highlight the program you wish to delete and tap on Remove.

Problems With Screen Brightness

If you are having trouble seeing the screen, you will need to readjust the settings to accommodate your needs. Remember, though, the brighter you make the screen, the more battery life it uses. Therefore, you may want to place the setting only as bright as you need it to see the screen, especially if you are concerned about your battery power. To verify the brightness setting, follow these steps:

1. Go to Start.
2. Select Settings.
3. Select the System tab at the bottom of the screen.
4. Locate and select the Brightness icon and adjust the slider to your preference.

Problems With Beaming and Connections

If you try to beam to another PDA and are not able to do so, first check to be sure that the beam function is enabled as follows:

1. Start
2. Settings
3. Connections
4. Beaming—be sure the beaming capability is checked

Another cause of this problem may be low battery power. Check your battery power by doing the following:

1. Go to Start.
2. Select Settings.
3. Select the System tab at the bottom of the screen.
4. Locate and select Power to check your battery power level; generally, a power level below 70% will not permit beaming. Charging your battery will correct this problem.

Lost Books or Data

If you find that your PDA is not operating properly or, when you tap on an e-Book or tool, the application does not work or is missing key components, first try doing a soft reset. If that does not work, you can easily get back up and running *if* you have a recent backup on your memory card or PC. To resolve this problem, follow these steps:

1. Do a hard reset on your device (this will wipe out all programs, returning your device to factory default settings). The steps required to perform a hard reset vary among devices. Please consult your owner's manual for the procedure to perform a hard reset.
2. Perform a Data Restore function:
   a. On the Today screen, tap on Start and select Programs.
   b. Select Data Backup and tap on the Restore tab at the bottom of the screen.
   c. Select the backup you wish to restore and tap on Start.
3. When the system restore is completed, you should be "up and running."

If you have not performed a backup for some time, first perform a data backup by following these steps:

1. On the Today screen, tap on Start and select Programs.
2. Select Data Backup and in the Select Backup to: option, select your memory card. If a card is not available, you can back up to your PC or the main memory of your PDA. (Note that if you have a lot of applications on your PDA, you may not have enough memory on your PDA main memory to do a complete backup.)
3. Give the file a name that is meaningful, for example, today's date.
4. Tap on Start to begin the backup.

When the backup is complete, complete the previous steps 1–3 to resolve the problem of lost books or data.

Lost Data After Complete Battery Loss

If you have lost all power to your device and, consequently, lost all installed applications and data, you can quickly get back up and running *if* you have a recent backup. First, be sure to fully charge your PDA and then follow the procedure for restoring your device as listed previously.

If you do not have a recent backup or any backup at all, you will have to manually reinstall all missing applications. This situation is a clear (and painful) example of why performing regular backups is a good idea.

For more troubleshooting information, consult your device owner's manual or go to the manufacturer's Web site to access the knowledge base for your particular device.

Fatal Error Message

If you see a fatal error message on your PDA screen, it is likely that the application you were attempting to use is corrupted and has lost critical files required to operate properly. In this event, if a soft reset does not correct the problem, you may need to uninstall the problematic application and reinstall it. If the fatal error message persists, you may need to contact the application developer for support.

Problems With Palm

Device Not Operating Properly

On occasion, your device will stop working properly, freeze, or display an error message. The best thing to do in these instances is a soft reset; it is the most common "fix" for problems associated with your PDA. So, before you try anything else, perform a soft reset, which is the equivalent of rebooting your computer and will not result in any data loss. In most cases, this simple action is sufficient for resolving the problem. Usually, a soft reset involves inserting your stylus into the reset button, a small opening on your PDA. To perform a soft reset, you should consult your owner's manual to determine where the reset button is for your particular device.

On occasion, a soft reset will only get you back to the same error message, perhaps because the problem application is looping. This problem is commonly referred to as a boot-loop error. In this event, you will need to do a system reset, or warm reset. A system reset tells your device to stop what it is doing, allowing it to reboot normally and bypass any problematic system extensions. Usually, a system reset is necessary to resolve problems that emerge after installation of a new third-party application. In this event, you will need to remove that application; otherwise, the same loop error will occur the next time you try to use that application.

Data Loss After Soft Reset

A soft reset is a procedure that shuts down all currently running applications—the equivalent of restarting your computer. If you find that you have lost your data and applications after performing a soft reset, it is very likely that you have a more serious problem and may need to send your PDA in for repair. Before you do this, try the following steps:

1. Make sure to fully charge your PDA.
2. Perform a hard reset on your device (see instructions for performing a hard reset later in this chapter).
3. Connect your PDA to your PC (be sure that both the PC and PDA are turned on).
4. Perform a HotSync by either
   a. Pressing the HotSync button on your cradle or
   b. On your PC, select Start ➜ Programs ➜ Palm Desktop ➜ HotSync Manager.

The HotSync operation will restore all previously installed files; it may take a few minutes, so be patient. Once you have all of the applications reinstalled, perform a soft reset again. If you lose all of your data again, you will need to send your PDA in for repair. If you still have your data and applications, hooray! You are good to go.

Problems With HotSync

If you are having trouble with syncing, be sure that HotSync has been installed and that it is turned on. If HotSync still does not work, complete the following steps:

1. Perform a soft reset.
2. Verify that the HotSync Manager is turned on.
3. Remove the device from the cradle. Be sure the cables are clean and connected properly. If you are using serial ports, verify that the correct

serial port (either Com1 or Com2) is connected. (Note: If you are like many people and have just guessed which serial port you plugged the cable into, you may have entered the incorrect port at this juncture. So, if you find that the HotSync is not working, right-click on the HotSync icon in the desktop and change from Com1 to Com2 or vice versa.)

4. Place the device into the cradle and press the HotSync button. Be sure the Palm is firmly placed in the cradle. Note: *Do not* perform a Hot-Sync until you have the Palm in the cradle.

5. You may want to look at the Palm Web site (http://www.palm.com) for additional concerns.

Palm will distribute updates for the Palm Desktop program on a regular basis. This will correct any "bugs" and often add increasing functionality and stability to the syncing process. Therefore, you should check the Palm Web site (http://www.palm.com/us/software/desktop) for updates on a regular basis.

Device Freezing

Your device may "freeze" and stop responding to your stylus taps. In this event, perform a soft reset by inserting your stylus tip into the reset button of your device; this is the equivalent of rebooting your computer and often corrects the underlying issue. Device "freezing" can occur if a network connection was improperly terminated. Usually, your PDA will reset itself after about 30 seconds, but, if it remains frozen, perform a soft reset according to your owner's manual.

Beaming Problems

If you are having beaming problems, be sure that the beaming functionality is enabled. To check this, follow these steps:

1. Select the Home icon.
2. Select System.
3. Select Preferences.
4. Under General Preferences, be sure the device setting to Receive is turned on.

Sometimes when attempting to beam, you may receive a message telling you that your device is out of memory. In these instances, perform a soft reset and try again.

Problems With Stylus Accuracy

Occasionally, you will find that your stylus taps on your screen are not accurate and, as a result, your PDA does not perform properly. This problem may mean it is time to open the digitizer and realign your screen tap settings. To do this, follow these steps:

1. Tap on Home icon.
2. Then tap in the top right corner of your screen.

3. Select System.
4. Select Prefs (Preferences).
5. Select Digitizing.
6. Follow the target and realign your screen; this should fix the problem.

Problems Turning Off the PDA

If you are having problems turning off the Palm, you may need to do a soft reset. To do this, you will need to locate the soft reset button on your device (described on page 400). If this procedure is not successful, try to do a system reset (warm reset) described earlier in this section.

Problems Charging the PDA

If you find that your PDA is not holding its charge, first be sure that the connections are secure when charging. If you are charging the device using the cradle, be sure that you have placed the device *securely* in the cradle and that it is plugged into an electrical outlet. If you are using the adaptor to charge your device directly, check to ensure that the connections are secure. You may also want to check to see whether there is debris in the area where your device connects to the cradle. In addition, examine your cradle and cables; are there any broken areas? If so, this may be the cause of the problem. If the PDA is still not charging, do a soft reset and place the device back into the cradle. For the most part, these simple measures will resolve any charging difficulties.

Problems With Screen Brightness

If you are having problems with the brightness, you may have tapped on the brightness icon in the graffiti section and altered the brightness. Therefore, look in the graffiti section of the screen and find the brightness icon, tap on it, and use the toggle to adjust the brightness to your needs. Remember, the brighter the screen, the more battery use.

Forgotten Password

If you forget your password and your device is *not* locked, you can use a password hint to remember your password to get into your device. If you do not have a password hint or the hint does not help, do the following:

1. Perform a HotSync to back up all of your data.
2. Next, use Security to delete the password. Go to Security and select Forgotten Password; this action will delete not only the forgotten password, but also any entries you have on your PDA that are marked as private.
3. You can restore your private files by performing another HotSync.

If you forget your password and your device *is locked,* you must do a hard reset. The hard reset will wipe out all data (applications and files), but you can reinstall applications by performing a HotSync with your computer. Your recovered data will be as up-to-date as the last time you performed a HotSync operation.

Lost Data After Complete Battery Loss

If your Palm device completely loses all power, you will have lost all of the applications and data that you have previously installed. If you have performed a HotSync with your PC at least one time before, you can quickly restore all files by following these steps:

1. Be sure to fully charge your PDA.
2. Connect your PDA to your PC (be sure both the PC and PDA are turned on).
3. Perform a HotSync by either
   a. Pressing the HotSync button on your cradle or
   b. On your PC, select Start ➔ Programs ➔ Palm Desktop ➔ HotSync Manager.

The HotSync operation will restore all previously installed files. This may take a few minutes, so be patient.

Fatal Error Message

Sometimes you may get a Fatal Error message when you try to open a recently installed application. This error usually happens because the new application is not compatible with your Palm device. In this event, you should contact the developer of this application to see whether there is an update or patch available for your device. If none is available, you will need to remove the program from your device.

HotSync Crashes When Syncing Date Book

On a rare occasion, you may get the following error message: "This program has performed an illegal operation and will be shut down." This problem may be due to a corrupted date book data file. To solve this problem, you will need to either reinstall the current Palm Desktop application onto your PC or go to the Palm Download site (http://www.palm.com/us/software/desktop) and download the most recent version of Palm Desktop.

Summary

We have provided some troubleshooting tips for commonly occurring problems with your PDA. For the most part, these tips are sufficient to get you up and running quickly; however, sometimes you will need more detailed support from your particular device's manufacturer (see Box 19.1). In addition to accessing the knowledge base available at the manufacturer's Web site, be sure to check to see whether any updates for your device have been posted. These updates may help you in preventing future problems. It is a good idea to check the other Web sites listed in Box 19.1 as well. Often sites that are maintained by special interest groups, such as those listed, can be a valuable resource in helping you troubleshoot and manage your device.

Box 19.1   **WEB RESOURCES FOR TROUBLESHOOTING**

Manufacturers' Web Sites

PALM OS

Palm	http://www.palm.com
Sony	http://sony.com

POCKET PC OS

Asus	http://usa.asus.com
Casio	http://www.casio.com
Compaq	http://h18000.www1.hp.com
Dell	http://www.dell.com
Fujitsu-Siemens	http://www.fujitsu-siemens.com
Hewlett Packard	http://www.hp.com
Sony	http://esupport.sony.com/perl/select-clie.pl?template=EN http://sonyelectronics.sonystyle.com/micros/clie
Toshiba	http://www.toshibadirect.com

Other Web-Based Support Links

BOTH PALM AND POCKET PC

American Thoracic Society	http://www.thoracic.org/palm/palmtips.asp
Geek.com	http://www.geek.com
PDATopSoft.com	http://handspring.pdatopsoft.com/tips
PDASupport.com	http://www.pdasupport.com/PocketPCSupport.htm

POCKET PC

A Few Pocket PC Tips, Tricks and Links	http://bevhoward.com/ASync.htm
Pocket PC FAQ	http://www.pocketpcfaq.com

PALM

The Palm Tipsheet	http://www.palmtipsheet.com
InterPUG: Palm User Group	http://www.interpug.com

Tips From the Experts

- A quick fix for an "uncooperative" device is to perform a soft reset; this is always the first thing to do and often solves minor problems.
- If you are having problems getting your PDA to connect with your PC, first check to make sure that all cables are securely connected and that your device is properly placed in the cradle.
- Check to make sure your device is fully charged. Forgetting to charge the device is a common error.
- If your device has a lock mechanism, be sure to check this first if you find that the device will not work; this is an easy mistake to make because the lock mechanism will lock your device at any point, so it may appear that it is frozen or completely dead. A soft reset will only take you back to the same screen again and again.
- If you see low battery warnings, charge your batteries *immediately* even if there is an error message onscreen.
- Be sure to sync your PDA regularly so that your data is current to minimize the risk of losing important contacts, appointments, and files in the event of a power loss.
- Do a system backup routinely. At a minimum, you should do a backup before installing new applications and then again after you decide that the newly installed application is working satisfactorily.

 WebLink. | Visit http://thePoint.LWW.com/cornelius for supplemental information and activities.

Internet Resources

This section provides you with links to additional resources that may be useful. These links are organized into broad categories, which include support sites, user groups, evidence-based practice resources, as well as freeware and shareware resources. Many of these resources have been discussed throughout the book as well. These lists are by no means all-inclusive but can serve as a good starting point for you. Because handheld technology is very dynamic, it is also a good idea to do a search periodically, using an Internet search engine to locate new and potentially useful PDA resources. Joining a PDA user group like the ones listed here is another very good strategy, particularly for the novice PDA user, because user groups can provide extensive expert advice and troubleshooting support; they are also a good way to network with other users and to keep up with the latest resources, tips, and tricks.

Manufacturer Support

Palm Devices

Palm support	http://www.palm.com/us/support
PalmSource	http://www.palmsource.com/index.html
Sony	http://esupport.sony.com

Pocket PC/Windows CE

Asus	http://support.asus.com
Casio	http://www.casio.com/support
Compaq	http://www.hp.com/country/us/en/support.html
Dell support	http://www.support.dell.com
Fujitsu-Siemens	http://www.fujitsu-siemens.com/support/index_start.html
Hewlett Packard support	http://welcome.hp.com/country/us/en/support.html
Microsoft Windows Mobile	http://www.microsoft.com/windowsmobile
Sony	http://esupport.sony.com
	http://sonyelectronics.sonystyle.com/micros/clie/support
Toshiba	http://www.csd.toshiba.com/cgi-bin/tais/su/su_sc_home.jsp

Other Support Sites

Palm and Pocket PC/Windows CE

PDA Support.Com   http://www.pdasupport.com/PalmSupport.htm

Palm Devices

American Thoracic Society	http://www.thoracic.org/palm/palmtips.asp
Ectopic Brain	http://medicalpda.net/basics.html
Geek.com	http://www.geek.com
Handheld-Tie-Net tips	http://handheld.tie.net/tips/default.htm
Helphand's Not So FAQs	http://www.geocities.com/Heartland/Acres/3216/favorites.html
InterPUG-Palm User Groups	http://www.interpug.com
Palm/Palm Pilot: Personal experiences and tips	http://www.faughnan.com/palm.html
The Palm Tipsheet	http://www.palmtipsheet.com
PDA TopSoft.com	http://handspring.pdatopsoft.com/tips
PDA Support.com	http://www.pdasupport.com/PocketPCSupport.htm

Pocket PC/Windows CE

Pocket PC tips, tricks, and links	http://bevhoward.com/ASync.htm
PDA Support.Com	http://www.pdasupport.com/PocketPCSupport.htm
Pocket PC FAQs	http://www.pocketpcfaq.com/faqs/pocketpcsupport.htm
Windows Mobile	http://www.microsoft.com/windowsmobile/help/pocketpc/supportsetup.aspx

Evidence-Based Practice Resources

Palm and Pocket PC/Windows CE

Centre for Evidence-Based Medicine	http://www.cebm.utoronto.ca
Clinical Evidence	http://www.clinicalevidence.com
DynaMed	http://www.dynamicmedical.com
Dr. Alper's useful links	http://www.myhq.com/public/a/l/alper
Evidence-Based On-Call	http://www.eboncall.org
First Consult	http://www.firstconsult.com
InfoRetriever	http://www.infopoems.com
JournalToGo	http://www.journaltogo.com

National Library of Medicine,   http://www.nlm.nih.gov/portals/healthcare.html
   National Institutes of Health for
   Health Care Professionals
National Guideline Clearinghouse   http://www.guideline.gov/resources/pda.aspx

Palm

PDA-MD Healthy Palm Pilot   http://www.healthypalmpilot.com/Research_Tools/
                                        Evidence_Based_Medicine
The Pediatric Pilot Page   http://keepkidshealthy.com/pedipilot.html

Pocket PC/Windows CE

A Student's Guide to   http://denison.uchsc.edu/SG/PDA.html
   Medical Literature

Freeware or Shareware

Palm and Pocket PC/Windows CE

5 Star Shareware   http://www.5star-shareware.com/PDA
About Electronics and Gadgets   http://palmtops.about.com/od/freewaredownloads
Handango   http://www.handango.com/
PDA Street   http://www.pdastreet.com/software.html
Tucows   http://www.tucows.com/downloads/Windows/PDA
Wireless Information System for   http://www.nextcentury.com/HostedProjects/WISER
   Emergency Responders (WISER)
National Heart, Lung, and Blood   http://hin.nhlbi.nih.gov/bmi_palm.htm
   Institute BMI Calculator
American College of Cardiology   http://www.acc.org/clinical/palm_download.htm
   Foundation

Palm

Freeware Palm   http://www.freewarepalm.com
Centre for Evidence-Based   http://www.cebm.utoronto.ca/palm/ebmcalc/ download.
   Medicine EMB Calculator   htm?agree=I+Agree+to+Disclaimer

Pocket PC/Windows CE

CeBeans   http://www.cebeans.com/free-pocket-pc-programs.htm
Freeware Pocket PC   http://www.freewareppc.com
Healthcare Resources for   http://www.umkc.edu/lib/HSL/JFY/pocketpc-healthcare-
   Microsoft Windows Powered   resources.htm#ebm
   Pocket PC
PocketGear   http://www.pocketgear.com
Snapfiles   http://www.snapfiles.com/pocketpc

PDA User Communities and Special Interest Groups

Palm and Pocket PC/Windows CE

PC Today PDA   http://www.pctoday.com/services/PDAGroup.aspx?GUID
PDA Cortex   http://www.pdacortex.com

Palm

New England Palm User Group   http://www.ne-palm.org/pug.htm
   Directory
PDA Wiki User Group Directory   http://thepdawiki.com/PDAUserGroups/view

Pocket PC/Windows CE

Ontario Pocket PC   http://www.onppc.com/forum
Pocket PC Thoughts   http://www.pocketpcthoughts.com/links.php?cat_id=
           23&manage_links
Smartphone and Pocket PC   http://www.pocketpcmag.com/_top/User_Groups.asp
   Magazine Directory
Chris De Herrera's Directory   http://www.pocketpcfaq.com/faqs/usersgroups.htm

PDA Readers

Palm and Pocket PC/Windows CE

Adobe Acrobat Reader   http://www.adobe.com/products/acrobat/readstep2.html
Mobipocket   http://www.mobipocket.com/en/DownloadSoft/default.asp

Palm

Documents to Go   http://www.dataviz.com
Palm Reader   http://www.ebookmall.com/palm-reader.htm

Pocket PC/Windows CE

Microsoft Reader   http://www.microsoft.com/reader/downloads/ppc.asp

 Visit http://thePoint.LWW.com/cornelius for supplemental
information on available resources.

Glossary

ActiveSync • Computer program by Microsoft used to synchronize a Windows-based handheld device with a computer

Algorithm • A specific rule (or set of rules) or step-by-step procedure that details how to solve a problem or accomplish a goal

Applications • Software or programs that run on your PDA or PC

Bar code • A group of lines of varying width printed on the label of a product; the common term for Universal Product Code

Bar code scanner • A data capturing device that "reads" bar codes and then communicates the data to computer systems

Beam (Beaming) • To send information via the infrared port between two PDAs or to a printer or other infrared-enabled device

Block Recognizer • A Pocket PC/Windows CE tool that mimics Palm Graffiti as a means for entering text or data, using the same unique shorthand alphabet developed by Palm

Bluetooth • A short-range (about 33 feet or 10 meters) wireless connection protocol for cellular phones, mobile PCs, and other portable devices; it can also be used to send information between two PDAs or to send information to a printer

Boot-loop error • An error message that continues to emerge even after a soft reset. This error occurs because a problem third-party application is looping

Calendar button • A button on the lower right side of the handheld device that, when pressed, provides quick access to the calendar

Categories • Organizing tools that enable the user to sort information into separate folders to help locate information (appointments or contacts) quickly

Clinical Decision Support (CDS) • A class of computerized information systems or software that uses database resources to assist users in decision-making activities, including patient care options, by providing structured (rules-based) information on diagnoses and treatments

Compact Flash (CF) • Memory chips enclosed in a small plastic case that retain data after they are removed from the system; commonly used in handheld computers, cell phones, digital cameras, and audio players to expand memory and functionality

Conditional logic • Programming strategy used in decision-making tools in which specific actions or responses will occur, depending on which conditions are met

Configure • Setting options of built-in tools/features to user preferences

Contacts button • A button on the lower right side of the handheld device that, when pressed, provides quick access to the contacts

Cradle • The base that the handheld device can be set in for the process of synchronization or charging

Default install directory • The location of memory in the handheld device that is automatically selected for the download of programs

Download • The process of transferring data or applications from a server to a computer or handheld device

Drag and Drop • The process of right-clicking on an application, dragging it into another area, and "dropping" it for downloading

Drop-down text menu • A list of preset text options available to speed up text entry on the PDA

e-Book • A book published in electronic form that can be downloaded to computers or handheld devices

e-Journal • An electronic format of a journal available via the Internet

Ethernet • A local area network (LAN) connecting several computers; it allows computers to transfer data over a communications cable

Fatal error • An event that occurs for any number of reasons while operating a computer or PDA and often causes the system to shut down or "crash," resulting in the loss of any unsaved work

Foldable external keyboard • A device that attaches to your PDA either directly or via infrared (IR) and allows you to type as you would on your desktop

Folders • In Pocket PC/Windows CE devices, places where you can organize and store items (documents, images, and applications) for easy access

Freeware • Software that is developed, usually by individuals or small companies, and distributed at no cost to the user, usually via the Internet. Individuals can freely use this software, and the developer/owner retains the copyright

GPS (Global Positioning System) • A system of satellites and receiving devices used to compute, with great accuracy, positions on Earth; GPS is used in navigation

Graffiti • Palm's original Graffiti writing software that provides a quick way to enter text or data, using a unique shorthand alphabet

Hard reset • A system reset that effectively stops all currently running programs, removes all third-party applications or tools, and returns the device to original factory settings; it is used only when the system has crashed so badly that soft reset or "reboot" does not work

Highlight • A technique of using the stylus to select specific text to be quickly deleted and permitting cutting and pasting text from one area to another

Hotspot • A connection point for a Wi-Fi network, supported by a small box (hub) that is hard-wired into the Internet

Infrared (IR) • An invisible radiation wavelength used to transmit data

Infrared (IR) port • A sensor that allows exchange of data between PDAs, a PDA and a printer, or a PDA and another IR-enabled device; the range capability is about 3 feet

JPEG (Joint Photographic Experts Group) • A type of picture image (filename.jpeg) required for viewing pictures and images in IPAQ Image Zone; the default image viewing program for Pocket PC. JPEG is a compression method standardized by ISO

Keyboard • Built-in data entry tool for both Palm and Pocket PC/Windows CE devices that resembles a miniature keyboard. Using a stylus, you can tap on the letters to form the word

LAN (Local Area Network) • See *Ethernet*

Letter Recognizer • A Pocket PC/Windows CE tool using conventional printed letters, numbers, and symbols to enter information into the PDA

Linux • A very stable, open source version of UNIX operating system, available at no charge

Media files • The nature or type of media file; this is found after the title of the file (e.g., song.mp3 is an MP3 media file). Plenty of variations of media files exist, but only Windows media and MP3 files work in the default Pocket PC media player

Mode • The function or form used to enter information into the PDA

Modem • A device that allows digital data to be transmitted over a phone line (The term is an abbreviation of the words *modulator-demodulator*)

Operating System (OS) • Software that is the foundation enabling programs to run on a PDA, for example, Palm OS and Pocket PC OS

Palm • An operating system for PDAs created by Palm, Inc.

Palm Desktop • Palm computer program for use with Windows operating system

Personal Digital Assistant (PDA) • A small handheld computer that organizes information; also known as handheld, palmtop

Pocket PC • A Windows-based operating system for PDAs created by Microsoft; also known as WinCE

RAM (Random-Access Memory) • Temporary storage of PDA files that enables PDA applications to run

ROM (Read-Only Memory) • Used for static memory on a PDA; typically the space where the operating system is stored or where fixed Personal Information Data applications are shipped with the standard PDA OS

Search tool • Imbedded program that enables users to quickly locate information on the device; both the calendar and contact manager offer this feature

Secure Digital (SD) card • Memory chips enclosed in a small plastic case that retain data after they are removed from the system; for memory data storage only

Secure Digital Input/Output (SDIO) card • An interface, similar to CF cards, that extends the functionality of devices with SD cards by allowing data to be transmitted both into and out from a device

Serial port • A port on the computer where an external modem, a serial printer, or other device that uses a 9-pin serial connector can be attached

Shared folder • The folder on the computer desktop that permits Pocket PC/Windows CE users to access and edit, on the computer, documents housed on the PDA (Notes, Word, Excel)

Shareware • Software that is distributed for free on a trial or limited basis, with the understanding that the user may need or want to pay for it later. Sometimes shareware has a built-in expiration date so the software stops working; other shareware is distributed in a "lite" version of the application with some key functionality becoming operational only after the product is purchased. This strategy often entices users to purchase the full version of the program

Skin • External appearance of your media player; the theme for your media player

Soft reset • The same as rebooting a computer; a soft reset stops all currently running programs but does not result in any loss of third-party installed applications or tools

Stylus (**Stylus pen**) • The input device for a PDA—the user touches the screen with a stylus to execute commands

Syncing • Establishing a connection/partnership between the PDA and the computer in which files and programs are shared

Template • A set of predesigned formats for text and graphics used to eliminate the need to recreate the same forms repeatedly; using a template saves time by speeding up the data entry process

Theme • Determines the color scheme and background picture of the PDA and allows the user to personalize the PDA to his or her specific tastes

Transcriber • A Pocket PC/Windows CE tool that allows you to enter data, using your own handwriting

Trilateration • A geolocation technique used by a GPS that involves calculation of the distance of a specific location from four or more Earth-orbiting satellites

Universal Serial Bus (USB) • An interface between a computer and add-on devices, serving as a way to connect peripheral devices to computers; allows you to connect multiple devices concurrently and replaces the functionality of serial and parallel ports, including keyboard and mouse ports

URL (Uniform Resource Locator) • The "address" of a particular document/resource on the Internet that functions similarly to a house address; URLs begin with "http://" on the World Wide Web

USB port • A port on the computer where devices that require a Universal Serial Bus connection, such as a mouse, a scanner, a printer, or a PDA can be attached

WAN (Wide Area Network) • A network that interconnects geographically distributed computers or LANs, such as across two campuses or libraries located across town

Warm reset • A system reset that tells your device to stop what it is doing, allowing it to reboot normally and bypass any problematic system extensions (boot-loop error)

Wi-Fi • An abbreviation for "wireless fidelity;" a high-frequency wireless local area network (WLAN) that uses radio signals to transmit and receive data over an area of about 200 feet; allows handhelds, desktops, and other wireless devices to exchange information at up to 11 mbs (megabytes/sec) at several hundred feet; also known as 802.11a, 802.11b, 802.11g

Windows Media Player • The default media player that comes as a standard feature for Pocket PCs

Wireless • A feature that allows you to read, transmit, or receive information via the Internet without your PDA or PC being physically connected by a cable

WLAN (Wireless Local Area Network) • A wireless network that uses radio frequency technology to transmit network messages through the air for relatively short distances, interconnecting devices in an office building or a college campus

Writing area • The area on Palm devices, below the screen, where you enter data (text, numbers, or symbols)

Zip file • A folder that contains multiple files that have been compressed or "zipped" to take up less space

Index

Page numbers followed by letters *b* and *f* indicate boxes and figures, respectively.